à la Carte

Lean Meats

ROAST BEEF, VEAL OR LAMB, BROILED STEAK, PAILLARD OF VEAL
VEAL SCALOPPINI, LAMB CHOPS GARNI
BEEF IN VEGETABLE WREATH, BROILED HAMBURGER
BROILED CALF, BEEF or CHICKEN LIVER

Fowl, Wild and Domestic

ROAST HERBED CHICKEN
ROAST TURKEY WITH VEGE-NUT DRESSING
CORNISH GAME HEN OR WILD FOWL STUFFED WITH WILD RICE

Curries Indienne

CHICKEN, LAMB, SEAFOOD, EGG, AVOCADO, LENTILS, VEGETABLE

Fishes from the Seven Seas

FILET OF SOLE OR FLOUNDER, GRILLED HALIBUT, BAKED SALMON
RED SNAPPER IN PARCHMENT, BROILED LOBSTER TAILS
GOLDEN SHRIMP ON RICE, OYSTERS, CLAMS

Meatless Main Courses

PILAFF OF CRACKED WHEAT or RICE, WILD RICE HAMBURGERS
STUFFED GRAPE LEAVES, CELERY-NUT LOAF, BAKED SOYBEANS
EGGS A LA MODE

Garden-Fresh Vegetables Unlimited

SHORT-COOKED SHREDDED CARROTS, BEETS
CAULIFLOWER OR BROCCOLI, BRAISED ENDIVE OR CELERY
BEAN SPROUTS SAUTE, CHINESE SNOW PEAS
BAKED ONIONS WITH OREGANO, BROILED EGGPLANT
STEAMED ZUCCHINI, OLD-FASHIONED SALSIFY, BAKED PARSNIPS
LIGHT-HEARTED BAKED POTATOES
BROWN RICE, CRACKED WHEAT

MIRROR, MIRROR ON THE WALL

Mirror, Mirror on the Wall

INVITATION TO BEAUTY

by GAYELORD HAUSER

FARRAR, STRAUS AND CUDAHY
NEW YORK

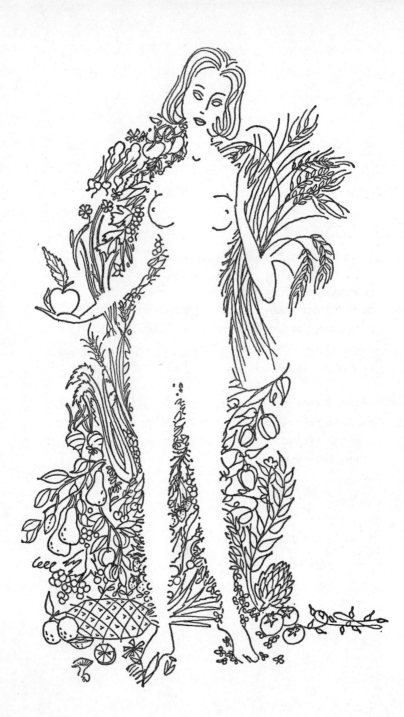

Eve

"And how beautiful the look of her face. And how fine is the hair of her head, how fair indeed are her eyes and how pleasing her nose and all the radiance of her face . . . how beautiful her breast and how lovely all her whiteness. Her arms goodly to look upon, and her hands how perfect . . . all the appearance of her hand. How fair her palms and how long and fine all the fingers of her hands. Her legs how beautiful and without blemish her thighs. And all maidens and all brides that go beneath the wedding canopy are not more fair than she. And above all women she is lovely and higher is her beauty than that of them all, and with all her beauty there is much wisdom."

From a parchment scroll written more than 2,000 years ago.

Contents

Foreword   xi

Part One: BEAUTY WITHIN YOUR REACH

 1. You Can Be Beautiful   3

 2. Beauty Is an Inside Job   8

 3. The Mental Climate of Beauty   18

Part Two: THE BEAUTY-FULL FOODS

 4. Your Cosmetic Diet   29

 5. Your Day of Beauty-Full Eating 39

 6. Your Beauty Alphabet of Vitamins and Minerals 63

 7. Romantic Foods   78

Part Three: YOUR HIGH ROAD TO BEAUTY

 8. Contours of Beauty: Your Figure 99

 9. These Pains Can Be Pleasure: Reducing 118

10. The Quick and Happy Way to Exercise   127

11. Beauty's Sheath: Your Skin   138

12. Beauty's Facade: Your Face   149

13. Beauty's Jewels: Your Eyes   173

14. Frame for Beauty: Your Hair   185

15. Gateway to Beauty: Your Mouth   193

16. Beauty in Your Hands   200

17. Pedestals of Beauty: Your Feet   205

18. Your Beauty Sleep   210

19. Exquisite Cleanliness   221

Part Four: AT HOME WITH BEAUTY

20. The Family Dinner Table   227

21. A Beauty Spa in Your Bathtub   235

22. Your Man   243

23. Your Beautyfarm   262

24. Au Revoir   277

Part Five: BEAUTYFARM COOKERY

25. Out of the Frying Pan   283

26. Cosmetics from Your Kitchen Shelf   351

Foreword

*"Mirror, mirror on the wall,
Who is the fairest one of all?"*

It all began eons ago in the Garden of Eden, where a snake looked around for someone to talk to. It was not Adam but Eve, the lady of the garden, whom the snake chose because he found Eve subtle, eager and much more curious than her Adam.

But no sooner had the lady of the garden fallen for the new-fangled apple (there are those who say that the snake won the argument when he told Eve that the apple was good for her complexion), than she turned on her persuasive feminine charms and said to Adam: "Take a bite, dear, it's good for you!" And we read that Adam promptly ate thereof.

Whether or not we believe the story of the Garden of Eden, one thing is certain. Ever since then, Eve has had tremendous power over Adam and her whole family. It is always Eve who tries new things first; her curiosity about better ways of living is greater than her man's—probably because she bears the day-to-day responsibilities for the well-being of her family.

And so, thousands of years after the famous episode in the Garden of Eden, I address myself directly to you, Eve. I know that all your life you have looked for the kind of beauty that does not come off at night, an inner beauty that is your birthright. I know you have tried many things. I have seen you cut your hair, shorten your skirts, paint your cheeks. Time and again you have stepped up to your mirror, asking the ancient question:

"Mirror, mirror on the wall,
 Who is the fairest one of all?"

In the old fairy tale, the mirror answered the queen that, indeed, she was the most beautiful of all. But life is not a fairy tale; all too often your mirror tells you that you are not so beautiful as you would like to be. But does it also tell you that you *can* be beautiful? You see, to read your mirror is a certain art, and I want to teach you this art. I want to show you how to satisfy the hunger for true beauty—a beauty that can come only from within. I want to show you how to bring out your inner beauty, how to make you come alive with verve and vitality, how to make the most of your beauty potential.

Once you are on your way to your own radiant perfection, then I ask you to use your womanpower to help your Adam. A great many Adams are worried today, not so much about their looks as about their hearts and their vitality. You can help immeasurably—not only your man but your whole family.

For woman's beauty is not imprisoned by her skin; it permeates her entire home, creating warmth, love and harmony, and often it radiates far beyond her own four walls.

You never realize the great importance of beauty until you are in a place where it does not exist. The inspiration to write this book came to me in Moscow, of all places, while walking down Gorki Street. It was a sad experience: no happy faces, no bright complexions, no shining hair, no laughing eyes, no gay colors, no smiles! Here was the bitter proof of what happens when a people make the best of their machines and the worst of themselves. I realized then and there that I must shout from the housetops, that I must tell women of the Free World and especially American women, that they are unbelievably lucky, that they must take advantage of their great riches and their many freedoms and must make the best of themselves.

The thought that struck me so forcefully there was: "Beauty is duty."

Part One

BEAUTY WITHIN
YOUR REACH

CHAPTER 1

You Can Be Beautiful

I say this with confidence even though you tell me that your
nose is too long, your mouth too wide, your forehead too high or
low for ideal beauty. For you could have the most perfect features
and still not be beautiful. Of all the great beauties of history, there
was probably not one whose features were perfect!

No doubt, you have on your dressing table a full assortment of
beauty products, which you use diligently. The Cold Cream
Queens of Fifth Avenue and Wilshire Boulevard have taught you
a great deal about beauty care. They have provided sweet-smelling
creams and lotions, and cosmetic artifices that help you to look
your best.

But I am not talking about beauty that comes off at night.

BEAUTY UNIQUELY YOURS

I am talking about your individual kind of beauty. Real beauty
is a combination of many qualities. And there is a particular
combination that is uniquely yours, which belongs to no one else
in the world but you, if you will only learn what this combination
is!

Beauty is within your reach *today*. Whether you know it or not,

3

you live in the greatest golden age of beauty that has ever existed. Never in the history of womankind has there been such an abundance of opportunities for the attainment of beauty.

In ancient Egypt, only a woman of a royal or wealthy class could afford oils and unguents, and a slave to rub them on her tawny, sun-dried skin. Beauty did not come easily in days of old, and sometimes it cost heavily. Just to keep herself decently clean, a woman needed wealth and a staff of slaves.

In the Middle Ages there were no private baths, and women might not bathe for years. When knighthood was in flower, those romantic castles reeked of stale perspiration which the most pungent perfumes could not override.

Sometimes a woman literally paid in blood to be beautiful. If her complexion was too ruddy, she summoned a midwife or physician to bleed her for the sake of a fashionable pallor.

Our American pioneer woman barely had a breath to spare for the pursuit of beauty; she was too busy trying to survive. Yet she yearned for beauty. She created it in her spotless home and sparkling pots and pans.

The hardships of those days roughened and wrinkled a woman's hands and face. Her frequent childbearing, without proper nutrition, rest, or medical care, often made her old and misshapen before she was forty.

Do you know how lucky you are?

YOUR BEAUTY POTENTIAL

Today, with our modern scientific knowledge, there are no limits to a woman's beauty potential.

The simple, stunning truth is this, and I tell it to you out of my many years of experience, observation and constant study.

Every woman, no matter how modest her endowments, can be beautiful. She need not be rich, noble, or high-born. She need not be blessed with perfect form or features. All she needs is the *will* to beauty, plus the gift of feminine perception.

And to what an astonishing degree women possess this gift! My amazement and admiration for woman's intuition is never-ending. I like the way H. L. Mencken put into words this special gift of women:

"Women are the supreme realists of the race," he said. "Women decide the larger questions of life correctly and quickly. They see at a glance what most men could not see with searchlights and telescopes; they are at grips with essentials of a problem before men have finished debating its mere externals. Apparently illogical, they are the possessors of a rare and subtle super-logic."

You women of today have even more than this. You have curiosity and a sense of adventure. You know the value of material things, but you also know that things of the spirit are more important.

You know that your body is a valuable instrument. In times of great exaltation you are inclined to forget it, as indeed you should. But in your day-to-day living, which takes up most of your lifetime, do you give your body conscious care based on scientifically derived information?

WATCH OUT FOR BEAUTY THIEVES

We live in a golden age of science, but it has its dark side.

Dr. Paul Dudley White speaks of America being malnourished, not because it is poor, but because it is rich. We, as a nation, are suffering from *malnutrition* due to *overnutrition*. We eat a diet of 40 to 50 percent fat, when a good diet would have 25 to 30 percent fat.

As a nutritionist, who has spent a lifetime studying this problem of the rich but inadequate American diet, I agree.

I even go a step farther. Not only do we eat too much fat, we eat too little of the good, the life-giving, the *beauty-giving* foods. We have refined the vitamins and minerals out of our clean, sanitary, packaged foods. We have put in additives that do not replace the natural good that we have removed. And we have put in other additives that may keep our food from spoiling—for that is the purpose of them—but do us harm that we hardly know.

There is another beauty thief in our way of life, and that is nervous tension. You can see its ugliness in your mirror. It steals your beauty and your health. Listen again to Dr. White:

"There's no reason why we should be unhealthy," he said, "simply because we're prosperous. . . . We are born to use our muscles, it must be. And we know there's a beneficial effect not only on the circulation, but on the digestion, and *on the nerves.* You know, the peripatetic philosophers used to walk along the stoa, or promenade, when they philosophized. I think they realized that with good use of the leg muscles you also get better circulation in the brain."

Prosperity is a two-way street. It can provide you with the finest technology the world has ever known for the enhancement of your beauty. But it can also rob you of your treasure in the subtlest and sneakiest of ways.

LOVE YOURSELF

Modern psychiatry tells us that all the riches of Croesus can do nothing for a woman who does not love herself. Do I hear you protesting that I advocate selfishness? The fact is that I do. I believe in the selfishness that leads us to make the most of ourselves. The psychiatrist Erich Fromm tells us that love of others is impossible without love of self.

Beauty is a duty. Love of self, as reflected in the care of your person and the enhancement of your looks, is an expression of a healthy personality. The opposite is also true. Neglect of your person and the carelessness of beautifying habits is a symptom of mental illness.

Love is the great vivifier. It is the inspirer of new life, new freedom, unending youth. How long it takes for this simple truth to be learned! The time to learn is now.

If love is the great vivifier, then health is the greatest fuel of beauty. Now do not give in to a false sense of security. Health does not mean beauty, and beauty does not inevitably flow from bodily health.

By physiological standards, the people I saw in Russia were healthy people. They have built their country with their own sweat and brawn, but in doing it, they have made the worst of themselves. They seem to have lost respect for their own healthy bodies, to have forgotten their own faces. They attach no importance to the uniquely individual personality. That is the result when the rights of the individual do not count.

Come along with me

Perhaps you cannot see the forest for the trees. This is where I come in. I want to lead you through the maze of information provided by scientific effort, to interpret for you our vast fund of knowledge about the human body, the personality. I want to show you how the mysterious aura of beauty may be created by modern methods and creative new regimens.

I want to guide you away from the outdated and outworn notions of beauty culture, and show you new goals to strike for. Some of them are astonishingly easy, but somehow elusive. I want you to join me in this expedition to discover the secrets of beauty. I want you to see the relationships between the science of nutrition and the art of beauty, and how the breakdown of beauty can result from an ignorance of proper foods. I want you to see the all-too-human errors of overindulgence for what they are: the hidden hungers of body and mind.

I want to clear paths for you to make the attainment of beauty not a burden but a happy experience in good living.

Accept my invitation. Discover that beauty is not only an art, but also a science and a beautiful way of life.

CHAPTER 2

Beauty Is an Inside Job

The people who make your lipsticks and eye pencils, the hairdresser who waves your hair—they talk a beauty language that you can understand. Their language does not even need words. You can see its meaning in the mirror, right there in the beauty salon.

But their kind of beauty still comes off at night. And even during the day, it cannot always cover up the weary lines of fatigue and low energy, the sagging posture of a body that has poor muscle tone. They cannot give you that radiance from within that illuminates even a plain face and an ordinary figure, and makes them exceptional.

Oh, yes, that store-bought, manufactured beauty *can* put a moment's glow on your cheeks, a shine on your hair. With a skillful coiffure, clever makeup, a well-fitted girdle, you can look attractive when you go out. Cinderella looked beautiful, too, on her way to the ball. But you know what happened when the clock struck midnight.

At what hour does your particular midnight strike? Does your part-time beauty fade when the clock strikes nine?

To me there is only one true beauty foundation, whether for your complexion or your hips. It is manufactured inside your own remarkable body.

8

Your laboratories of beauty

It is produced in thirty trillion tiny laboratories, each one a living breathing part of you. Some of them are so small that they have to be magnified 50,000 times by the electron microscope before they can be seen. Yet your beauty begins with those thirty trillion microscopic factories. They will manufacture your beauty if you will only give them the right materials.

Those thirty trillion factories are the cells of your body, the living units of which you are made. They are of many kinds—they are specialists. Each one is an expert at its own line of work. Bone cells, brain cells, the skin cells that keep making new skin for you, the nail cells and hair cells that keep growing new nails and new hair—they are your beauty factories; and those very special cells of your glands, they make magic, contributing to your good looks via their various hormones. Here is just one example:

Beauty magic

A ten-thousandth of a gram is an infinitesimal amount. You cannot even see it. Yet a few ten-thousandths of a gram of iodine can make the difference between a beautiful woman and a pitiful cretin.

Your thyroid gland needs that iodine. It is an essential ingredient of the thyroid hormone, thyroxin. Thyroxin goes out in your blood stream to all your cells, and stokes their tiny metabolic furnaces. It stimulates them to turn your food into energy. That is what we mean by metabolism.

When your thyroid gland does not have enough iodine, it cannot supply enough thyroxin to keep up the rate of your metabolism. When your metabolic rate is low you are likely to be tired, dull, sleepy a good deal of the time. You may become bloated, because your body keeps too much water. You will probably tend to be overweight.

And note this. You can see the loss of beauty in your mirror. With your thyroid working below normal, your skin becomes coarse and rough, your hair dull and lifeless.

There are parts of the world that are poor or completely lacking in iodine, where centuries of erosion have leached it out of the soil. In those lands, health and beauty both suffered. People grew accustomed to ugly necks thickened with the growth of goiter until science discovered that lack of iodine was the cause.

We are fortunate. The sea and all its delicious gifts are rich with this precious, beauty-giving element. Every fish and shellfish, all the sea greens of the oceans are bountiful in their supply of iodine and its beauty magic.

That is why on my lists of beauty-full foods you will find these gifts from the sea. That is why I invite you to eat plentifully of these foods, as the Oriental peoples have done for thousands of years. I invite you to take beauty from the sea.

That is one example of what I mean by beauty from the inside.

And so it is with all the other fifty-odd nutrients that I am forever urging my students to use. Each of them makes its small but essential gift to your beauty, the beauty that can be yours not part-time but around the clock—the beauty that begins with the cell.

The wonder of the body

Let me share with you my wonder at the miracle of the body. I have never lost my sense of awe at its marvels. Let me tell you why you should never take it for granted, simply because it is familiar. Let me persuade you to treat it with the love and respect it deserves.

I do not like to compare this living miracle with mechanical devices. But we live in a machine age and sometimes it helps us to visualize the body's mysterious ways by comparing it to familiar things.

So now, think of your body as the most remarkable piece of automatic machinery in the world. It has automatic heating and cooling systems that respond to the most sensitive thermostat. It has automatic communication systems that make an IBM machine seem like a child's toy.

Your body has an automatic distribution system bringing raw materials and carrying away waste products. What can be more marvelous than the blood stream, your beauty stream, that carries the means of life and beauty to every cell, to your bones, your

nerves and muscles, your skin, teeth, fingernails, and each and
every hair of your head!

Most wonderful of all is your body's power to turn steaks and
chops, cheese or asparagus or green salad into the raw materials
of life. Your digestive system, with its auxiliary organs, the liver
and kidneys, is an amazing chemical laboratory.

THE DIS-ASSEMBLY LINE

Let me be your guide through this chemical plant.

It is a long journey that the food takes, sometimes fast and
sometimes slow. Some foods that you ate five or six hours ago are
still being worked on in your small intestine, and some remain in
your large intestine ten hours or more. The alimentary canal is a
hollow tube twenty-five or thirty feet long—more than five times
your own length from chignon to shoetip.

It is like an assembly line, this tube. At various points, all along
the way, different processes go on, different physical and chemical
treatments are performed on the food. But we find that although
it works in stages like an assembly line, in fact it is a dis-assembly
line. For the work of this plant is not to put the food together but
to take it apart.

Every bit of food that you eat has to be broken down into its
separate chemical components. Every bit of plant stuff and animal
stuff has to be dis-assembled, so that the body can re-assemble it
into human stuff.

This plant begins working on your food the moment you put it
into your mouth. You yourself begin to break it down as you chew.
(And please chew it well; you will be satisfied with much less
food, and it is your best insurance against overeating!) As you
chew and chew, the saliva moistens the food for its journey, and
a wonder-working enzyme in the saliva, called ptyalin, begins the
chemical conversion of starches into sugars. This is the first step
in the transformation of foodstuffs into the stuff of human energies
and muscles and bones.

The stomach is a very active station, a muscular churn that
grinds and mixes the food, and at the same time pours into it
powerful chemicals like hydrochloric acid, and enzymes like pepsin
and rennin that break down proteins. The stomach is only a wide

place in the alimentary canal, holding a quart or a quart and one-half, but it has thirty-five million glands supplying digestive juices!

Despite the stomach's many glands, most of the work is done not there, but in the small intestine. This winding, coiled tube is perhaps twenty-one feet long. But it is lined with small, closely set, bud-like projections, called *villi*, and through these villi the food substances are absorbed into the blood, molecule by molecule, as they are separated from the digestive mixture. There are about five million of these little budlike mouths. Thanks to them, your small intestine has an absorptive surface of one hundred square feet, just imagine, almost as big as the nine-by-twelve rug on your living room floor!

One of the marvels of this chemical plant is its economy. With so large a surface, the intestine can extract from the food every bit of its nourishing value. That is a wonderful thought for thrifty housewives, who do not like to see food wasted. But it is a warning if you want to stay slim and trim.

When that old devil, Temptation, urges you to take second helpings, remember: Your efficient small intestine, with its millions of hungry little villi, will not let this extra food go by. Your body will store every bit of it away as fat.

INTESTINAL GARDENING

In the large intestine are the friendly bacteria, and they look rather like flowers under the microscope. We call them the intestinal flora. They are microscopic plants; actually they are parasites, but they do important work for us. They manufacture some essential vitamins of the B family, although not in large enough quantities for the body's entire needs, and also vitamin K, so necessary for blood clotting when the body suffers an injury.

The intestinal bacteria also help to keep in check other parasites that are not friendly. Some of the fungus infections that spoil the skin are regular inhabitants of the body that run wild when the intestinal bacteria are reduced and lose their control. For keeping up the vigor of the intestinal flora, there is one wonderful, easily available food, one whose praises I have been singing for years: yogurt.

Yogurt, kumiss, acidophilus and all the cultured milks are the valuable nutrients for this microscopic beauty garden of the intestines. Wise folk in the Balkan countries and other parts of the Old World have thrived on them for centuries. They knew these were health-giving, beauty-giving foods, although they did not know why.

The "liquid" you

As long as the nutrients remain within the digestive system, they might as well be in a jar on your pantry shelf. Nutrition is not within the body, not within reach of the cells, until it is in the blood.

The great poet Goethe called the blood stream "that very special fluid." It is very special indeed. It is your body's river of life, and it is your river of beauty as well. It carries the raw materials of your beauty to every cell. It is so important that it is regularly filtered and purified by the kidneys, and the liver watches over what comes into it from the intestines.

Once passed by the liver, the blood goes on its way, rich with the good nutrients for the cells. In the lungs it takes on its load of oxygen. And then it makes the circuit of the body, sparkling with oxygen and laden with foodstuffs—a glowing river of energy, vitality and beauty.

As for speed, every two minutes by your watch, this glorious beauty stream travels through your body from top to toe and back again. It is a continuous, ever-running stream of life. There are about ten pints of it, eighty percent water, carrying a freight of red and white blood cells, oxygen and food, plus its own very special minerals and proteins with which it does its work.

As Dr. Alexis Carrel used to say, it "does it all in silence." The chemistry of the blood is a science all by itself, tremendously interesting, but also tremendously complicated.

Let me give you an illustration. The blood must have a certain balance of mineral salts in order to carry out its subtle chemical exchanges with the cells. Calcium is one of these components, and a certain proportion of it in the blood is essential. If there is not enough, the bones and teeth will give up some of their calcium to the blood to maintain its vital calcium balance. The blood, dealing with all the vital chemistry of the body, has priority over separate parts.

Thus the chemistry of your blood becomes the most vital part of your beauty. In order to maintain the well-knit bones of a graceful body, in order to keep your teeth healthy and beautiful, you must supply, *in your food*, calcium enough for all—for bones, for teeth, and most of all for blood.

BEAUTY'S RAW MATERIALS

Remember this: Luckily, your digestive system can throw out many of the worthless foods you eat. *But it cannot put in what is not there.* The body can assemble the human stuff of which you are made, but not unless you give it the essential ingredients.

It must have *all* the building blocks of its necessary proteins, *all* the amino acids out of which it can make new cells for your skin and hair, new red blood cells to keep up your oxygen supply, new cells to replace old ones everywhere in the body.

It must have whole, natural sugars with their own supply of B vitamins that are necessary to turn sugar into energy. Otherwise the sugar you eat will steal B vitamins from other functions in the body, and your beauty will suffer from their lack in many subtle ways.

Your body must have the natural unsaturated fats that emulsify readily in the digestive system, and provide the essential fatty acids to keep your tissues and especially your skin young and supple.

Your body must have the special substances that it cannot create, the vitamins and minerals necessary for its own special products, its enzymes that preside as catalysts over the chemical life processes, and the hormones that stimulate and regulate the body in its cycles and its adaptations to environment and stress.

These are the essentials, the raw materials of your beauty. If you faithfully provide them, your body's own marvelous chemistry will do the rest.

In the last analysis you eat for your cells. It is your cells that have to be fed. The entire digestive system, that amazing chemical plant that we have just explored, exists only for the service of your cells.

YOUR NERVES AND YOUR LOOKS

And now, consider that most remarkable, most formidable, most human system, your brain and nervous system. A nerve cell is very tiny, but it puts out long branches, some of them three or four feet long. Every time you learn a new skill, millions of nerve cells put out new branches linking up with other nerves. Thus they form the new nerve pathways that coordinate your thoughts and actions, whether for figure skating, knitting or cooking a good dinner. Every time you memorize something—a poem, a name, a telephone number, a recipe—your brain cells make new connections so that you can call up the memory by association when you want it.

Your quick, responsive nervous system is a living part of your beauty. Because of it your body moves with grace. Your face lights up with the glow of interest and intelligence. Your human brain and nervous system make you not a clod of earth but a woman sensitive to her world and the place she fills in it.

What has your nervous system to do with the food you eat? A great surgeon, the late Dr. Sterling Bunnell of California, who did so much to save and restore the damaged bodies of men in World War II, told in his textbook on hand surgery of how the all-important nerves of the hand repair themselves after injury, even if they have been severed, if they are surgically sutured. The nerves heal, he said, remarkably well, *but only if they have good nutrition.* To a surgeon, good nutrition means a good supply of nourishing blood, rich with oxygen and with the nutrients on which the cells feed. Most important of these for the nerves are that whole big family of B vitamins.

EACH DAY A NEW YOU

When you suffer injury or infection, your body swiftly calls up an army of millions of cells of very special kinds. There are armies of repair cells, some for skin, some for bone and other kinds of tissue, that knit up the damage. There are divisions of fighting cells that attack the infecting germs or viruses and literally devour them —eat them up! There are battalions of scavenger cells that come to dispose of the dead germs and dead cells and clear the area for a return to normal activity.

All this happens when you have even so small a blemish as a pimple on your skin. And when it is all cleared up, your skin cells, in the growing layer underneath, push up new cells to make a smooth new surface, replacing the scarred surface where you suffered the damage, and presently your skin is as good as new. Indeed, it is literally new.

Where do you suppose all these busy, efficient cell armies come from? They are made in the bone marrow and the lymph vessels and the spleen and a number of sites called, all together, the connective tissue.

But they are not made out of thin air, or beautiful thoughts, they are made out of the food you eat. You have heard that your body renews itself every seven years. That is not true. *It renews itself all the time, every moment.* Not long ago the United States Atomic Energy Commission verified through studies with isotope tracers that ninety-eight percent of the atoms that make up the blood and bones and body tissues are replaced in *just one year*. They are replaced by new atoms which our body processes, taken from the food we eat, the fluids we drink, the air we breathe.

Think what it means, this wonder of change. When you look in your mirror, never say again, "This is the face I was born with; this is the skin I must put up with, all my life."

THE WONDER OF THE UNIVERSE

The living cell is the ultimate wonder of your body. It is the marvel of the universe. The Harvard astronomer, Dr. Harlow Shapley, says there is no substance anywhere in the universe to compare with the substance of living matter.

They can get along, those wonderful metabolic marvels. They can perform their miraculous sleight of hand to change the foods you give them into the substances they need. But only to a point. Some substances they cannot make. They need not only proteins but certain highly complex protein combinations called the amino acids, some of which they cannot make themselves. They need those other complex combinations, the vitamins; we call them *vita*mins because they are *vital*, essential to life. And they need the minerals.

BEAUTY UNLIMITED

In nutrition we talk of the daily minimum requirement of these essential substances that the cells must have. The minimum requirements are an average subsistence level, the minimum that will do to sustain the body without incurring deficiencies.

The cells can get along on a subsistence diet. But for vitality and beauty they need that something extra, an abundance of the health-giving, beauty-giving foods. That is why my Cosmetic Diet is fortified with extra amounts, not a minimum but a maximum, of complete proteins, vitamins and minerals.

We are an omnivorous species. We can eat almost anything, and live. Our marvelous chemistry makes human stuff out of the most amazing variety of diets around the world. Rice eaters, fish eaters, eaters of nothing but animal flesh, people who live on nuts and roots and berries, and the walking lady from Great Britain to whom I gave an interview after my lecture in London, and who claims to live almost entirely on grass—all of us live and work and play, think and function as human beings, because our marvelous body chemistry can convert all these strange diets into human tissues and human energies.

While it is true that on such strange diets human beings have survived, they have not thrived. They have suffered disease, deformity and early death. Often their bodies and even their minds have been retarded by deficiencies in their diet. We have all seen pictures of their misshapen bodies, their prematurely old faces.

These peoples eat as they do because that is the best that their environment provides. But our food supply is unlimited.

At your command is the greatest variety of foods any nation in history has ever enjoyed, and the science of nutrition to guide you in its use.

CHAPTER 3

The Mental Climate of Beauty

Laugh and the world laughs with you; laugh and be healthy, advised the Illinois State Medical Society not long ago. Laugh and live long, said the famous Dr. Sara M. Jordan of the Lahey Clinic in Boston.

Laugh and be beautiful, I say.

Modern doctors will tell you how closely your mind and your body are interrelated. Your beauty is created by neither one alone. It is the product of both.

You have heard the saying, Ugly goes to the bone. Well, so does beauty. Body and mind nourish each other, and both of them nourish beauty.

Alas, they may also starve, or even poison each other. And that is always fatal to good looks.

Look about you, and you will quickly see what I mean. Stand on any Main Street and watch people pass. You will see repression and constraint. In most women you will see a departure from the natural and true. You will see tension, the backward pull of lines and muscles, the lips hard and thin, the brow ridged with lines, the hands clenched. The whole posture is stiff, angular, harsh.

Then notice people's gestures. The gestures of a tense person— of an unhappy person—are stiff and angular. But a happy, relaxed person's movements are rounded, circular, embracing, as though to include the whole world in his or her happiness.

LOVERS OF LIFE, OR ACCOUNTANTS

In a long and interesting life I have discovered that some approach life as lovers and some approach it as accountants.

The lovers of life also have some sad moments, but as a whole they usually find something to be excited about. Their lives are predominantly happy ones and these people are not tense, but the accountants of life are forever balancing the checkbook of life, belittling it with ifs, buts and troubles. The accountants of life are forever complaining or anticipating troubles; no wonder they are tense.

Naturally we cannot always be relaxed. Sometimes we must mobilize all our power, like a runner at the Olympics. An athlete is tense in every muscle and nerve. His is the tension of action, the tension for which the human body is built. When the race is over, then nerves and muscles let go in complete, harmonious relaxation.

There is tension of the mind and spirit, too, that is natural and beautiful. The mind is tense when it is at work on a challenging problem. The emotions are tense in moments of strong feeling. But then the moment is over, or the job is done. Then, like the athlete, you let go. Mind, body, spirit—all relax.

How long is it since you enjoyed the feeling of relaxation, like a gentle wave washing away the ugly lines and angles of tension?

" 'Beauty is truth, truth beauty,' that is all ye know on earth, and all ye need to know," Keats wrote as he contemplated the beauty and harmony of a Grecian urn.

THE PHYSIOLOGY OF HAPPINESS

No intelligent human being can question the interdependence of beauty and happiness. Beauty does not always make one happy, but happiness always brings a kind of beauty. A bride is always beautiful. Many women are beautiful in pregnancy, and when nursing a baby. Happiness, love, the knowledge that she is nourishing life—all these shine in the loveliness of a woman at these great moments in her life.

Because I am a man writing this, perhaps you will say that like all men I am sentimental about brides, and about mothers and babies, and that I see beauty where there is actually only an aura created by my own imagination. And if I tell you that the great painters of the Renaissance all preferred to use models who were pregnant, you will perhaps say that they were sentimental, too, and they painted that radiance in the forms and faces of their women because they imagined it there.

But you are mistaken. The radiance is really there. Because happiness is literally translated into physical beauty. Happiness brings a glow to the skin, brightness to the eyes, a spring to the step, grace to the body. It creates all these elements of beauty in terms of body processes that it stimulates and energizes. The cells, the multitude of small lives that make up the life of your body, are quickened by happiness.

And the cells are also dulled and slowed by a dull, torpid spirit or by a mind that is not interested in anything.

The ancients understood that body and mind are one. *"Mens sana in corpore sano"*—a healthy mind in a healthy body, wrote the Roman poet, Juvenal. The ancients knew this through intuition, but we know it through science, the science of endocrinology.

We know today that mind and body are closely tied together by the mysterious endocrine glands. Everything that happens to you, from the outside or the inside, calls forth a reaction from these glands. Every change in your state of mind is communicated directly to your body by these glands.

If you are anxious or joyful, excited or depressed, your glands send the message throughout your body. Their messengers are the hormones, which they pour directly into the blood stream.

LAUGH AWAY TENSION

Why does Dr. Sara Jordan recommend laughter? Because when we are *upset* emotionally, we are out of balance. And at such moments it is laughter that breaks the strain, snaps the tensions, and quickens these glands to their work.

The whole function of these glands is to keep our inner climate in balance. They work as partners: one set of hormones quickens your heartbeat, another slows it down. One speeds up your metabolism, another tones it down to give your system the rest it needs.

Dr. Jordan says, "There is plenty of evidence that glands like the pituitary, adrenals and others—with their hormonal secretions —exert their beneficent influence in this way."

These glands work together with your nervous system, to keep your inner climate in balance.

THE WISDOM OF THE BODY

Professor Walter B. Cannon, the great American physiologist, named this system of adjustments "the wisdom of the body." Through the endocrine glands your state of mind is translated into body language. You blush when you are embarrassed. Your heart thumps when you are excited. And when you are happy your cheeks are pink, your eyes shine, your circulation speeds along, and you feel alive in every limb. That is when you are at your most beautiful.

Your state of body is also translated into a state of mind. When your body is well nourished and supplied with all its essential foods, when it is active and in good tone, you feel happy!

That is why a sure cure for the doldrums is to step out in a brisk walk, head up, arms swinging in rhythm, lungs swelling with deep breaths of good fresh air. You cannot take your depression with you on such a walk. Try it, the next time your spirits are low.

The posture of happiness creates the mood of happiness!

But the mechanism works both ways. A lift of the body can lift the spirit, and a depression of the body can depress the spirit. A poorly nourished body, a sluggish circulation—inevitably these create a low state of mind. And whether the first cause is physical or mental, your body shows the effects.

MOTHER NATURE'S STEPCHILDREN

If we lived in a state of nature, the wisdom of the body would automatically take care of the ups and downs of the mind and spirit. But we live very far from the natural state. We are no longer Mother Nature's children—we are rapidly becoming her step-children!

In our cities of steel and concrete, in our automobiles and jet planes, in our air-conditioned homes, we cannot respond in simple, direct ways as people did when they lived close to earth and growing things and weather. Our world is complex, and its impact on us is a mixture of signals.

We moderns rarely experience a simple surge of emotion or of tension, and then return to a state of balance. We assume emotional attitudes for life, and we become their prisoners.

Dr. Franz Alexander of Los Angeles, the great teacher of psychosomatic medicine, has written and lectured for years on the damaging effects of these emotional strait jackets in which most of us unconsciously spend our whole lives.

If ever you have a chance to hear him speak, do not miss it. From him you can learn how a repressed need for love can lead to ulcers, and how repressed hostility and aggression can lead to crippling arthritis, hypertension, even heart disease.

If these hidden emotional attitudes can have such destructive power over our health, what must they do to your looks!

Long before serious symptoms of illness appear, the damage is evident in face and figure, in complexion, in the loss of easy, graceful movement and glowing vitality.

EMOTIONAL POSTURE

I am not suggesting that we can always be happy. Happiness is not a free gift of life. It is rare and fleeting, and it almost never comes unalloyed. But we must be ready to grasp it when it comes our way, and we must be able to seek and find it.

Many things in life are beyond our power to change. But we can change our emotional posture—our attitude!

You may have heard me tell this story in my lectures:

Two workmen were tearing up the pavement. Asked what they were doing, one answered:

"Digging holes."

The other said:

"We're building a cathedral."

THE COURAGE HORMONE

By the time we are adult, most of the large decisions in our lives have been made. Work, marriage, a way of life are fairly fixed. The rest is living day to day.

You can live it dully, ploddingly, perhaps resentfully. Or you can live it eagerly and fully.

If there is trouble to be borne—as there is in every life—you can let the burden bow you and wear you down. Or you can face it with spirit and courage and either overcome difficulties, or if that isn't possible, perhaps they're God's problems and you must forget about them.

In the wonderful wisdom of the body, there is even a Courage Hormone! Yes, the Courage Hormone of the adrenal glands, which races through the blood stream, mobilizing energy to do what must be done.

Only inanimate objects let themselves be worn down by the forces of nature and life. Only mud and stones get pushed around. Your living cells are organized to overcome trouble.

Sigmund Freud, whose name has been used to cover many confusions, was nevertheless a very wise man. He believed that there were two great forces within each human being, the creative force which he named Eros, or love, and the destructive force which he named Thanatos, or death.

It is hard to believe, but we are all self-destructive at times. We are self-destructive when we give in to false appetites, when we eat, drink and smoke too much, when we burn the candle at both ends, even though we know better. And, of course, we are also cheating mind and spirit when we starve ourselves of mental nourishment.

A willingness to sit and let others do the thinking and entertaining for us seven days a week, as so many do before the television set, is self-destructive. A willingness to be a passive spectator and let life go by is also self-destructive.

Chronic boredom is an illness, says a distinguished psychosomaticist, Dr. Arnold A. Hutschnecker, in his book, *The Will To Live*.

G. K. Chesterton, a wise and witty man, found that this willingness to be a spectator instead of a participant is "the one main modern defect." He said, "To amuse oneself is a mark of gaiety, vitality, and love of life. To be amused is a mark of melancholy surrender and a potentiality of suicide. The former means that a man's thoughts are attractive, artistic, and satisfying; the latter means that his own thoughts are ugly, unfruitful, and stale."

To let others do our reading, dancing and playing is like engaging someone to make love for us. It is like requiring the priest or parson to say all our prayers. The human being who has never made love, never prayed, never danced is hardly better than the jellyfish floating in the sea.

The millions of years of life, struggling to achieve a soul, are wasted on such a person. His own fabulous body and the mind that dwells in it are wasted on him.

LOVE, LOVE, LOVE

Love is the best of all cosmetics. Love is nature's most magical beauty potion.

Cinderella is not only a favorite childhood heroine—she is constantly being revived in modern dress by novelists, playwrights, and motion picture producers. You and I are not screen writers but we could write this script ourselves. Remember the drab little librarian, hiding her shyness behind big spectacles, her hair pulled back in a tight bun. Enter the hero, and what happens? The glasses come off, the hair is freed to fall softly around the face, a white collar perks up the dreary dress, the heavy "sensible" shoes are replaced by attractive pumps. A dash of lipstick, a touch of rouge, and *voilà!* out of the cocoon emerges a butterfly!

And what has caused this miracle? What else but love!

You have seen the miracle take place in your own home town, in the office where you work, perhaps in your own family. We have all seen it happen in the life of England's beloved young Queen Elizabeth. Before her engagement to Prince Philip she was a rather plump and plain young girl. By the time of her marriage she had become a slender, regal, genuinely beautiful woman.

It is no secret that Queen Elizabeth fell deeply in love with her handsome Prince Charming. Love, and the desire to be beautiful in the eyes of the loved one, can work miracles of beauty.

That feeling of floating on air when you fall in love is more than a dream. It is a biological fact. Through the marvelous connections between mind and body, love heightens all the body processes. The nerves and the endocrine glands send their electrifying message to every organ and muscle; the blood carries the happy news to every cell. A woman in love hardly needs the touch of rouge to bring a glow to her face and a light to her eyes. Love does it for her. Love creates her beauty from within better than any cosmetic can do it from without.

And if love is fortunate, and finds its natural sexual fulfillment, then this beauty is constantly renewed. The act of love is nature's perfect mechanism for release from tensions, all kinds of tensions whether they are in the mind, the muscles, the nerves. Sexual fulfillment frees all the energies from the ugly prison of tension.

Most beautifying of all is the knowledge of being loved, that someone finds you beautiful and desirable. Through those loving eyes a woman can see herself as beautiful and she begins to feel and act *as if* she were beautiful. And that is an important step to beauty.

CAN YOU FIND LOVE?

You will tell me that not all of us are so fortunate as to find this marvelous, beauty-giving love, and that is true.

Sometimes life seems to withhold this most precious gift. But I believe that when love comes, it does not come by accident. Before you can discover love, you must learn to love yourself.

I have said earlier in this book that self-love is not the same as selfishness. Nor is it the same as vanity. Selfishness and vanity are the weaknesses of people who do not truly love and value themselves.

Selfish, vain people are people who, in the depths of their hearts, do not believe themselves worthy of love. That is why they must hungrily demand so much for themselves. That is why they parade their looks and accomplishments before others. They are forever in need of reassurance that they are worthy of love. They feed on admiration, a poor substitute for love. They are driven to "protest too much," like the lady in Shakespeare, in the effort to convince the world—but most of all themselves—that they are worthy.

To love yourself means to value yourself, and if you value yourself you are not afraid to give of yourself to others. You are not afraid to love. And remember, the surest way to win love is to give love, love without strings attached, to a man, a child, a friend.

To love yourself also means that you consider yourself worthy of your own care and development. You do not condemn yourself because you are not perfect—instead, you value your goodness and find it worth your while to struggle with your weaknesses.

If you love yourself, you can look in your mirror without hating yourself for the imperfections you see there. You can quietly contemplate your image and make the most of your possibilities, your Beauty Potential.

Cultivate love. Read the inspiring book, *The Art of Loving,* by the famous psychoanalyst and philosopher, Dr. Erich Fromm. It will give you new insights into this most sublime of human emotions. It will show you that you do not need to wait for life to bring love to you.

Love, with the beauty that it brings, is a gift you can create for yourself.

BEAUTY IN THE MIND

If you have found your life dull and boring, ask yourself why. Perhaps the dullness is not outside, but within.

You were not always bored. Everyone has known moments of aliveness, when the world was freshly created every morning and there was never enough time to do the things one wanted to do. The world of children is like that. When did you let this joy in life become dull and stale?

For each of us there are still such moments and such opportunities. The smell of the woods or the mountains may be the magic to make you forget tiredness. Good news can make a sufferer forget his pain. Music can stir the glands to pump their beautifying hormones into the blood stream.

For each one, there is a key to unlock the beauty that springs from within the mind.

Enthusiastic activity for others, or the immersion of the self in a project for its own sake, may loosen the bonds and give the body its freedom. Love gives it.

If we have no enthusiasm for God or God's creation then we are stagnant. Stagnation is not living. "Because thou art neither cold nor hot I will spew thee out of my mouth," says the Book of Revelations.

Part Two

THE BEAUTY-FULL FOODS

CHAPTER 4

Your Cosmetic Diet

Why a Cosmetic Diet?

Every day of our lives we use food to build us up or build us down. Most women know the value of the right kind of food when it comes to reducing. They have experienced it themselves or they have seen their friends transformed by diet. But to say that food is only for the perfecting of the figure is like saying "water is only for bathing."

I must admit that back in 1922, when I first started to teach nutrition, I too did not understand the beauty-giving power of foods. At that time I was only interested in health; I knew a great deal about that, because it was through food that my tubercular hip finally healed. I wanted the whole world to know about it. I lectured, taught classes from coast to coast, wrote books and a nationally syndicated column, "Your Food and Your Health." I did a national radio program, and later a television program. I believe I made Americans more and more food conscious, and after I wrote *Diet Does It*, my first best-seller, I went on a lecture tour of Europe; wherever I went the halls were not big enough to hold the eager people interested in nutrition.

And then I made a discovery: Whether it was in Paris or San Francisco, Berlin or London, women by the thousands would invariably thank me for what my diets did—not for their health, but for their looks! I have heard it thousands of times and in many languages: "My skin is like new, I never have any more trouble with dryness." "Now my hair is alive, it is so easy to handle." "I am also proud of my nails." "I have no new cavities since I eat your way; my dentist could not get over it."

And usually they would add: "And I feel and look so much better!"

Finally in 1938, Ann Delafield attended one of my lectures in New York City, and asked me to arrange an *Eat and Grow Beautiful* food program and supervise the diets of the ladies on Elizabeth Arden's beauty farm in Maine. I was delighted with the opportunity to see at first hand just what beauty-full foods could do even for spoiled rich ladies who could afford to spend from $300 to $600 a week.

That beauty farm was successful; so was Miss Arden's second one in Arizona, where Mrs. Eisenhower was a guest, and the beauty farm movement has been growing ever since.

BEAUTY-FULL FOODS MAKE
BEAUTIFUL PEOPLE

Where does beauty begin?

The question is a fascinating one. In every city I visit, on this continent or in Europe, or in South America, I find new evidence to support this belief: that beautiful human beings grow on the things that are free and unsophisticated. They flourish on sunshine, air, water, and natural, unrefined foods.

A London physician, Sir Robert McCarrison, corroborated my belief most dramatically on his return from a small country at the northern tip of India, the land of a people called the Hunza. There are no more than perhaps 20,000 of the Hunza, but every one of them is unusually good looking, remarkably healthy. The men are strong, virile, lean, none under six feet tall. The women are petite, with golden shimmering skin, pearly white teeth, jet-black hair. They are virtually free of disease, and rarely prey to the nuisance ailments that plague today's civilized societies.

Why has nature been so kind to the Hunza people?

Why do they enjoy long and vigorous life?

Above all, why are they so *beautiful?*

This distant land, isolated in its mountains, is almost the last place left on earth where man's modernism and sophistication have not yet penetrated. The Hunza neither refine, nor blanch, nor bleach, nor color their food. Their produce is raised in naturally fertilized soil and taken directly to their cook-houses to be prepared for eating. There are no intermediate packagers, processors, to rob the foods of their good proteins, vegetable oils, vitamins and minerals. The peelings of fruits and vegetables are not thrown out as garbage. Nothing is boiled to death and nothing is wasted.

And here is another strange true story: Dr. Weston Price, a Cleveland dentist, closed his office in Cleveland and traveled around the world to find out for himself why there are so many deformed mouths and decayed teeth. He came back from his travels with the report that as long as people ate non-refined, simple foods their bodies and faces were handsome; their facial bones were broad, not pinched, their eyes were wide apart, the cheek bones high and well developed; the lower third of their faces was wide and the jaw bones were sufficiently large to permit the teeth to grow evenly without crowding; their chins were strong and broad, never receding.

Dr. Price's descriptions of the healthy human beings he photographed almost sound like a Hollywood makeup man's dream: eyes wide apart, high cheek bones, good mouth, strong white teeth and a strong chin—and all this was the gift of nature, the result of eating their own natural simple food. You can see Dr. Price's remarkable pictures for yourself. They have been put on slides and can be obtained from the American Academy of Applied Nutrition, Los Angeles, California.

What does a gardener do when he wants to raise the most beautiful flowers? He uses the best soil, fortifies it with nitrates, vitamins, minerals, humus that is rich in organic fertilizers. When a farmer sets out to raise sleek prize-winning cattle or poultry he does the same thing. He feeds them diets that have been scientifically formulated, full of the essential vitamins, minerals, and nutrients, grains and greens.

I think it is about time we fed our people as well as we feed our livestock and our flowers. Surely your beauty is worth as much care as that of a plant, a cow, or a chick!

Now you know the reasons behind this Cosmetic Diet that I have devised for you and all women who not only wish and long for beauty, but will do something about it. The Greek word from which we take our word "cosmetic" means *to adorn*, and this is what the diet of beauty-full foods will do. It is the science of nutrition applied to beautifying the body, with special emphasis on those significant points of beauty, the skin, hair, nails, teeth, eyes, and the contours and carriage.

The diet is built on those three essentials of any sound human diet, which I call the Big Three: proteins, carbohydrates, and fats. You eat all three of these every day, but do you choose the right ones, and in the right proportions? There is a world of difference. When it comes to your looks, no less than your health, you should no longer guess. You should KNOW.

THE MAGICAL PROTEINS

Protein is magic—protein is beauty—protein is proud posture. Yes, from your shining hair down to your pink toenails and the trillions of cells in between, every cell needs protein.

In a biological sense, human life, in fact all life, is protein. A new biology is about to be born, based entirely on the discovery of how the living cell synthesizes its own proteins out of the foods we eat. This is an exciting front in biological research today. Out of it more and more secrets about your health and good looks will emerge.

What has this to do with your personal beauty?

Virtually everything! Every cell in your body clamors for protein. Not just any protein, but the complete proteins containing all the essential amino acids, the building blocks out of which the cells can make their peculiarly human proteins. Your blood, bones, muscles, glands, organs, your skin, hair, nails crave these essential protein foods. And any lack of them takes a proportionate toll of your beauty potential.

Protein is the foundation of our Cosmetic Diet, because it is the foundation for all health and good looks.

Here is a list of the most complete proteins. All of them contain the eight essential amino acids, the building blocks that your body cells need for their own protein synthesis: lysine, leucine, isoleucine, tryptophan, phenylalanine, threonine, methionine, valine. You need not remember their strange, rather difficult names; only remember the foods that contain all these amino acids, the beauty-full proteins.

Milk, in all forms: buttermilk, yogurt, acidophilus, kumiss, powdered milk.

Cheese, particularly lean cottage cheese, Cheddar, American, Roquefort.

Eggs, of all fowl.

Liver, of all kinds.

Beef, the leaner the better: veal, lamb.

Fish, especially salt water varieties, rich in iodine.

Chicken, and all lean fowl.

All these complete proteins are derived, as you see, from animal sources. Together they are your magic key to beauty, and at least one of them should be eaten at every meal.

If your pocketbook permits, take most of your proteins from animal sources. They are richest in the beautifying amino acids and they contain one in particular—lysine, which is of monumental importance. Lysine, by its peculiar biochemical magic, increases and elevates the protein content of the less expensive vegetable proteins in your meal. Many nationalities have known this intuitively. The Chinese combine their vegetables with a bit of meat, the Mexicans serve their beans with chopped meat; the Italians serve their pasta with meat sauce and cheese. In our Cosmetic Diet protein is the tissue rebuilder par excellence. We need it to prevent or repair so many beauty defects: sagging muscles, limp skin around the neck, drooping tissues of the face, soft abdomens and expanded waistlines, drooping breasts in young women—all these point to a lack of protein in your diet.

You do not automatically get enough protein every day; you must take pains to do so. You should be getting half as many grams of protein daily as your body has pounds of weight: for 140 pounds, at least 70 grams. If your husband's weight is 200 pounds, he needs 100 grams.

Check your intake with the table of protein foods on page 44. You will probably be surprised. Most women do not get sufficient protein and therefore they wrinkle and age prematurely.

BEAUTYFARM MAGIC

Since animal proteins are the most costly of all foods, and not plentiful in some parts of the world, I have included some of the less expensive vegetable proteins in my Cosmetic Diet. Through the magic of the complete proteins, especially the component, lysine, which is contained in all animal foods, the vegetable proteins in soya beans, grains, nuts and seeds can be made into valuable building foods by combining them with the animal proteins. For instance, you increase the protein level of any food by adding comparatively inexpensive dry skim milk powder. Powdered skim milk is one of the most valuable beauty boosters, and so is the inexpensive lean cottage cheese.

Beans, gelatin (also an incomplete protein) and grains are boosted into valuable beauty-building protein when eaten with a bit of milk, meat or cheese. Take advantage of this astonishing chemical fact if you have a family to feed. Combine the more expensive animal proteins with the less expensive vegetable proteins. If you are a vegetarian for aesthetic reasons, you can now buy lysine in concentrated form to fortify your vegetable proteins, and derive twice the benefit. Still better, buy yourself some liver tablets. I recommended these to George Bernard Shaw. He took them grudgingly, but I believe they kept him going when everything else failed. There is magic in protein and liver is the number one protein.

"E" IS FOR ENERGY (CARBOHYDRATES)

In our fast-moving, get-up-and-go culture, quickly summoned energy is as important for our bodies as it is for jet planes. Your body can turn the proteins we just discussed into energy too, but a man of average size would have to eat nearly four pounds of meat a day to provide his body with the energy it needs, even at rest, and almost four times that quantity for heavy work.

The Eskimos actually eat such huge quantities of protein food and a good proportion of fat, but most of us do not work as hard as Eskimos. It is much cheaper and wiser to obtain our energy from the large family of carbohydrates—the starches and sugars.

Yes, that is what I said. But I mean the right kind of starches and sugars as nature provides them, still beauty-full and not emptied of their beauty-giving nutrients.

I am and shall forever be the sworn enemy of the foodless confectioneries, pastries, and all such denatured sweets which bring you nothing in terms of health and beauty. They do not necessarily give the quick energy you expect of them. Many of them, on the contrary, slow up the body functions. In addition they rob your precious vitamin store for their metabolism, since they bring no vitamins with them. And finally they come to rest without shame or mercy around your waistline, chin or buttocks.

I am convinced that much of our overweight problem is due to the many empty foods which the human body is not able to use and so deposits as fat.

On the other hand, there are magnificent vitamin-rich, mineral-rich, starch and sugar foods which your body will metabolize with brilliant success. These will give you the quick energy you need, and in addition they will bring new wealth to your beauty treasury.

You will find such starches and sugars in whole grain kernels, whole bread, root vegetables, sweet fruits, vegetables and their beauty-giving juices. When it comes to nature's own energy-giving sweets, you can select from these delicious sugars: golden honey, dozens of different flavors; real maple syrup; rich dark molasses; natural brown crystal sugar; the new-found sweet of the carob tree; real licorice, and all the sun-dried fruits such as apricots, figs and dates.

With the Cosmetic Diet you can strike from your beauty budget forever the sugary concoctions so massively consumed in our country today—more than eighteen pounds of candy a year for every man, woman and child! Also, the many sweetened soft drinks, truly empty food which have no place in an *Eat and Grow Beauty-full* regime; they can do you no good.

These overrefined sugar products are the real trouble-makers; they come to you emptied of vitamins and minerals. To metabolize them, to burn them into the energy which is all they are good for, your body must use its precious B vitamins garnered from all the other foods you eat. These empty sweets charm you with their white smiles, dupe you with the illusion of nourishment, and then proceed to rob you!

When you need a sweetener, take the honest companionship

of pure honey. You will be surprised at how well it "marries" with other foods. Do not be deterred from this delightful, beauty-rich food by the fact that it is sticky. Buy a glass container like the one you use for maple syrup, which cuts off the flow without a drip. For your elegant guests, do as many of my students do: offer them honey from a silver beehive honey jar and watch them enjoy a gourmet treat. Use it in your tea and for all sweetening purposes. If you have ever eaten ripe strawberries sprinkled with golden honey, you will never use sugar and cream again.

QUICK ENERGY

Here is something you should know about quick energy. When you are low in energy and reach for a sweet, your impulse is correct. You are tired, usually, because you are low in blood sugar. But the sweet that you reach for—what does it do for you?

In a curious condition called hyperinsulinism, the reverse condition to diabetes, the pancreas manufactures too much insulin and the blood sugar characteristically falls so low that you may suffer from palpitations, light-headedness, and other disturbing symptoms in addition to fatigue and consequent depression and irritability. The interesting fact about this for all of us, as Dr. E. M. Abrahamson points out in his book, *Body, Mind and Sugar*, is that the quick-energy sweet does more harm than good. It sends the blood sugar up in a sudden rise and, then by stimulating the pancreas to produce even more insulin, it ends by depressing the sugar level even lower than it was before and you are back where you started.

This is something for beauty-seeking Eves to remember. You cannot conquer fatigue with its drawn look by the quick sweet alone, not even by the whole and wholesome sweet of natural sugar. The energy values of carbohydrates are part—but *only* part —of your Cosmetic Diet. Only proteins, the complete proteins with all the essential amino acids, can form the solid, dependable foundation of your health and beauty and give you sustained energy for hours by keeping your blood sugar level high. (See page 44.)

Select your beauty-full, high-energy foods from the following: grains, such as buckwheat (kasha), whole wheat, oats, brown rice, whole grain bread; fruits and their juices; vegetables and their freshly made juices.

Recommended sweets: unheated honey, unsulphured molasses, dark brown sugar crystals, real licorice, St. John's bread, fresh or in powdered form, dried fruits of all kinds.

THE BEAUTY-FULL FATS

Contrary to what you may have heard, the right kinds of fat can make you beautiful. This truth in body esthetics may surprise you: a thin layer of fat beneath a woman's skin provides a surface for the radiation of light. Against it, outside sources of light and color are cast with transforming beauty. The greatest painters of nudes, from Botticelli and Raphael to Renoir, knew this principle. They never painted a model so thin that her skin had no underlayer of fat.

So take a hint from the great painters. If you have struggled for a slim figure and have tried to avoid all fats, change your policy. Shun only the hard, saturated animal and hydrogenated fats, they are the troublemakers, for you and even more for your man. Instead, use those fats which contain the valuable unsaturated fatty acids. These you find in the golden vegetable oils.

Some years ago a German chemist, who approached statistics with a poet's passion, estimated the fat content of a beautiful woman as eleven percent of her total volume. It seems an odd way to measure beauty, but he was not inaccurate. He was referring to the fatty acid called linoleic acid.

Experiments have shown that animals deprived of this nutrient developed dry and scaly skin and their fur became rapidly dry and thin. When the important linoleic acid was returned to their diet, skin and hair thrived again.

There are many sweet-tasting liquid oils that contain this essential skin and hair nourisher. These oils can be used singly or combined in delicious salad dressing or mayonnaise. Even when reducing, you need at least one tablespoon a day of these oils to keep the skin glowing. Thousands of women told me that their complexions took on a new radiance when they began to use vegetable oils in place of the saturated hard fats. I believe that within a few weeks after using these golden oils with all the essential fatty acids, you too will become enthusiastic about the beauty-giving fats. Take your choice of these golden natural oils:

LINOLEIC ACID PERCENT

Safflower	70	Cottonseed	50
Poppyseed	62	Sesame	41
Sunflower	57	Peanut	25
Soybean	53	Linseed	20
Corn	53	Sardine	15
Wheat Germ	50	Olive	8

FRESH BUTTER

You will note that in my Cosmetic Diet I have not ruled out butter. Fresh butter has a high content of vitamin A, valuable to beauty, but it contains insignificant amounts of the beauty-building fatty acids, compared with the vegetable oils. Yet it improves the flavor of so many foods and, as Alice Toklas says, "Butter marries so well," that it would be a great deprivation to give it up entirely. We can use fresh butter sparingly on bread and toast.

And for shortening, the best solution I offer to you beauty cooks is to combine the golden vegetable oils with fresh butter, half and half. In this way we gain the benefits of the fatty acids in the liquid oils, and the wonderful flavor and vitamin A content of fresh butter.

I have learned about this combination from my Roman students. You can barely taste the difference between all butter and half and half, especially if you use one of the milder oils such as sesame or sunflower.

Beauty-seeking cooks should use only margarine which is made wholly of vegetable oil. Shun the hard, hydrogenated fats. The label on the package will tell you whether or not it is hydrogenated. If so, it is not for you.

CHAPTER 5

Your Day of Beauty-Full Eating

If we relied on our natural appetites we would never make a mistake in eating. In the brain there is a built-in regulator for thirst, hunger, appetite, and when the body needs a certain kind of food, that built-in regulator creates the appetite for that particular food.

Perhaps you have heard of a famous experiment that was made years ago with a group of healthy toddlers, still young enough to follow their natural appetites. Every day, at every meal, these babies were set down before a table loaded with all kinds of simple, natural foods, and they were allowed to eat what they wished—and somehow, they selected the foods which they needed.

Yes, nature would regulate our eating for us, if we would only allow her to do so. To show you how easy it is, here is a day that I have planned for you, a single day of natural, *beauty-full* eating. Try this experiment with me.

BREAKFAST

Breakfast is your vitality and beauty determinator for the day. I say that positively. Whether you will begin your day tired or glowing with energy is no longer a matter of guesswork. It is simple arithmetic.

When your blood sugar is at 90, you are comfortable. At 80, you are slowing down. At 70 you are hungry and your lassitude becomes fatigue. At 65 you are craving for sweets and your insides are grumbling, and if the level continues to drop you may suffer headache, weakness, wobbliness, heart palpitations, mental confusion, nausea and worse. And your nerves, which feed only on the sugar supply in your blood, suffer first and most from this needless starvation!

Now let us see what happens when you begin your day with your habitual breakfast. It is about twelve hours since your last meal, and the average level of blood sugar after twelve hours of fasting is between 90 and 95. In a famous study which was reported some years ago by the United States Department of Agriculture, two hundred volunteers ate various kinds of breakfasts, from black coffee alone or "coffee-and" to a classic breakfast of juice, oatmeal with sugar and cream, bacon, toast with butter and jam, coffee with sugar and cream.

With only coffee, the blood sugar went steadily down during the morning, and the volunteers became more and more irritable, nervous, headachy and exhausted.

HIGH VITALITY ALL DAY LONG

For those who had taken good protein with their breakfast, either eggs or fortified milk, the blood sugar rose to a vigorous 120 and remained at that level through the morning hours.

But here is the most remarkable part of this remarkable story: all through the day, no matter what those volunteers ate, those who had eaten a breakfast without protein continued to have low blood sugar, with all its miseries. And those who had taken good protein with their breakfast enjoyed high blood sugar, high vitality, high efficiency and high spirits all day long.

Now do you understand why I say that breakfast is your vitality determinator for the day? As for your looks, when you are irritable, nervous, fatigued, how do you imagine you look? Your mirror has shown you, many times. When your blood sugar falls, everything falls—including your face.

Now I know what you will say—I have heard it so many times: "But I *can't* eat such a big breakfast!" My answer to you is, you *will be able* to eat it and enjoy it too. Begin by eating and drinking a bit less the night before.

Do you realize what upside-down people we have become? We give our bodies the biggest load of food at night, before going to sleep, exactly when we need it least. And then we cheat ourselves at breakfast, the meal with which we begin the day's working and living, just when we need food most.

BREAKFAST AND YOUR LOOKS

You can change that. You will want to change it, when you remember that it is the foods you eat at breakfast, when the day is young, that determine how much verve and vitality you will have all day, how much sweetness and light you will give to those around you—yes, and what kind of face you will present to the world.

Would you choose to be pale and tired and drawn? Or would you prefer to be glowing with inner warmth and well-being? It is yours to choose a good day or a poor one: it is as clear as though it were written on the breakfast menu.

I am thinking especially of the fifteen million Americans who try to look and feel their best on a breakfast of cold cereal which gives them only three grams of poor-quality protein. And another fifteen million, the "coffee-anders," who eat an empty white-flour roll with their heavily white-sugared coffee. Half an hour after such a miserable meal the blood sugar dives to a new low.

Forgive me if I refer to the Russians again. I have seen their system with my own eyes and I detest it thoroughly. But dictators can give orders, and they realize, more than we of the free world, that a people must rise or fall by what they put into their stomachs. If you have ever seen the vitality and drive of the people of Moscow as I have seen them, you understand why I point to them again.

And what has breakfast to do with the Russians? Just this: nowhere else in the world does a whole nation get up in the morning and eat dinner at breakfast time.

No cold cereals or "coffee-and" breakfasts will do for them. They eat a main dish of meat or fish, with vegetables—cooked cabbage, if you please. I went to the Institute of Nutrition in

Moscow and Dr. Menshikov himself outlined the Russian regime for me. Furthermore, I saw the people eat such breakfasts with gusto.

CHOOSE YOUR OWN BEAUTY-FULL BREAKFASTS

I do not ask you to eat cooked cabbage for breakfast. Even though I have given you menus, they are suggestions for you to sample, illustrations of a principle. Ours is not regimented eating. Ours is a world of fabulous choice. We have so many good proteins, such a wide variety of golden grains in breads and cereals, an array of fresh and frozen fruits in our refrigerators from all our sunny lands. No king or queen, czar or rajah, in all the world's history, and no people, ever had such a wealth of beauty-full foods, and such freedom to choose among them. For you, women of the free world, this crucial first meal that will keep you at your best all day can be different for every day of the month.

Some of you, I know, are small eaters. For you I offer this suggestion: if you really find it difficult to manage a substantial breakfast each day, then make sure to have a mid-morning booster that will keep your blood sugar at high level—not an empty deceptive snack like coffee or cola and a doughnut but a fortified milk drink, a bit of bread and cheese, a sweet fruit with a handful of nuts or tasty sunflower seeds.

BLUEPRINT FOR BEAUTY-FULL BREAKFASTS

First: Fruit juice or whole fruit.
Second: Large helping of protein.
Third: Helping of whole grain bread or cereal.
Fourth: For enjoyment and more protein, enjoy one or two large cups of Swiss coffee (hot coffee with foaming hot milk).

Now let us set a buffet on a big long table so you can see the tremendous variety to choose from. I have listed the most popular breakfast dishes; you need not have ham and eggs every day of the week. They are a fine protein dish, but actually we need variety. The English people like fish, South Americans eat steaks, the Swiss people enjoy their famous cheese. These are all first class proteins. I urge you to try them. The mark of a modern woman is her willingness to extend her food horizons. Soon we will be traveling in space and I predict that concentrated protein breakfasts will become a must for all strenuous tasks. I suggest you start now. See how lucky you are; in this land of variety a clever woman can prepare a different breakfast for every day in the month.

I have tried to give you average helpings and good portions of protein dishes. Animal proteins are best; fresh and dried milk, lean cottage cheese and dried chipped beef are extremely high in first class protein. Use them generously to get your protein quota of 20 grams in every meal.

Breads and cereals are disappointingly low in protein unless you fortify them with soya flour, powdered milk or food yeast. But we *need* one good helping of carbohydrate to help keep energy and spirits high all day long.

I also urge you to learn to enjoy Swiss coffee in place of the beauty-destroying, heavily sugared and creamed beverage. Swiss coffee for breakfast is much to be preferred to black coffee; the milk adds extra protein, plus milk sugar for extra morning energy.

A FRESH BEGINNING

Each morning, as you begin your day of beauty-full eating, you will be creating fresh beauty for yourself. But now I want you to take my words literally, and make a fresh beginning with each meal. By this I mean: begin each meal with something fresh whenever you can.

This is a very new beauty secret, and also a very ancient one. Those of us who for many years have begun each meal with a fresh fruit or vegetable have always believed we were following the latest dictates of scientific nutrition—and so we were. But the truth of the matter is that, even without the aid of modern science, the wise Greeks practiced this rule 400 years before the birth of Christ. More than 2,000 years ago, the Greek physician Diocles Carystos wrote, "Eat your raw fresh vegetables first of all and follow with cooked food as your second course, and let fruit be the end of your meal."

In California and Florida and the sunny Mediterranean lands

Beauty-full Protein Foods	Amount	Grams of Protein
Beef	Average helping, 3 oz.	20
Beef, dried	Average helping, 3 oz.	30
Chicken	Average helping, 4 oz.	20
Heart, beef	Average helping, 3 oz.	14
Kidney	Average helping, 4 oz.	20
Lamb chops	2 small	20
Liver, all kinds	Average helping, 4 oz.	20-25
Steak, sirloin	Average helping, 4 oz.	20
Lean Ham	1 slice, 4 oz.	20
Lean Bacon	5 slices	10
Lean Veal	1 slice, 4 oz.	20
Turkey	Average helping, 4 oz.	23
Milk, whole	1 quart	34
Milk, dry skim	½ cup	22
Yogurt, fortified	1 cup	10
Cottage cheese, lean	½ cup	20-25
Swiss cheese	2 thin slices	20
1 Fresh egg	Large	7
Fish, broiled lean	4 oz.	20
Salmon	3 oz.	22
Tuna fish	3 oz.	15
Shrimp	10 medium	12
* Almonds	½ cup	15
* Pecans	½ cup	5
* Peanuts	½ cup	20
* Peanut butter	½ cup	24
* Seeds	½ cup about	20
* Walnuts	½ cup	10
* Lima beans	½ cup	5
* Navy beans	½ cup	6
Soya beans, dried	½ cup	37
Soya flour	½ cup	35
* Lentils	½ cup	10
* Peas, dried	½ cup	20
* Mushrooms	½ cup	8
* Buckwheat	½ cup	10
* Rice, brown	½ cup	8
* Wheat germ, fresh	½ cup	20
* Gelatin, plain	1 tablespoon	8
Yeast, food	1 tablespoon	10

* These foods become more valuable in our Cosmetic Diet when combined with animal proteins. Remember to repair the daily wear and tear and to keep tissue integrity at its firmest, you should have ½ gram of protein for each pound of your ideal weight (not your overweight). If your correct weight is 120 pounds, your daily protein needs are 60 grams. If your man weighs 180 pounds, his protein needs are 90 grams. Never forget that the complete proteins are made up of the health and beauty-giving amino acids.

of Europe it has long been a custom to begin a meal with something fresh, melon or fruit cup, or the crisp raw vegetables of French hors d'oeuvres and Italian antipasto. The lively fragrance and flavor refresh the taste buds, start the digestive juices and set the body's wonderful chemistry going for the rest of the meal.

SCIENCE TELLS US WHY

We know all this scientifically today. One of the great scientists of the last century, Dr. Rudolf Virchow, discovered and proved that there are physiological reasons for eating fresh foods at the beginning of a meal. He observed that cooked food called up a great increase of white blood corpuscles in the blood, the same reaction that the body makes to disease germs and bacteria. This is the wonderful defense system of the body, the "immune reaction" that protects us against disease. But it was Virchow's astonishing discovery that the body makes this same defense against processed foods! Then he found that when he fed his patients fresh, unprocessed food *first*, this rise in white blood corpuscles did not occur. Even more important, his patients *then* could eat their cooked meal without causing this irritable reaction of the blood.

I believe I am the first American nutritionist to apply Virchow's discovery in an Eat and Grow Beautiful Plan. In Europe, Dr. Bircher-Benner of Zurich and Dr. Werner Kollath of Hanover for many years have prescribed fresh fruits or vegetables at the beginning of breakfast, lunch and dinner.

The fresh color and flavor will set the "appetite juice" flowing even while you are enjoying it on your palate. And I have discovered other wonderful advantages to this agreeable custom.

Fresh things, eaten at the beginning of the meal when appetite is keenest, satisfy that first sharp hunger and prevent overeating.

Your salad, with its mildly acid dressing, also stimulates all the digestive processes and contributes bulk to encourage those muscular intestinal walls that might otherwise become lazy.

Finally, and most important for beauty, large fresh salads are our best vehicles for the skin-beautifying essential fatty acids. We get them in large amounts in the golden liquid oils of our delicious salad dressings.

Thus your fresh beginning for each meal serves beauty, health and a slim waistline, as well as appetite and the pleasure of eating.

LUNCH TIME IS SALAD TIME

More and more women are not only taking care of their homes, but also holding responsible jobs, and are away from their handy kitchens at lunch. And those who stay at home caring for young children also have a full-time job, and tend either to skip this important meal or to eat whatever snack is handiest, without regard to whether it meets the body's needs at midday.

And then there are the otherwise lovely ladies of leisure for whom luncheon is a social occasion with friends—but too often they make it a "stuff and gossip" session, abetting each other in crimes against their good looks with fatty sauces, pastries and sweets.

For you, whichever of these three you are, I have devised what I call a meal in a salad bowl—tempting, compact, not too expensive, and above all nourishing enough to keep energy at a high level all through the afternoon.

I am convinced that much afternoon tiredness and mental letdown which costs Big Business millions—or at home leads to short tempers and five o'clock storms with the children—can be prevented. So can the cost of your good looks as the afternoon wears on.

And you social lunchers can be just as charming—and much prettier—on delicious protein salads in place of fat-sodden entrées, and refreshing fruits and compotes instead of beauty-thieving pastries.

YOUR BOWLFUL OF BEAUTY

Whether you order this salad at your favorite restaurant or are lucky enough to make it yourself, here are its essentials:

For a base, cut up the freshest, greenest, crispest vegetables (at least a cupful): add to this a good portion, not less than twenty grams, of your favorite stick-to-the-ribs protein food (see list, page 44), and toss it all together with a golden oil dressing.

You can be generous with this oil dressing, for in it are the valuable unsaturated fatty acids which put a glow and bloom into your complexion. I believe there is nothing—and I mean nothing— which can do more for your skin than these fatty acids. European nutritionists call them Vitamin F, and they are as essential as all other vitamins. Without them the skin is dry and hungry.

On beautyfarms, salads like this are served in great bowls with a choice of half a dozen different kinds of dressing. The salad it- self can be different every day, with the endless variety of delicious fresh things we have to choose from, all the year round. And there need never be monotony in the dressing with the many golden oils providing their different nuances of taste.

I urge you to try them all, individually and in combination. Mix these oils, two or three different kinds in one dressing, the less expensive to extend the more costly ones, and by all means add a little of a good grade of olive oil. Olive oil is not rich in the unsaturated fatty acids, but it is richer in flavor than any of the other oils and it gives an elegance to salads which no other oil can. (See beautyfarm salad dressing, page 337.)

Good oils deserve good vinegars, and again we have a wealth of them to choose from.

Shun the white synthetic kind, which contributes neither good- ness nor flavor but only an edge sharp as a knife. It is just as easy to use cider vinegar with its mellowness of ripe apples, or if you have a French or Italian taste, flavorsome wine vinegar (but use it more sparingly). A salad must never have an outright acid or sour taste; sheer sourness is so strong and dominating that it kills all other flavors. It is best to follow the classic French proportions of two-thirds oil and one-third vinegar.

ADD THESE SMART FLAVOR NUANCES

For a milder and fresher-tasting dressing, use lemon juice, rich in vitamin C, in place of vinegar; I know some excellent cooks who sprinkle a few drops of lemon juice over all salads, especially fish salads, no matter what dressing they use. And to give their salads of other kinds a bit of mystery and soften any sharpness in the dressing, they use their imagination and spice them with various flavors—vegetable salt, salad herbs, or something unexpected like a drop or two of honey, wonderful when fruits are in the salad. You can be a true gourmet and do as they do on a French beautyfarm: make your own delicately flavored honey vinegar (see recipe, page 337).

No matter what you may have heard or read, take my word for it that fats are necessary even when you are reducing or weight-watching. The excess of hard animal fats and the many hydrogenated fats in the diet of most Americans has given a bad name to all fats, including the ones that are necessary to keep skin and hair beautiful.

REMEMBER YOUR BEAUTY-GIVING OILS

It is true that the health and beauty-giving values are destroyed when manufacturers shoot hydrogen into otherwise good oils so that they can stand in warehouses and on market shelves for a long time without spoiling. But why should you pay that hidden price in health and beauty? I believe that much of the excess fat which thirty million Americans carry around their waists is in part due to these fats. The human body is not equipped to metabolize such quantities of inert fats, so they are deposited where circulation is slowest—around the middle!

But with the fresh, unsaturated, liquid oils it is quite a different story: they are untreated by heat, and so they have not lost their abundance of the essential fatty acids, especially linoleic acid, and most of the antioxidants. Liquid oils are easier for the body to metabolize; they are not deposited as excess fat unless you are overeating generally.

So whether you are keeping your ideal weight or reducing, do not have less than a tablespoon of your favorite oil a day, *every* day, in some form; use it in cooking, in plain salad dressing or in your own delicious homemade mayonnaise. Real mayonnaise, made with unheated fresh oil, a fresh egg yolk and a dash of vinegar, is a splendid complexion food, a delicious inner and outer cosmetic. The oil furnishes your body with the beautifying fatty acids, your skin vitamin; the fresh egg yolk contributes softening lecithin, also vitamin A for your skin, and the vinegar adds flavor, speeds digestion and externally protects the acid mantle and makes the skin unbelievably soft.

BLUEPRINT FOR BEAUTY-FULL LUNCHEONS

First: A fresh start with any and all fresh green salad vegetables, broken up or chopped, the more the merrier (at
least a cup).

Second: Your favorite salad protein, 20 grams, never less than
half a cup. Have lean cottage cheese, shredded meat or
fish. Toss salad with golden oil dressing or mayonnaise.

Third: A carbohydrate for prolonged energy. A muffin, a slice
of protein, rye or wholewheat bread, lightly buttered.

Fourth: For enjoyment and stimulation, a glass of milk, yogurt
or your favorite beverage with milk.

YOUR CHOICE OF PROTEIN SALAD BOWLS

Cottage cheese salad bowl
Chicken salad bowl
Cheese salad bowl
Lean ham salad bowl
Tongue salad bowl
Lobster salad bowl
Shrimp salad bowl

Tuna salad bowl
Eggs, hard-cooked
Left-over meat
Soya bean salad bowl
Gelatin meat or fish salad (aspic)
Fruit and nut salad

FOUR O'CLOCK BEAUTY SAVER

One of my challenging Hollywood assignments was to keep the
glamor girls from looking wilted by mid-afternoon. Making motion pictures is the cruelest, most strenuous kind of work; after
a few hours of repetitious "takes" in stuffy air, under hot Klieg
lights, even the brightest and fairest of stars began to droop, and
the sharpest of all eyes, the movie camera, caught every listless
line.

Once at the Hal Roach studio my task was to sustain the
gorgeousness of twelve showgirls who really deserved the word
"gorgeous"; the picture was *The All-American Coed* and Frances
Langford was its lovely star. Lady Mendl was my guest in Beverly
Hills at the time, and since she was interested in all phases of the
theatre (she actually began her career as an actress for the great
David Belasco) I took her along to see how drooping glamor girls

can be revived without benzedrine and other pep pills. I knew it would be inspiring to the girls, too, to see how an internationally famous hostess kept her glamor and vitality undimmed even at the age of eighty. All went well through lunch and after, until in mid-afternoon those long-stemmed American beauties began to fade visibly.

THE BEAUTY BAR

My answer was to set up a beauty bar, the first in Hollywood. At three o'clock sharp the camera stopped turning, and all those beautiful girls came to the bar to replenish their beauty. For fifteen minutes, in their gold and silver lamé gowns, they sipped my booster cocktails and nibbled at the beauty-full proteins laid out for them on platters.

They had their choice of these cocktails: orange juice with fresh egg yolk beaten into it; soluble skim milk flavored with orange-blossom honey; chilled yogurt fortified with dark molasses; and Lady Mendl's own favorite, which I call my Hi-Vi Booster, cool glasses of lushly red tomato espresso, spiced with one or two heaping teaspoons of celery-flavored food yeast and a teaspoon of lemon juice. On the platters were the more solid Hi-Vi beauty treats: crisp whole wheat crackers with cubes of cheese; non-hydrogenated peanut butter; avocado slices spiced with vegetable salt and lime juice; and that ever-wonderful, ever-popular standby, Hi-Vi cottage cheese with parsley, chives, basil and all the fresh herbs we could find in the Farmer's Market (see Between-meal beauty boosters, page 61).

After a few days of our beauty bar refreshment the girls and even the director saw the difference. More important, the day's run of film showed the girls as fresh-looking and their dancing as crisp in the afternoon as it had been in the morning.

LEISURELY DINNER TIME

All over this great land, dinner time is home-coming time, the end of the working day and the beginning of evening leisure; in many homes it is the one time when families can sit down together to a meal. The wise modern woman realizes the importance of this meal to her own and her family's happiness, and she refreshes her spirit and her appearance with a bit of rest and relaxing care for herself in preparation.

She knows that the man of the house needs a chance to unwind, too, before sitting down to dinner. The American cocktail before dinner can be a relaxing custom, but it is too often misunderstood and abused. I am sorry to see people pickle their stomachs with martinis, killing their natural appetites and all sense of taste of food. It is then that most people tend to overeat, not knowing *what* they are eating and getting no pleasure from savoring their food.

UNWINDING BEFORE DINNER

Intelligent people need not be slaves to strong cocktails simply because that is the custom. Occasionally why not try nature's own cocktail, a tall glass of cool vegetable espresso, flavored with fragrant garden herbs and spices, or a foaming glass of freshly made fruit juice.

After a busy and perhaps a tense day, such a drink does wonderful things. It helps to unwind taut nerves; it quickly erases fatigue with its high content of natural sugars; most important, it raises the blood sugar level to the point where you will have no wish to overeat.

On beautyfarms they make good use of this discovery. Half an hour before dinner the guests are served vegetable and fruit juice cocktails. Afterward at dinner they find that they are quite content with one good helping and do not want a second.

Perhaps you are one of the many, many people who unconsciously try to relieve their inner tensions by overeating, even stuffing themselves. Many women—and men, too—would see their weight problems vanish if somehow they could manage not to bring their tensions to the table. There is a way to do this: do the swing-sway and slump relaxation, then have a glass of fresh vegetable or fruit juice. Sipped slowly, preferably through a straw, it is amazingly relaxing; the good natural fragrance and flavor seem to melt away tensions, and their magic is physical as well as psychological, for in fluid form these perfect nutrients which the body needs so badly are almost immediately absorbed into the blood.

Now when we come to dinner itself, even though I have already talked about the Russians and their big dinner-breakfasts, I must talk about them again. For whether we like it or not, they are an impressively vital people, and even with their comparatively poor selection of food they are determined to be the world's leading nation. And this is what I have to tell you now: the Russians eat their lightest meal in the evening.

In my Town Hall Lectures I have told audiences all over this country: "The Russians are the only people in the world who get up in the morning to eat dinner, and eat breakfast before they go to bed." And it is the absolute truth.

MODERN DINING IS LEAN DINING

Dinner too should be nutritious and light and lean; about twenty grams more of good protein in lean meat, fish, or fowl, with a green short-cooked vegetable, an occasional baked potato or kasha or brown rice, and always a crisp salad. For pleasure and digestion, there is a bowl of fresh fruit or a honey-sweetened compote, occasionally an open-face fruit pie, a custard or for variety a tangy cheese.

BLUEPRINT FOR BEAUTY-FULL DINNERS

Your Choice:
> Fruit cup
> Green salad
> Vegetable espresso
> Hot or cold jellied broth

Your Choice:
> Broiled lean meat
> Liver
> Fish
> Nut loaf

Your Choice:
> One or two short-cooked vegetables
> Light-hearted baked potato
> Kasha
> Rice

Your Choice:

> Fresh fruit
> Honey compote
> Custard
> Open face fruit pie
> Cheese
> Yogurt
> Café espresso
>   or
> Your favorite beverage

COSMETIC DIET

Beauty is not a *part* of the body, but of all the thirty trillion cells together. That is why beauty begins with a Cosmetic Diet, including all the important nutrients for the entire body. There follow some menus to guide you. If you like them, use them, or if you prefer, make up your own. Eating, as we have learned, should be fun and not regimented. I thoroughly agree with Dr. Margaret Mead when she says: "The present phase of American 'dieting' and 'slimming,' counting *calories*, has something of the same pathetic rigidity that accompanied early bottle feeding. Eventually bottle feeding was modified according to the needs of 'self-demand' or 'self-regulation.' "

It is this self-regulation we must strive for so that we can once and forever say goodbye to all diets, including those of Gayelord Hauser. For the present, all I ask of you is to remember that in the Cosmetic Diet we cut down on all unfriendly fats, we eat fewer starches and sugars, but we eat more proteins and we include as many fresh fruits, vegetables and unprocessed foods as possible.

I have said very little about the few "skinnies," those lucky ones who would like to gain weight. They can follow the same principle, perhaps eat smaller meals and between meals enjoy the rich milk shakes made with very ripe bananas. A French physician says that with greatly underweight people it is not so much a question of eating more as it is a matter of learning to relax so that they assimilate their food better. His recommendation is to relax ten minutes before meals and five minutes after meals. This certainly is a simple procedure and I suggest that you underweighters eat in the modern manner and apply the French doctor's advice.

Since breakfast to a very great measure determines how a woman feels and looks throughout the day, let me give you a few sample menus. I ask you only to have a protein-rich breakfast for ten days. If you do not like the proteins in my breakfast menus, select those that you like better. Just see to it that you get twenty grams. If you do not feel and look much better after these ten days, then go back to your limp and empty "coffee and" combinations.

Since protein foods are the most expensive of all foods, I suggest that you with small budgets obtain a large part of your proteins from the inexpensive Hi-Vi lean milk (half a cup, nine grams), cottage cheese or homemade cream cheese (two tablespoons, five grams). Your good bread—wheat germ or soya muffin—can add another three to five grams of protein to your breakfast.

MILLION-DOLLAR EYE OPENER

If you are a slow riser, easily irritated or naturally mean in the morning, a small eye opener can help you to get going, make you more amiable and attractive. The minute you jump out of bed, drink a small glass of your favorite fruit juice. It must be naturally sweet, never sugared, orange juice, pineapple juice, apple juice or papaya juice. The natural sugar in any unsweetened fruit juice, taken on an empty stomach, performs the magic. It raises your blood sugar level promptly and makes everything, including you, look more rosy at the breakfast table.

YOUR COSMETIC DIET

MONDAY

BREAKFAST: Orange juice
1 scrambled egg, fortified with milk
1 slice lean ham
1 slice wholewheat toast, lightly buttered
Choice of beverage: coffee, tea or milk
Preferably Swiss coffee: half hot coffee
    and half hot foaming milk

MID-MORNING: If hungry: Your choice of Beauty Snacks

LUNCHEON: BOWL FULL OF BEAUTY: Cottage
                    cheese on bed of dark green lettuce
                    Golden Fruit Dressing
                    1 Slice 100 percent wholewheat bread,
                    buttered lightly
                    Fresh or honeyed fruit, if desired
                    Choice of beverage: mint tea, English tea,
                    papaya tea, coffee, milk or yogurt

MID-AFTERNOON: If hungry: Your choice of Beauty Boosters

DINNER: Mixed salad bowl
                    Golden oil dressing
                    Large lean hamburger
                    Steamed zucchini
                    Apple Snow
                    Choice of beverage: demitasse, milk or
                    tea

BEFORE RETIRING: Baby yourself with a calcium-rich hot
                    milk drink

TUESDAY

BREAKFAST: Half grapefruit
                    Your favorite cold cereal à la mode
                    (Sprinkled with 2 tbsp. wheat germ, 1
                    tsp. honey)
                    Served with half cup Hi-Vi lean milk
                    3 slices crisp lean bacon
                    Choice of beverage: coffee, tea or milk
                    Preferably Swiss coffee: half hot coffee
                    and half hot foaming milk

> ### EAT AND GROW BEAUTIFUL RITUAL
> Breakfast time is the best time to take your vitamin-mineral concentrates and be fortified for the day ahead.

MID-MORNING: If hungry: Your choice of Beauty Snacks

LUNCHEON: BOWL FULL OF BEAUTY: Half cup
    shrimp on bed of romaine
Golden oil dressing
One wheat germ muffin, buttered lightly
Fresh or honeyed fruit, if desired
Choice of beverage: mint tea, English tea,
    papaya tea, coffee, milk or yogurt

MID-AFTERNOON   If hungry: Your choice of Beauty Boosters

DINNER: Red apple and red cabbage salad
Favorite oil dressing
Lean pot roast of beef
Short-cooked shredded beets
Kasha
Yogurt with honey
Choice of beverage: demitasse, milk or tea

BEFORE RETIRING: Baby yourself with a calcium-rich hot
    milk drink

WEDNESDAY

BREAKFAST: Applesauce, sprinkled with 1 tbsp. wheat
    germ and 1 tsp. honey
Chipped beef, simmered in Hi-Vi lean
    milk
Served on 100 percent wholewheat toast
Choice of beverage: coffee, tea or milk
Preferably Swiss coffee: half hot coffee
    and half hot foaming milk

EAT AND GROW BEAUTIFUL RITUAL

Breakfast time is the best time to take your vitamin-mineral concentrates and be fortified for the day ahead.

MID-MORNING: If hungry: Your choice of Beauty Snacks

LUNCHEON: BOWL FULL OF BEAUTY: Shredded Swiss cheese on bed of watercress and lettuce
Green yogurt dressing
One slice Milwaukee rye bread, buttered lightly
Fresh or honeyed fruit, if desired
Choice of beverage: mint tea, English tea, papaya tea, coffee, milk or yogurt

MID-AFTERNOON: If hungry: Your choice of Beauty Boosters

DINNER: Raw tender spinach salad
Golden oil dressing
Tender broiled liver
Baked onions with oregano
Broiled grapefruit Caribbean
Choice of Beverage: demitasse, milk or tea

BEFORE RETIRING: Baby yourself with a calcium-rich hot milk drink

THURSDAY

BREAKFAST: Large slice of melon
Your favorite hot cereal à la mode
(Sprinkled with 2 tbsp. wheat germ and 1 tsp. honey)
Served with half cup Hi-Vi lean milk
Choice of beverage: coffee, tea or milk
Preferably Swiss coffee: half hot coffee and half hot foaming milk

---

EAT AND GROW BEAUTIFUL RITUAL

Breakfast time is the best time to take your vitamin-mineral concentrates and be fortified for the day ahead.

MID-MORNING: If hungry: Your choice of Beauty Snacks

LUNCHEON: BOWL FULL OF BEAUTY: Chunks of tuna fish or chicken on bed of lettuce and celery
Favorite oil dressing
One slice high protein bread
Fresh or honeyed fruit, if desired
Choice of beverage: mint tea, English tea, papaya tea, coffee, milk or yogurt

MID-AFTERNOON: If hungry: Your choice of Beauty Boosters

DINNER: Carrot and pineapple salad
Golden mayonnaise dressing
Lean, broiled minute steak
Braised celery
Light-hearted baked potato
Fruit compote, Lady Mendl
Choice of beverage: demitasse, milk or tea

BEFORE RETIRING: Baby yourself with a calcium-rich hot milk drink

FRIDAY

BREAKFAST: Pineapple juice
Finnan-haddie, poached in Hi-Vi lean milk
One slice old-fashioned rye toast, buttered lightly
Choice of beverage: coffee, tea or milk
Preferably Swiss coffee: half hot coffee and half hot foaming milk

EAT AND GROW BEAUTIFUL RITUAL

Breakfast time is the best time to take your vitamin-mineral concentrates and be fortified for the day ahead.

MID-MORNING: If hungry: Your choice of Beauty Snacks

LUNCHEON: BOWL FULL OF BEAUTY: Chopped
                   hard-boiled eggs on bed of dark green
                   lettuce
                   Green-Gold dressing
                   One soya, sesame muffin, buttered lightly
                   Fresh or honeyed fruit, if desired
                   Choice of beverage: mint tea, English tea,
                   papaya tea, coffee, milk or yogurt

MID-AFTERNOON: If hungry: Your choice of Beauty Boosters

DINNER: Celery-carrot espresso
                   Grilled halibut
                   String beans with slivered almonds
                   Fresh fruit gelatine
                   Choice of beverage: demitasse, milk or
                   tea

BEFORE RETIRING: Baby yourself with a calcium-rich hot
                   milk drink

SATURDAY

BREAKFAST: Sliced orange
                   One boiled egg, spiked with herbal salt
                   Two slices lean Canadian bacon
                   One wheat germ or soya muffin, buttered
                   lightly
                   Choice of beverage: coffee, tea or milk
                   Preferably Swiss coffee: half hot coffee
                   and half hot foaming milk

EAT AND GROW BEAUTIFUL RITUAL

Breakfast time is the best time to take your vitamin-mineral concentrates and be fortified for the day ahead.

MID-MORNING: If hungry: Your choice of Beauty Snacks

LUNCHEON: BOWL FULL OF BEAUTY: Chilled fish or meat salad on bed of crisp greens
                    Green yogurt dressing
                    One slice El Molino bread, buttered lightly
                    Fresh or honeyed fruit, if desired
                    Choice of beverage: mint tea, English tea, papaya tea, coffee, milk or yogurt

MID-AFTERNOON: If hungry: Your choice of Beauty Boosters

DINNER: Avocado and grapefruit salad
                    Golden fruit dressing
                    Roast herbed chicken
                    Short-cooked shredded cauliflower
                    Peas with fresh mint
                    Honey ice cream
                    Choice of beverage: demitasse, milk or tea

BEFORE RETIRING: Baby yourself with a calcium-rich hot milk drink

SUNDAY

BREAKFAST: Fresh berries
                    Cottage cheese pancakes
                    With honey or maple syrup
                    Three slices lean crisp bacon
                    Choice of beverage: coffee, tea or milk
                    Preferably Swiss coffee: half hot coffee and half hot foaming milk

EAT AND GROW BEAUTIFUL RITUAL

Breakfast time is the best time to take your vitamin-mineral concentrates and be fortified for the day ahead.

MID-MORNING:	If hungry: Your choice of Beauty Snacks
LUNCHEON:	BOWL FULL OF BEAUTY: Waldorf salad on bed of tender lettuce
	Lean whipped cream dressing
	One square cornbread Carrotte, lightly buttered
	Choice of beverage: mint tea, English tea, papaya tea, coffee, milk or yogurt
MID-AFTERNOON:	If hungry: Your choice of Beauty Boosters
DINNER:	Yogurt and vegetable soup, Persian style
	or
	Watercress and nasturtium salad
	Golden oil dressing
	Chicken curry Indienne
	Fluffy brown rice
	Fresh pineapple or persimmons
	Choice of beverage: demitasse, milk or tea
BEFORE RETIRING:	Baby yourself with a calcium-rich hot milk drink

Between-Meal Beauty Boosters: You may not be hungry between meals, but if you are, do not hesitate to enjoy a booster. Any time you feel hungry or have a sense of letdown, have one of the following mid-morning beauty snacks: a glass of lean milk; for those who enjoy a coffee break, Swiss Coffee; the new delightful Caruba drink; if you need something more substantial, have a fresh egg yolk beaten into a cup of hot broth or a nutritious glass of yogurt. Whenever possible, have one glass of fresh vegetable espresso. (See also page 50.)

To Prevent Mid-Afternoon Letdown: You can choose from any one of the following beauty boosters: a frothy eggnog; fortified tomato juice; a cracker with cream cheese; a cup of instant Swiss Broth or a delectable carrot and apple espresso.

For Sleeping Beauty: Check up on your protein intake. Remember, for lasting loveliness you need half a gram for every pound of your ideal weight. (If you weigh 120 pounds, you need 60 grams.) You can make up any protein deficit at bedtime. Nothing is as soothing and conducive to deep sleep as warm, protein-rich calcium drinks. And so that there is no possible chance of missing any of the beautifying vitamins and minerals, this is the time to take the capsules with the entire spectrum of all known vitamins and minerals prescribed by your doctor, unless you have already taken them in the morning. Here is your choice of bedtime beauty boosters: cup of warm milk with honey; hot Swiss Broth; Milk Lassie; hot tomato juice with a teaspoon of food yeast. If needed, take two bone flour calcium tablets with cup of warm milk so that you won't have to count sheep.

CHAPTER 6

Your Beauty Alphabet of Vitamins and Minerals

In my home in Hollywood hangs a watercolor by the famous sculptor-painter, Rodin. Every time I look at it, I think of his wise description of beauty. He said, "Beauty is but the spirit breaking through the flesh."

I believe the spirit of which Rodin spoke has two components; they show in all his masterpieces. The first is vitality, the captivating glow of physical energy. The second is a quality that we cannot call physical; I like to describe it as an inner aliveness. Both these qualities emanate from within, from the physical and emotional harmony of a fully functioning human being. When they are filtered through the unique personality, every woman assumes her unique kind of beauty.

An entire history of woman's beauty could be based on her daily bread. It was woman who led the way to the greatest revolution in human history, the beginning of agriculture. While her Stone Age Adam hunted fresh meat, she gathered fruits, nuts, berries that often saved the tribe from starvation when game was scarce. She discovered that the grains of wild grasses, growing season after season near the watering places, were good to eat.

She learned the beautifying and strength-giving effects of whole grains even before her man learned to write down the record of wars and conquests. The first food staple of civilization was cereal porridge made of pounded whole grains. Later—many hundreds of years later—came the art of baking that nutritious ground grain into bread.

Most bread you eat today is a poor excuse for that rich, nutritious bread of prehistoric Eve, or, for that matter, the bread your great-grandmother ate in the last century. A slice of whole-grain bread contains about one-tenth of a milligram of vitamin B-1. A slice of modern bread, stripped of its germ grains, contains about one-sixtieth of a milligram of B-1 and even less of the other B vitamins. No wonder you complain of dry skin and try every moisturizer that you can apply from the outside; actually this anti-drying, anti-sagging, anti-wrinkling skin vitamin should be in your daily bread.

Creams and lotions have their place, of course, but creams cannot replace this beauty vitamin in your body chemistry.

The French call vitamin B-1 or thiamine, *joie de vie*—the joy of life vitamin. The British call it the morale vitamin because of the boost it gave to their health during the war. I call it your number one beauty vitamin.

Some years ago in southern Italy, where I now make my home for part of the year, thousands of people became afflicted with a mysterious skin disorder. Hospitals were crowded with patients who, besides their severe nervous and intestinal symptoms, suffered from a baffling condition of rough, dry, leathery, brownish skin. No medication or ointment helped them. After painstaking investigation it was found that the spaghetti and bread that formed the major part of their diet had been entirely depleted of vitamins, especially vitamin B-2, riboflavin. When processors learned to retain the germs of their grains and flours, the widespread skin affliction quickly disappeared. Science learned the word *pellagra* from the Italians. It means dry skin.

Commercial bread bakers everywhere complain that we are eating less and less bread. Can it be that you modern Eves are learning that ordinary bread is empty of essential nutrients? That it adds only starch and wraps a roll of fat around the waistline?

Dr. E. V. McCollum of Johns Hopkins University says about so-called "enriched" breads and flours:

"In the manufacture of wheat flour, a score or more of essential nutrients present in significant amounts in the wheat kernel are removed. To give such a flour, supplied with three vitamins and iron, so good a name as 'enriched' is misleading."

Many women have found their own answer to the sad decline of bread in our time: Bake your own bread. Use whole grain or at least unbleached flour, and boost it with extra wheat germ, milk solids, and yeast, as recommended by the outstanding nutrition studies of Cornell University. You will find that such home-baked bread is a treat to the palate, and of tremendous value to your health and beauty. You will never want to return to commercial, empty bread after baking your own.

And if you are just too busy (or too lazy) for the whole operation of baking good bread, here is good news: a small mill in California has perfected a 100 percent whole grain loaf mixture, including everything, even the bread pan! All you do is add water, mix it and put it in the oven. The bread is utterly delicious and so satisfying that all you want is one fragrant, nourishing slice. Please don't underestimate the value of good bread.

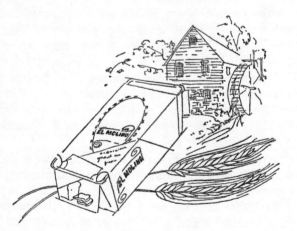

How can you be sure?

The most beautiful woman in the world is no more than a composite of the chemicals that make up her bones and flesh and skin. But she is also no less than those chemicals, the precious beauty-giving elements in the foods she eats. How can you be sure that nature's honest beauty has not been lost from the foods that come to you over the long route from field to processor to warehouse, from warehouse to market and so to your dinner table?

I therefore urge you to fortify your foods and enrich your diet with vitamins and minerals. Today, as you know, we have the new menace of sprays and insecticides, so that we are advised to peel our vegetables, and in this way lose so many valuable minerals and vitamins that are in the skin or just beneath it. And so, though you market expertly and cook with the greatest care, you still must lose a great part of the value of your foods. For beauty and full vitality you want not minimum but *maximum* requirements, and abundance of beauty-giving nutrients.

Here then is my beauty alphabet of vitamins and minerals, the reasons why they are essential to your beauty, and the ways in which you can make sure to have them in needed amounts, each and every day throughout your long and beauty-full life.

The Beauty Alphabet of Vitamins

Vitamin A

This is the vitamin which Dr. Henry Sherman of Columbia University frequently refers to as "the long life vitamin"; and a well-known New York dermatologist treats his stage and film star patients with high potency vitamin A for youthful, radiant skin. This vitamin could be called an inner skin lubricant par excellence. It nourishes the layer of fat underneath the skin which helps to keep the skin firm. A deficiency can cause dull and strained-looking eyes, even night blindness, rough skin, cracking nails, dry and brittle hair and dandruff.

Foods richest in vitamin A: Fish oils, liver, eggs, whole milk, cream cheese, carrots, dark green leafy vegetables, apricots, cantaloupe.

Also in concentrates: Vitamin A is available in capsules supplying 25,000 to 50,000 International Units. Where fat digestion is a problem, and in acne, physicians often recommend water soluble Vitamin A. It is unwise to take more than 50,000 units daily, unless recommended by your physician.

Vitamin B Complex

The beauty values of this group of vitamins are so many and varied that it is difficult to list them all. They are essential to the energy-producing metabolism of sugar. Most interesting is their close relationship to the health of your nerves. Nervous tension, irritability, which produce lines of tension in the face, an apprehensive expression in the eyes, unattractive distortions of posture, generally gain relief with increased consumption of the B complex.

Of particular interest to women approaching middle years is the helpful effect of B complex through the period of menopause; the addition of B complex nutrients to the diet eases the tensions of this process of glandular change and doctors often give very high potency injections of the needed B vitamins.

The B vitamins occur together in nature and are best taken in their natural combination. Those of the 15 B vitamins most closely affecting your looks are discussed separately.

Foods richest in vitamin B complex: Liver, brains, heart, oysters, cottage cheese, fortified skim milk, wheat germ, food yeast, whole grains, soya bean, peas, watercress, asparagus. To preserve the vitamins from vegetable sources, short-cooking in a minimum of water is essential, otherwise vitamins are lost in the liquid.

Also in concentrates: Capsules combining most important B vitamins are readily available.

Vitamin B-1 (Thiamin)

A high proportion of this B vitamin serves as a buffer against stress and strain. Fatigue, depression, lack of the joy of living is often traceable to a deficiency of B-1; with the deficiency eliminated or prevented, a smile comes more easily to illuminate a woman's face.

Foods richest in vitamin B-1: Wheat germ, liver, whole grains and breads, food yeast, milk, salad greens, egg yolk, meat, oysters, nuts, seeds, soya beans.

Also in concentrates: In tablets from 25 to 100 milligrams; also in lesser amounts in vitamin B complex preparations.

Vitamin B-2 (Riboflavin)

This vitamin contributes to healthy skin, bright eyes, calm nerves, and the hemoglobin content of blood, which makes for a glowing complexion. In mild deficiency there may be troublesome symptoms of burning eyeballs and eyelids, photophobia or sensitivity to light, poor adjustment to sudden light changes. Fissures at the corners of the mouth may be caused by more serious deficiency of this and other vitamin B factors. Beauty-seekers on reducing diets should have adequate B vitamin reserves if they want to avoid a tense, harried expression.

Foods richest in vitamin B-2: Milk, meat, cottage cheese, yogurt, liver, eggs, green leafy vegetables, almonds, soya beans, food yeast, avocados, peas.

Also in concentrates: In tablet form from 5 to 10 milligrams.

Vitamin B-6 (Pyridoxine).

This vitamin must be supplied daily. It is a vitamin of the first order. Many film and television stars can thank this vitamin for their blemish-free complexions. It is known in medical circles as the *anti-dermatitis* factor, of particular value in skin disorders, dry scalp, oily skin. It is an important agent in the metabolism of fats and fatty acids so necessary to the skin's health and beauty. A diet rich in Vitamin B-6 foods has a soothing effect on the nerves and helps to promote restful sleep.

Foods richest in vitamin B-6: Liver of all kinds, food yeast, wheat germ, whole grains and breads, soya beans, nuts, egg yolks, milk, green vegetables, unsulphured molasses.

Also in concentrates: In tablet form supplying 10 to 25 milligrams.

Vitamin B-12

This is the miraculous "anti-anemia factor," first discovered in liver, then isolated from the B complex, which has transformed pernicious anemia from a fatal disease to a condition that can be controlled with comparative ease. Many medical authorities believe that this vitamin is inadequately provided in the average diet low in animal foods, and strict vegetarians often have a vitamin B-12 deficiency.

Foods richest in vitamin B-12: Muscle meats, liver of all kinds kidney, eggs, milk, yogurt.

Also in concentrates: From 5 to 15 micrograms, and in single tablets of 25 and 50 micrograms.

Niacinamide (Niacin)

This vitamin was the missing clue in pellagra, which devastated populations in southern Italy and in the American South, with high mortality, in the early 1900's. It was believed to be an inherited disease, or one caused by bacterial infection, until Dr. Joseph Goldberger traced the connection with the lack of animal proteins in the traditional Southern diet of "grits and greens." One of the symptoms of pellagra was a terribly blemished skin. A medical belief today is that a marginal or sub-clinical pellagra may be common because of a generally low level of niacinamide (or niacin in the average diet. The vitamin is prescribed for skin, nerve, digestive disorders, and disfiguring conditions of the mouth and gums.

Foods richest in Niacinamide: Powdered milk, food yeast, fish, liver, heart, wheat germ, lean meat, peanuts, seeds, whole grains and bread.

Also in concentrates: From 50 to 100 milligrams.

Para Amino Benzoic Acid

This is one of the several members of the B complex that have been used to prevent graying of the hair in animal experiments. PABA, as it is sometimes called, is also helpful in allergies.

Foods richest in Para Amino Benzoic Acid: Organ meats as liver, kidney, heart; meats, food yeast, fish, fruits, nuts, whole grains.

Inositol

This vitamin is *lipotropic,* which means that it helps to break down fats in the body to their ingredient fatty acids, which are necessary to firm contours and in preventing the accumulation of cholesterol in the arteries. It is also helpful in the body's utilization of vitamin E. It is considered another one of the anti-gray-hair vitamins.

Foods richest in Inositol: Food yeast, wheat germ, whole grains, fruits, organ meats.

Choline

This vitamin, too, is an agent in fat metabolism, an aid to hair and skin beauty, and has an indirect but significant relation to beauty in its beneficial influence on the health of the glands. It is most available in the too rarely eaten organ meats.

Foods richest in Choline: Organ meats, seeds, food yeast, peanuts, wheat germ, corn germ, green leafy vegetables and lecithin.

Calcium Pantothenate

Probably the leading *antichromotrichia* (anti-gray-hair) factor in the B group, this vitamin is also of value in protecting the skin against dermatitis, and contributes to the health of the digestive system.

Foods richest in Calcium Pantothenate: Egg yolk, wheat germ, molasses, peanuts, food yeast, lean beef, liver, vegetables of the cabbage family, salmon, potatoes.

Biotin

Research in this vitamin is almost as new as space exploration. It shares in the B vitamin benefits to beauty of skin, hair, eyes, the health of glands. Severe deficiencies have produced skin lesions, grayish skin color, sleeplessness and muscle pain.

Foods richest in Biotin: Wheat germ, food yeast, liver, peanuts.

Vitamin C

This most familiar of vitamins is a star of the beauty firmament. It is essential to the firmness and health of gums and teeth; it is an aid to the health of capillary walls and thus to prevention of varicosities and the occasional small patches of broken surface capillaries or black and blue marks that mar the skin. It helps to guard against infections, colds, allergies. Recent research also shows that vitamin C is needed for the health of connective tissue which cushions bones and joints and gives suppleness to posture and grace to body movement. Remember that vitamin C must be taken every day since the body is unable to store it; also that it is a "factor of demand," meaning that what is enough for one person may be inadequate for another.

Foods richest in vitamin C: Rose hips are the richest natural source; citrus fruits, black currants, berries, pineapple, avocados, tomatoes, green peppers, beansprouts, all green leafy vegetables.

Also in concentrates: 100 milligrams ascorbic acid; or rose hips in tablet form, 100 milligrams to 250 milligrams per tablet.

Vitamin D

This, the sunshine vitamin, is essential for good bones and teeth. The body makes its own vitamin D in the skin, in sunshine, also in "skyshine" or the reflection of sunlight from water, snow, or light colored surfaces (but not through ordinary window glass). It promotes the body's use of calcium, in some way not yet understood. A deficiency shows in dental caries, more seriously in softening of the bones.

Foods richest in vitamin D: Irradiated milk, irradiated yeast, tuna fish, herring, mackerel, canned salmon. Best source is not food, but exposure to sunlight; moderate tanning, not so much as to dry and toughen the skin, serves for adequate vitamin D without detracting from skin beauty.

Also in concentrates: Fish liver derivatives, fish liver oils, up to 2,000 U.S.P. units.

Vitamin E

Long known as the anti-sterility vitamin, this is now being used by some gynecologists with the B complex to relieve menopause symptoms. It is also considered of value by some heart specialists, neurologists, and dermatologists. For those who cannot tolerate fats because of a gall bladder condition, it is available in fat-free form. At the Shute Clinic in Canada this vitamin was prescribed to keep my heart young, and I faithfully take my daily fat-free capsule of 200 I.U. of Alpha tocopherol with my other concentrates at breakfast.

Foods richest in vitamin E: Wheat germ oil, wheat germ, whole grains.

Also in concentrates: Never less than 5 International Units in multiple supplements; from 30 to 200 units in single concentrates.

Vitamin F (Unsaturated Fatty Acids)

This possibly unexpected letter in your beauty alphabet of vitamins stands for those essential unsaturated fatty acids which we talk so much about because of their value to the skin and in the layer of fat under the skin which helps to prevent fine lines. It is a grave mistake to eliminate these even when on a reducing diet. They are also essential to arterial and organic functions, the control of cholesterol levels in the blood, and body warmth. Meat fats and the hardened or hydrogenated fats in solid shortenings should be replaced by the unsaturated vegetable oils because they contain the unsaturated fatty acids.

Foods richest in vitamin F: All the natural golden vegetable oils, used internally and externally in salad dressings and cosmetic mayonnaise. Also available in capsules.

Vitamin K

This, the blood-clotting vitamin, is normally manufactured by the body itself, in the intestines. It plays a role in liver function and in blood manufacture, and is thus one of the beauty vitamins. It is usually adequate in a good diet.

Foods richest in vitamin K: Cabbage, cauliflower, spinach and all leafy vegetables.

Also in concentrates: Up to 1 milligram in multiple supplements.

The Beauty Alphabet of Minerals

Calcium

Good bones make possible an erect stature that is beautiful in anyone, male or female; good teeth that resist decay are a tremendous asset to beauty. Without added calcium during pregnancy a woman may suffer in her health generally and invite gum and dental disorders, not only for herself, but for the baby. Unsuspected dietary deficiencies of calcium have recently been revealed in this country among people of all ages; women and girls are the worst offenders against their own health and beauty in this respect. If you do not like fresh milk, by all means make use of the powdered skim milk, or supplement your diet with mineral tablets made with very fine bone flour, plus vitamin D.

Foods richest in Calcium: Milk, powdered skim milk, yellow cheeses, cottage cheese, yogurt, molasses, almonds, sesame seeds, turnip greens and broccoli.

Also in concentrates: Bone meal tablets with Vitamin D.

Iodine

The thyroid gland must have iodine to make its hormone. When iodine is lacking in the drinking water, as it is in the Alps and in some areas of the United States, endemic goiter may develop with its ugly swelling distorting the throat. Hypothyroidism, or low thyroid function, may also develop with its accompanying dry skin, dry brittle hair, and beauty-destroying sluggishness. Some persons may require a higher supply. A simple precaution is to vary your diet often with iodine-rich fish and seafood and add sea vegetables to your vitamin-mineral supplements.

Foods richest in Iodine: Fish, shellfish, iodized vegetable salt, sea water.

Also in concentrates: Sea greens made from sea vegetables. One single tablet contains the daily iodine ration.

Iron

Without sufficient iron in your beauty stream the pallor of anemia robs your face of its glow and your lips of inviting redness. Iron promotes the body's whole economy. It clings magnet-like to other nutrients, helps vitamin A to protect your eyes, vitamin C to nourish gums, teeth and connective tissue. It encourages the B vitamins and the iodine of thyroid hormone to give beauty to your skin and luster to your hair. Iron raises the body's energy level and brings you glow and well-being.

Foods richest in Iron: Liver of all kinds fresh or desiccated, oysters, sweetbreads, eggs, food yeast, unsulphured molasses, soya beans, lentils, avocados, grapes, raisins, apricots.

Also in concentrates: From 10 milligrams. In nutritional anemia formulas, 180 milligrams.

Phosphorus

The sea at night glows and flashes with phosphorescent light. In the body it glows more quietly, combining with calcium to make the hard material of teeth and bones. Phosphorus is essential to the chemical balance of the cells. It stimulates brain function, soothes nerves, quickens muscular response.

Foods richest in Phosphorus: Fish, lean meat, poultry, eggs, whole grains, lean cottage cheese, milk, yogurt.

Also in concentrates: Multiple mineral supplements made from very fine bone flour with vitamin D.

Sulphur

Tradition connects sulphur and molasses with the first robin of spring. Chemistry connects it with healthy shining hair and strong fingernails. It is an essential part of the protein molecule and is indispensable, though in small quantities, to the body's health and good looks.

Foods richest in Sulphur: Peanut butter, wheat germ, eggs, lentils, cheese, beef, clams.

Trace Minerals

(Copper, Magnesium, Manganese, Zinc)

These are the tremendous trifles of beauty. Only the merest trace of each is needed, but even so they are indispensable to health and good looks. By biochemical magic they activate the vitamins, enzymes, amino acids and the other minerals in maintaining the subtle balance that creates health and beauty.

The trace minerals are found in many foods, but sea water, salt water fish and sea vegetables are the richest sources of all.

Fluorine

All over the United States there is great controversy about fluoridation of our drinking water for the protection of our teeth, and people become very emotional and violent on the subject. I personally believe it is always safest to follow the concepts of old Mother Nature and eat plenty of fish and seafood of every kind. These gifts of nature provide us with the right kind of fluorine to protect our teeth. Sicilians usually have excellent teeth, probably because a large part of their diet comes from the sea. Where tooth decay is rampant many dentists now recommend the addition of bone meal flour, a rich source of fluorine and of calcium, to the daily diet. (See what a Swedish dentist did with finely ground bone meal flour, page 193.)

WHY EXTRA VITAMINS?

Some of the world's leading nutritionists believe that vitamin and mineral concentrates are an excellent protection not only against the stresses and strains of the jet age, but against the over-refining, overcooking, peeling, straining, draining, storing and reheating of foods, and also against excessive smoking and drinking. And so why should we take a chance, when the whole spectrum of vitamins and minerals in small and scientifically compounded capsules can be taken with our breakfast? I myself have not missed taking them one single day in the past twenty years, and countless thousands of my students the world over consider their morning vitamin and mineral ritual their best health and good looks insurance.

To settle this question of extra vitamins and minerals in your diet once and forever, listen to what Dr. Tom Spies has to say. Tom Spies is the man who performed modern nutritional miracles with thousands of people in his clinic in Birmingham, Alabama. I saw the results of his work with my own eyes when I was his guest at the Birmingham Hospital. Here is what he has said about vitamins: "The expensive way to use vitamins is to avoid them, develop nutritional failure, lose your job." Dr. Tom also said the cost for extra vitamins he prescribed for the thousands of patients he treated at his clinic "was less than the price of cigarettes."

And here is what Dr. Norman Jolliffe, Director of the Bureau of Nutrition for the New York City Department of Health, has to say: "Some patients may try sincerely to eat a satisfactory diet, but fail because of business, working or home conditions, or for other causes beyond their control. Others, in spite of pleading, cajoling or verbal spanking, will not eat a satisfactory diet because of habit, fads or fancies, lack of necessary information or sheer obstinacy; others have real food allergies. When, under these conditions or whenever a satisfactory diet cannot or will not be regularly consumed, practicality dictates an appropriate dietary supplement." And in the Public Affairs pamphlet No. 69-A, "Vitamins and Health," written by the distinguished William Rubin, is the following line: "Taking vitamins should be considered like buying insurance."

WHAT VITAMINS SHOULD YOU TAKE?

If you are anxious about your good looks and the well-being of your family, you will always make sure that your meals are basically sound. All the tablets in the world cannot take the place of good meat, wholesome bread, golden vegetable oils and, above all, the fresh foods: our fruits, vegetables and juices. My forty years in nutrition have taught me that good health and good looks can be achieved and maintained only when the diet is rich to extravagance in all the vital food factors upon which the body depends for its soundness.

So I must repeat: Much of the food we eat today no longer comes from the fields into our kitchens like the food of the lucky Hunza and other primitive peoples. There are many losses in the storage of foods, in handling and shipping. Minimum amounts of nutrients are not sufficient in our plan for beauty-full eating. We must strive for maximum, not minimum amounts of all the vital food factors.

As you read the Beauty Alphabet of Vitamins and Minerals in these pages, you no doubt discovered that you may be short of many food factors and you wonder how to cover them. Perhaps you are really below par, physically and nutritionally. In such a case, there is only one thing to do: consult your doctor. He may have to give you higher potency injections of vitamins and other nutrients, including liver and vitamin B-12. By all means follow your doctor's prescription, otherwise how can you expect him to bring you back to health?

In our Eat and Grow Beautiful regime, I address myself not to sick people, but to the millions of wise women who are well and who want to stay well. The kind of beauty I want you to have is built upon the cornerstone of health, and the simplest way to protect yourself against any vitamin or mineral deficiency is to include in your daily schedule a balanced concentrate containing the entire spectrum of vitamins and minerals. These are best taken with your meals, preferably at breakfast time to give you added vitality for the day ahead.

One of the newest and simplest ways to select the right kind of concentrate for yourself is on the basis of your approximate age group: as a young adult, up to age 35; for middle years, up to age 55; and for seniors, from age 55 on.

The healthy young adult woman who wants to protect her health and good looks should especially work against tiredness, one of the commonest beauty robbers. Nutritional tiredness is very prevalent among women in their thirties. You should investigate a vitamin formula which is well balanced with the vitamins A, B-2, B-6, vitamin C and vitamin D, and with these the necessary minerals. Such a balanced, inexpensive formula together with a balanced diet also helps to maintain good-looking skin, hair and nails.

For those in the middle years there is an increased need for vitamins to withstand the extreme pressures and strains which catch up around this time. A generous formula of all vitamins is best for the middle age group, but the B vitamins should be increased for their beneficial effect on the nerves and digestion. Also the lipotropic factors are needed for the metabolism of fat. A great favorite which many doctors now prescribe is a balanced inexpensive formula in a base of whole dried liver and food yeast. Perhaps your doctor has already prescribed such a formula for you. Be sure to take it regularly together with your good diet. The years between 35 and 55 are probably the most strenuous in every life and need all the support we can give them.

A good dietary supplement for the years after 55 should contain the whole vitamin and mineral spectrum, but it should also contain betaine, which acts to prevent fat in important organs. Diastase is also needed as an aid in overcoming discomforts of bloating. All geriatric concentrates should contain lysine, the miraculous amino acid which converts low quality proteins into high nutrition for the rebuilding of body tissues. Vitamin-mineral therapy has been so remarkable in recent years that regardless of how many birthdays you have had, you can make your senior years your happiest.

CHAPTER 7

Romantic Foods

In Paris, at an international conference on nutrition, I learned an astonishing fact: there are 250,000 kinds of vegetables and more than two million animal species in this world, on land and sea. Of all this overwhelming variety, the human race eats only about fifty different vegetables and the same number of meats and fish.

When you consider that each land and each nationality limit their choice still further by custom and tradition, and each family also has its habitual choices, you can see that we unthinkingly stint ourselves of a great wealth of eating pleasure and adventure in a world of such abundance. Many peoples are limited in their choice only to what their own region affords. But we are so fortunate—all the variety of our vast land, and of many other lands, is ours to enjoy.

Through the years I have introduced many new and unusual foods, and my wonder foods have gone around the world and have been accepted and enjoyed by people in many lands. Now I want to bring you, for your pleasure, some delicious additions to your repertoire of beauty foods. Some of these will be new to you, some are unusual and exotic, and some are old friends with a long and distinguished history.

Join me in this adventure among foods that will bring new enjoyment to your table and new beauty values to your menus.

Luscious avocados

Old Mother Nature outdid herself when she gave us the beauty-full avocado, sometimes called the alligator pear because of its rough skin and pear shape. In this single delectable fruit are combined the proteins of meat, the fat of butter, the vitamins and minerals of green vegetables, and the flavor of nuts—a six-course dinner in a green shell.

The avocado is a pear only in shape; it is actually a fruit of the laurel family of trees, a native of the semi-tropics that grows wild in the West Indies, Mexico and Hawaii. Luckily for us, it was transplanted to Florida and Southern California and it thrives in both regions, so that we can enjoy avocados throughout the year. In Europe they are scarcely ever seen, an imported luxury far too expensive to be enjoyed often, but in the United States at the peak of their season they sell for as little as ten cents each. Out of season they cost from twenty-five to fifty cents a piece, but they are worth it, for if ever there was a cosmetic food it is this wonder fruit growing on a tree.

Within its soft yellow-green pulp is a good protein, very little starch when it is ripe and practically no sugar. It is a gold mine of elements essential to good looks and well-being: calcium in high amounts, magnesium, copper, potassium, sodium, phosphates, iron and manganese.

Added to all this are its treasures in important vitamins, especially vitamins A, B-1, B-2 and C. That's enough for one single fruit to hold without bursting. Yet it does contain one more beauty treasure: almost twenty-five per cent of the avocado is oil, the very best kind, with all the unsaturated fatty acids so important for a glowing skin. It is this precious oil that gives the fruit its smooth texture and its nutlike flavor. Mexicans spread ripe avocado on their tortillas—they call it their "butter that grows on trees."

Avocados play a star role on beautyfarms, and they can be the star of your kitchen as well, because they are so versatile and lend themselves to so many tempting dishes. To begin with they make an ideal salad fruit, halved and eaten alone with a spot of dressing, or sliced into your salad bowl with other fruits and vegetables; they blend superbly with all your salad ingredients.

By themselves avocados make a delectable cream soup for which you need no butter. And avocado pulp whipped and mixed with lemon juice and herbs makes an ideal mayonnaise-like dressing or a cocktail dip.

BREAD IS LIFE

In sunny Sicily, where I write this, life revolves around three beauty-full foods: grains, grapes and olives. Most respected of the three are the golden grains, and bread made with Sicilian grains is regarded as a tangible sign of Divine Providence. To this day the peasants make their children kiss the bread before eating. The mother places a round loaf of her homemade bread in the center of the table and during the saying of Grace, the children keep their eyes fixed on it as the symbol of Divine Love materialized.

Sicily is a poor country and the people attribute godlike power to anything which nourishes them. Sicilian grapes, almonds, olives each have their patron saints, but the bread-grains have no patron but the Almighty Himself!

When I bite into a piece of solid Sicilian bread I have mixed emotions. First I am happy because it tastes so good and is so full of nourishment that one slice satisfies. Then, when I think of the stuff which millions of people eat every day, I am sad. I believe nothing has suffered more abuse than our beauty-full whole grains; they have been purified and tortured until nothing is left but empty starch. The germ which contains the life-force itself, the B vitamins, the minerals, all are gone by the time the empty loaf of bread reaches our table; it no longer tastes like *His* bread, as the Sicilians call it, but like cotton batting.

A few years ago, while lecturing in Hamburg, I witnessed a bread revolution. Several thousand German housewives marched with banners saying, "*Wir wollen gesundes Brot,*" "*Wir wollen kein Gift*" ("We want healthful bread," "We want no Poison"). Within a few weeks there were twenty-four shops, and now throughout Germany there are bakeries where they sell delicious *bauern brot*—peasant bread—whole grain breads with all the good left in.

In America we are against revolutions of all kinds, but I should like to remind every Eve of her woman-power. Use it! Keep demanding whole bread, made with the beauty-full whole grains, and soon your markets will carry nourishing bread like our Sicilian bread.

CAROB SWEET

In my Sicilian garden I have a Caruba tree which is said to be one hundred years old. The tree is immense; a hundred people could relax in its shade. Every fall I am the most popular man with all the little girls and boys on my hill. That is when the fruit, called Carob or St. John's Bread, ripens and sends its sweet aroma all over the neighborhood. When it is ripe, this ancient fruit looks like a bean pod four or five inches long, of rich dark chocolate color. Sicilian children can hardly wait to eat it.

The carob is the fruit of the honey locust, and it has been known since Biblical times. It is delightfully sweet, with an aroma all its own. Most of the supply comes from southern Europe, but since its healthful qualities have been discovered, carob farms have sprung up in the fertile groves around Vista and Escondido, California.

I invite you to try carob in its fresh or powdered form. There is no exact analysis of its nutrient values, but we know that carob contains protein, carbohydrate, some vitamins and minerals. Because of its natural sweetness carob powder, which can be bought in health food stores, can be used in place of sugar. Dried, ground and toasted, it makes a pleasant coffee substitute, especially popular in Germany. The hard brown seed kernels of the carob bean make an interesting bulk-producing, jelly-like substance which is used as a bulk producer (like agar) in some of the reducing products so popular just now. Our chief interest in carob is as an enjoyable food and natural sweetener.

CRESS

As long ago as the 16th century, watercress was known as a beauty-full food. Francis Bacon wrote, "The eating of watercress doth restore the wonted bloom to the cheeks of old and young ladies." Empiric knowledge often contains a kernel of truth; Lord Bacon could not know, as we know today, that the reason water-

cress is so good for the complexion is its high vitamin A content.
This refreshing salad green is a member of the mustard family;
hence its nippy taste. Besides its astonishing 21,450 International
Units of vitamin A, this attractive green contains approximately
885 milligrams of calcium, 209 milligrams of phosphorus, 9.1 milligrams of iron, some B vitamins, plus 93.6 percent water.

In case you find watercress a little strong by itself, try mixing
it with other salad greens. The English add sprigs of watercress to
give a lively taste to sandwiches, and the French make a Potage
Cressionnière, a delicious tangy soup of potatoes and watercress.

On beautyfarms watercress is added to vegetable juices for more
character and more vitamin C. At a cocktail party in Paris, I
made a combination of fresh pineapple juice with fresh watercress
juice in equal amounts. It was the Duchess of Windsor's favorite
and it is a particularly delicious combination. When served
chilled it makes a good first course for a festive dinner.

At the Four Seasons, New York's most elegant restaurant, nasturtium and watercress salad is a specialty of the house. Watercress is a familiar favorite, but the combination with tender,
young nasturtium leaves is a delightful new treat. The American
Indians used nasturtium leaves as a tonic vegetable and to this
day in the West they call nasturtium leaves Indian Cress.

GARLIC

Garlic is a romantic food everywhere in the world except with
Americans. It is as old as the Bible and in ancient times it was
even considered an aphrodisiac. It was fed to Roman soldiers to
make them brave, it was considered medicinal for sixty-one ailments, and to this day it is worn by Sicilians to keep off evil or
illness. We can ignore its supposed magic, for it has real though
mild antiseptic powers; the Russians call it vegetable penicillin. It
is botanically a bulb and a member of the lily family.

We use garlic not as a medicine, but as a seasoning, just a
soupçon as the French advise. Although it is an ancient earthy
spice, its use today is sophisticated. Use it fresh whenever possible.
Rub your salad bowl with a clove of it to give a lively tang to the
salad. A gourmet cook considers a small hand-size garlic press a
necessary kitchen accessory. Its advantage is that it squeezes out

of a single clove enough juice and oil to spice your dish, but not enough to spice your breath.

Eleanor Roosevelt mentioned in her charming book, *On My Own*, that her doctor recommended garlic tablets to improve her memory and I am told that she received many letters asking if it really had improved her memory. Mrs. Roosevelt answered modestly that her memory is nothing to brag about, with or without garlic tablets. I believe many more people would like to take advantage of the benefits of garlic, but they don't like to advertise the fact. A progressive chemist has now solved the "advertising" problem by making tablets of wild garlic tamed and disguised with a pleasant honey-mint coating, so that it leaves neither taste nor trace. Fresh garlic enthusiasts should chew a sprig of fresh parsley so they won't advertise.

HONEY

When Julius Caesar asked a Roman senator and honored elder statesman how he managed to live a hundred years, the patriarch's answer was, "Honey within and oil without."

Honey is made of pure glucose and levulose, the simplest natural sugars, and it is one of the most rapidly metabolized of all foods. It enters the bloodstream directly; hence it is an almost instantaneous source of energy. Athletes take spoonfuls of it before a contest. The ethereal ballerina, Alicia Markova, puts a tablespoonful of honey in her tea. The tremendous energy and velocity of the fabulous Bolshoi Ballet dancers may depend more than a little on the fact that they consume quantities of honey before going on stage. I am happy to report that in this year's Olympics, the wise trainers of our athletes put jars of honey on their prodigies' tables. I am convinced that this wonderful sweet helped the United States to win some gold medals.

As a source of pure energy, honey is unrivalled. It is a real "go" food and especially good for busy Americans. Honey also contains priceless ingredients that are essential for the functioning of tissues and organs: enzymes, minerals, organic acids and the bioses or growth factors. The darker honeys have even more mineral salts than the lighter ones.

Honey is wonderfully rich in vitamins, especially B-2, B-6, and

H or biotin, also numbered in the B group; K, the blood-clotting vitamin essential to healing, and the indispensable vitamin C that keeps capillary walls and connective tissues healthy. No wonder scientists, from the ancient Greeks to the modern Soviets, have prescribed honey to promote the healing of wounds! Incidentally the B-2 or riboflavin content of honey is almost equal to that of chicken, is sixteen times higher than in fresh apricots, fifteen times that of grape juice or fresh apples, five times richer than in lean cheese or raw carrots.

Russian physicians today are testing honey clinically for various therapeutic uses, particularly in respiratory, lung, heart, gastrointestinal, eye, skin, and nervous diseases. We may soon see honey a respected item in the modern medical pharmocopeia as it was with the ancients!

Hippocrates told the ladies of ancient Athens that honey would preserve the beauty of their complexions, and they obeyed his advice and used it not only as a beauty-full food but also as a base for facial masks; among the cosmetic formulas in this book you will find formulas for honey masks.

Tupelo Honey The queen of honeys is *tupelo*. It is probably the most delicately flavored of all the honeys; it is always clear and will not crystallize.

Florida is the state which provides us with this truly royal sweet. In its wild swamps grow thousands of tupelo trees, and in the early spring they are laden with the blossoms from which the bees suck the nectar for this matchless honey. Do you know that a single little bee must make perhaps 35,000 trips from hive to flower and back again, to provide just one pound of honey?

Tupelo honey is more expensive than other honeys but it is well worth the difference: more than forty percent of it is pure levulose or fruit sugar, and it gives almost instant energy. It is an ideal beautyfarm food because so little is needed for quick energy, and it can be used in salad dressings, custards, and a great variety of high energy drinks.

To break yourself of the empty sugar habit, use the natural sweeteners for a while. Soon you will discover that you need less and less sweetening; your awakened tastebuds will again be able to enjoy the true flavors of wholesome natural foods.

This single change can do more for your figure and good looks than you can imagine. While I speak of natural sugars, I must tell you that in France after the appearance of my book, *Vivez Jeune, Vivez Longtemps,* one of the biggest sugar refineries made a natural brown sugar cube with typical French flair. They added a bit of vanilla. My French students call it "Le Sucre Gayelord"; it tastes delightful and is a *succès fou,* especially in Paris. I wish we could have such a natural sugar cube in America. Sugar refineries, please note: I know it will be a sensation!

KASHA

I was sitting in the dining room of the Hotel Metropole in Moscow, and at a nearby table some Muscovites were eating with gusto something that looked like wild rice or lentils. I ordered some, and discovered that it was *kasha* and delicious. I vowed that I would do my best to introduce you to this delightful and nourishing dish. It makes a welcome change from rice or potatoes and has a great "satiety value"—meaning that it sticks to the ribs. Its protein value is quite high and it is rich in the important B vitamins. One helping contains about twelve grams of protein.

Talking to Russian nutritionists, I discovered that kasha is their favorite grain. I also discovered that there is a "kasha pot" in every Russian kitchen: they cook it in quantity and keep it on hand at all times. They eat it with milk or curds, as porridge for breakfast; they put it in their rich soups; they eat it with meat dishes like Beef Stroganoff. My guide from the Intourist Bureau said, "Kasha keeps us strong, it even helped us win the war!"

The American pioneers also loved kasha, which they called buckwheat grits; today it is almost forgotten, although it is a delightful cereal. Only the Jewish people still make many delicious dishes with kasha. My favorite recipe for kasha is ideal for a beauty-farm dinner. (See page 324.)

LECITHIN

Every beauty-seeking Eve should make the acquaintance of lecithin (pronounced less-i-thin). It is probably one of the most important food elements that scientists have discovered in the last few decades. We know that it is involved in nourishing the skin and the thin, beautifying layer of fat beneath. "The least it can do for you," says Dr. Lester M. Morrison, "is to improve your health and give you added vitality; it may even save your life."

While precious lecithin is supplied by egg yolk, liver, and brains, it is difficult to obtain sufficient amounts in other foods. Lecithin is one of the lost treasures of nutrition, stolen from natural foods by refining and processing. Many of the natural oils and cereals containing lecithin are refined or saturated, and this elixir of the fat family is either destroyed outright or neutralized.

I recommend that you taste this vital food in the available form of *soya bean lecithin*. It is temptingly delicious, nutty in flavor, and a very specific aid to beautiful, firm, luminous skin.

To know about its spectacular merits as a life-saving protection from cardio-vascular disease, I suggest that you read Chapter 22, *Your Man*.

LICORICE

Considerable mystery still surrounds this "sweet root," which is what its ancient Greek name means. European children know and love it as a sweet to chew on, and it has been both a confection and a medicine for almost 3,000 years. The early Egyptians used licorice as a sweetener and made a favorite drink of it. Experimental research at the Massachusetts College of Pharmacy has lately isolated some hormones from the licorice root, and a Dutch physician recommends licorice syrup to soothe irritated intestines. But what interests us most is the fact that real licorice is a very sweet, natural sweetener and very little of it is needed to add a new taste to food and drink.

For relaxing, good-night licorice tea, add a teaspoon of finely chopped licorice root to a cup of boiling water and strain. Licorice is a mild laxative, so use it sparingly. Plain licorice roots are a Godsend for those who are trying to give up cigarettes: carry some in your purse and when the urge overwhelms you, just chew on the woody licorice root. The taste is extremely pleasant and your hands will have something to do. Licorice root has helped many to overcome the cigarette habit.

NUTS

Millions of good homemakers sincerely try to plan well-balanced meals, and then with one fell swoop they destroy all the good of their carefully planned meals by serving a dessert loaded with sugar, starch, and fat, and entirely empty of proteins, vitamins, and minerals. Such concoctions add nothing to your good looks—on the contrary, they steal away beauty by what they do add, which is only pounds and a sluggish burden on your metabolism.

Why should dessert be such a stumbling block to your good planning? All you want, all anyone wants at the end of a meal is a taste of sweetness. Yet the world is full of delectable sweets. In the book, *The Anatomy of Dessert*, by the Englishman Charles Bunyard, there was not one recipe for these deceptive concoctions full of the two main destroyers of your good looks, the refined sugars and the saturated, high cholesterol fats. Instead he sang the praises of the lovely fruits and nuts growing in the English countryside, and there were more than enough of these natural sweets to fill a book!

Almonds, fresh from the trees, just before their shells harden, are a favorite dessert in France, Italy and Spain. In Sicily, with these fresh, juicy almonds they also make a drink fit for the gods, called *latte di manderle*, "milk of almonds," and this is how they make it: the fresh almonds are peeled and pounded to a fine pulp, to which is added warm, not hot, water; this is flavored with a dash of real, not synthetic, vanilla extract and sweetened with honey. Chill this, and serve it as a glorious dessert drink.

At the Bircher-Benner Sanatorium in Zurich, Switzerland, almonds have the place of honor. They are served instead of meat, whole or grated; for those with weak digestion the ripe, peeled almonds are made into a tasty almond milk. Here is the American way of making nourishing almond milk twice as nourishing and I recommend it highly as a nutritious in-between beautyfarm drink:

Put one cup of skim milk into an electric blender, add one heaping tablespoon of blanched almonds, one teaspoon of honey and a drop of real vanilla; mix for just one minute; the addition of milk to the almonds makes this a potent, high protein, delicious, building drink. Fruit juices can replace the milk for those who have an allergy to it, or just for an agreeable change.

Peanuts are called "earthnuts" in German because they grow like beans in the earth and not on a bush or tree, in fact they are a member of the bean family. Ripe, lightly roasted peanuts are an excellent food; they are cheap and available everywhere; they grow like weeds in all but the very cold climates. I planted some in my Sicilian garden and was astonished at how easily they grow. The protein in peanuts is not as complete as that in meat and milk, but they are rich in vitamins, minerals and an excellent unsaturated oil. I highly recommend the eating of peanuts, along with other nuts and seeds, for between-meal hunger in place of candies and such empty sweets.

Peanut Flour is becoming more and more popular; it gives a delightful flavor to all baked foods. One tablespoon of peanut flour can be added to each cup of wheat flour without changing the rest of the recipe. One-half cup contains 30 grams of protein. You will have to go to your nearest health food store or diet shop to get peanut flour, but it is a real find for your beauty pantry.

PAPAYA

This golden melon which grows on a tree is one of the most interesting and unusual fruits in our markets. Even the tree is unique: it has three genders, masculine, feminine, and neuter. The little tree grows extremely fast; planted as a sapling, it bears fruit within just nine months.

The Spaniards were the first to learn the great value of papayas. They discovered that when they ate too many fried fish, a few slices of papaya helped their digestion and even prevented stomach aches. Professor R. H. Chittenden of Yale University confirmed the extraordinary nutritional value of papaya. The golden melon is loaded with enzymes; they are those important beautifiers made up of a vitamin, a mineral and a protein which activates digestion. The most active enzyme is called papain, but the fruit contains many other valuable enzymes. Dr. Chittenden proved scientifically what the early Spaniards learned from experience; the combination of enzymes has the power to digest proteins, as well as some fats and starches. When the enzyme papain was placed in a test tube with such varied foods as salmon, codfish, dried beef, potatoes, bread, roast beef, cheese, within a short time these foods were completely digested and liquified and could be poured from the tube. Today papain is widely used as a valuable vegetable tenderizer of meat.

Dr. John Harvey Kellogg of Battle Creek fame placed the papaya at the top of nature's best alkalizing foods. It is an excellent source of the beauty-giving vitamin C and of vitamins A and B-2.

Papayas grow easily in tropical and subtropical climates; the best ones I ate were in Jamaica, where this wonder-fruit is so plentiful that it goes begging. A few years ago you would enjoy papayas only if you lived in Florida, California and Hawaii. Today they can be purchased in fine markets throughout the country. The juice and concentrate can be bought in all special food shops. Papayas make an ideal beautyfarm food.

A slice of golden papaya makes an ideal breakfast fruit; sliced papaya sprinkled with lime and honey is an exotic dessert. Papayas are also an aid to beauty from the outside; they make excellent beauty masks. The papain enzyme clears away all the old dead cells and leaves the skin soft and glowing.

PARSLEY

This humble, plentiful, inexpensive little green is indispensable to good French cookery and you might make it indispensable to your own. It is the ideal beautyfarm and beauty-full green; to use it only as decoration, as so many American cooks do, is to throw away a treasure of beauty-giving vitamin A and a fair supply of vitamins B and C, to say nothing of the freshest, most versatile flavor which marries with everything from salad to fish and poultry stuffing and eggs in every form. When you make your delicious fresh vegetable espresso, you can hardly omit the sweet sharp tang of parsley, and it adds its pungent touch to cooked vegetables as well. It blends into any background whether of meat, fish or vegetables and I recommend a good handful of it chopped and mixed with cottage cheese. A gourmet stuffing for fish or poultry is made with whole grain bread, onions, celery, beaten egg, and a whole bunch of parsley, chopped fine, enough to make the entire mixture freshly, beautifully green.

Parsley can take the place of all the chlorophyll preparations that supposedly sweeten the breath: chew a bit after dinner and your best friends won't know there was delicious garlic in your salad.

ROSE HIPS

A rose is not only a rose to be smelled and admired—far from it! The fruit or seed of the rose is also one of nature's richest sources of the beauty-giving vitamin C. I first learned about rose hips while visiting Russia in 1928. When I exclaimed in amazement at seeing miles and miles of roses along the highway, my Intourist guide informed me that these were "vitamin roses," grown only for their precious fruit, the rose hips. Imagine, one of our most beautiful flowers also produces one of our most beauty-full vitamins, vitamin C.

My second acquaintance with rose hips came when it was served to me as a "kernle's tee" (tea of dried rose hips, seed and all, steeped for five minutes) in one of the oldest sanatoriums in Switzerland. Since then the fame of rose hips has gone around the world. In England and Germany, rose hips are made into a delightful marmalade, even into potent wine. During the war, when the British could obtain no citrus fruits, they saved their people from vitamin C starvation by harvesting these fruits from the rose bushes in their gardens, and processing the crop as food.

What a potent beauty food it is! In 100 grams of orange there are 50 milligrams of vitamin C. But 100 grams of rose hips contain up to 6,000 milligrams—about 120 times the content of our most common vitamin C source.

In Europe I have enjoyed rose hip soup, rose hip jam, jellies, purées. Stir your rose hip preparation in fruit juices, or make a purée of it to eat with meat or poultry dishes as you would eat cranberry or other preserves.

There are many varieties of roses which produce these vitamin-rich rose hips, but the Rosa Rugosa is one of the richest and easiest to raise. If you have any ground at all, do become an active beauty farmer and plant a few of these bushes. If you can't raise your own rose hips, you can now get them in powdered and tablet form.

SEA GREENS

Our oceans contain a treasure of health and beauty that equals and even exceeds that of our farms. The seas are teeming, not only with thousands of nutritious fish and shellfish, but with thousands of nutritious plants, sea herbs and sea vegetables.

In lands that are favored with long seacoasts, the people harvest vegetables and greens from the rich garden of the sea. For thousands of years the people of China have eaten all sorts of sea greens, and the Japanese to this day are the world's largest consumers of sea vegetation. One-fourth of their daily food comes from the ocean. As you perhaps know, there are very few overweight Japanese, and goiter is practically unknown among them. They have catalogued more than a hundred sea green species.

In the British Isles and Ireland the favorites are Irish moss, dulse, and sea lettuce, so called because it is as green and tender as lettuce. New England housewives in colonial days thriftily gathered greens left along the beaches after the outgoing tide. One of many sea greens that we eat fresh in Sicily is spaghetti del mare, "spaghetti of the sea," which grows on the rocks in long streamers and looks like spaghetti. The fishermen eat it by the handful right out of the ocean.

In America only people who live along the coast—usually those of Irish birth or extraction—buy Irish moss and dulse in the fish stores, where they are sold right along with the fish. I doubt if either the storekeeper who sells them or the Irish-bred girls who chew them in preference to chewing gum (wise girls!) know that these green and dark red leaves with their pleasant briny taste are treasure houses of beauty-giving iodine and other vital elements.

I talked in an earlier chapter about the ugly goiter that is so common in lands where iodine is lacking in the soil. Perhaps you remember Mark Twain's tall tale about the man in the Swiss Tyrol who had such a huge goiter that he had to use a wheelbarrow to get about. I have never seen such a big one as that, not even in Switzerland (neither did Mark Twain). But a lack of iodine can cause other disfigurements besides goiters. It is often responsible for overweight, especially around the hips and legs. For years Dr. William Brady in his popular newspaper column urged his readers to speed up their metabolism and lose their blankets of fat with daily rations of iodine. Dr. Brady also pointed out a fact that is well known to doctors: dry skin and hair, thinness and poor growth of hair, pallor or a waxy appearance of the skin are common signs of iodine deficiency.

Since the foods from the ocean are the richest source of iodine, it is obvious that we should include more of them, both animal and vegetable, in our diet. In recent studies it was discovered that some sea greens are a thousand times richer in iodine than any other food, and that from 70 to 80 percent of their iodine is in the form of do-iodo-tyrosine, the very best form for the body's use. The thyroid gland has to make only one chemical change to convert di-iodo-tyrosine to the powerful hormone, thyroxine, and this hormone is poured into the blood stream, your beautystream, to keep your metabolism high, your skin and hair healthy, and your energies at a peak of well-being.

SEA WATER

While I talk about the riches of the oceans, let me report that plain, ordinary sea water is being successfully used in many countries. In Germany, bottled North Sea water is highly recommended by some doctors as a rich source of minerals. In France a movement has begun to use the benefits of the Mediterranean Ocean; in Cannes, near the Casino, the French government is spending millions of francs for a seaside spa where every kind of sea water treatment is given; in the women's department the salt water facials and salt water steams are especially popular.

I am delighted that at last those vast chemical riches of our oceans are being tapped for the health and well-being of our people. Sea water itself is now being investigated by scientists as an inexpensive and unlimited source of trace minerals. Recently in the *Miami Herald*, Dr. George W. Crane wrote about his experience with sea water brine (see page 336). Dr. Crane points out that all water-soluble chemicals are in the oceans; he claims that some twenty of these are now leached from our earth by frequent plowing and heavy rains, therefore many of our foods are chemically deficient. He reminds us, too, that only a trace of iodine, added to table salt since 1924, has eliminated almost all goiters. Will a trace of other vital chemicals insure us against cancer or diabetes or even gray hair and baldness? Modern medicine regards this idea as probably the most significant innovation since the sulfa drugs and antibiotics.

Dr. Crane also reports the remarkable case of a man in his ninety-eighth year, who 15 months earlier was dying, after months of being bedfast, disoriented and unable to feed himself. Now for the first time in years he hobbles around, comes to the table, and can cross his arthritic leg over his left knee to take off his shoe. Yet the only change in his regime has been one daily spoonful of concentrated ocean water which is given to him without his knowledge, thus his improvement is not due to suggestion. Ask your friends along the sea to ship you inlanders a little ocean water!

Remember, these are Dr. Crane's experiences, not mine, but I am going right down to the beach and get myself a big bottle of ocean salt water for free!

SEEDS

Seeds are the beginning of new life. They are filled with the promise of life and the precious food for life in the most concentrated form. Remember the beautiful verse from Genesis: "And God said, Behold, I have given you every herb bearing seed, which is upon the face of the earth, and every tree in which is the fruit of a tree yielding seed: to you it shall be for meat."

Small as they are, seeds are highly concentrated packages of proteins and minerals, especially phosphorus and calcium which are so necessary for the beauty of your teeth and the strength of your bones. You might call them Nature's tasty beauty tablets. That is why I recommend them for between-meal nibbling, to take the place of the nutritionless sweets that can only hamper your good looks with extra pounds.

Sunflower seeds, melon seeds, and *pumpkin seeds* are delicious snack foods, in the same class as nuts (which are also seeds) to satisfy that between-meal craving which may be true hunger or may be tension hunger. Because they give the hands something to do, they have been a wonderful help to many in breaking the cigarette habit.

Here are some other valuable seeds that can be used in cooking and a variety of ways:

Flaxseed was a great delicacy in ancient days and was thought to be a love potion; medical lore of long ago prescribed it for respiratory ailments, and for generations Europeans used it to help lazy elimination.

Today flaxseed is again coming into its own. I saw sugar bowls filled with ground flaxseed meal on every table in the dining room of the famous Buchinger Sanatorium in Uberlingen, Germany, to be sprinkled over food. It is as tasty as wheat germ and inexpensive. All flaxseed products contain those valuable unsaturated fatty acids, the vitamin F so necessary for a glowing complexion. In the health food shops all over Germany, you can also buy cold pressed flaxseed oil, rich in fatty acids.

A particular value of flaxseed is its mild laxative quality. Flaxseed mixed with your morning cereal makes a natural "bowel motor" for lazy intestines. Many of the health stores in the United States will accommodate you by mixing a handful of ground flaxseed with their whole cereals. This makes an excellent hot breakfast cereal for beautyfarms and for your own family.

Sesame Seeds are a beauty treasure that I first learned about from an Indian princess in Paris. The Princess Karputhala—Sita, as her friends called her, was the belle of Paris society. She had the largest eyes I have ever seen, her teeth were literally like pearls, and her skin had the texture and delicate glow of a sun-ripened apricot.

It was this fairy-tale princess from an ancient Eastern land who taught me the wonders of an ancient seed; she told me that for thousands of years this modest little seed has been used by Indian women as food, as oil, and as a favorite cosmetic. Every maharanee had her own heavily scented complexion oil, the base of which was pure sesame oil. Fortunately for the rest of the world, sesame seeds are becoming more popular and are now cultivated in other countries; they are now successfully grown in California.

Most people know sesame seeds only as a sprinkling on rolls or bread, but this unassuming little seed is an "open sesame" of nutritional treasures. It contains a good protein and B vitamins, but most of all it is a treasure trove for calcium, so badly needed for good teeth and bones. One hundred grams of sesame seed contains 1,125 milligrams of calcium, whereas two glasses of milk contain only 600 milligrams.

If you cannot find sesame seeds in your market, try your nearest health food store. If you have a garden, add sesame to your cosmetic flower bed; it is an attractive plant with pink flowers and the seeds keep for years if you dry them thoroughly. Toast them lightly before storing and use them for topping bread and cookies, in pie crusts, biscuits and all your baking. Most of all, sesame milk makes one of the most delightful beautyfarm drinks; it tastes like almond milk and is much cheaper. Here is the recipe:

SWEET SESAME MILK

1 Cup washed sesame seeds
2 Cups of water
2 Teaspoons honey
2 Drops vanilla extract

Put ingredients in liquefier-blender and mix until smooth. If too rich, add more water. Keep it in the refrigerator and serve it chilled.

Note to Beautyfarmers: Keep this delightful between-meal drink on hand at all times. A professional, smooth milk can be made by soaking the cup of seeds in 2 cups of water overnight and liquefying them in the morning, without pouring off the water.

YOGURT

I have been teaching and preaching the delights of yogurt in this country for years and I believe I have succeeded in popularizing it as a delicious and wonderful food. But the real pioneer who brought yogurt to the United States was Dr. Simon Baruch, the father of Bernard Baruch, the beloved elder statesman. He long ago recommended it to his patients and to this day in the Baruch home at cocktail time fresh yogurt is always served, no matter what other refreshments are offered to the guests.

You cannot do better than to make yogurt your staple beauty-full food at meals and between meals, in soups, sauces, and desserts and as a light and delicate snack. It is an ideal source of whole proteins plus good quantities of calcium and B vitamins, especially riboflavin, and it is recommended by physicians as a support for the valuable intestinal flora.

In this country yogurt is a cultivated, sophisticated food of gourmets who love it for its delicacy and the light, fresh flavor it contributes to a great variety of exquisite dishes. But in the rest of the world it is an ancient favorite; in fact it goes back to the Bible as one of the forms of cultured milk that all the peoples of the world developed, each from the milk of a different domestic animal. In faraway Cathay the dish made from the milk of mares in the royal stable was eaten only by the great Khan and his descendants, and it was a kind of cultured milk that Father Abraham gave to the three angels who visited him. How could we possibly call yogurt a fad food when it was eaten even in Biblical times?

True yogurt as we know it is the food of the long-lived Bulgarians. The famous Russian doctor Ilya Mechnikov believed that yogurt might be the secret of the Bulgarians' prolonged youthfulness and vigor. During his many years at the Pasteur Institute in Paris he introduced it to France, and the French called it the "milk of eternal life."

Yogurt is available now in dairy and food stores all over this country, but you can also make your own at home with little trouble and less expense. You can develop the taste of a true yogurt gourmet and enjoy its refreshing light taste and satin-smooth texture by itself, or mix it with fruit and honey, molasses or brown sugar as a tempting sundae. Mixed with golden oil and a little lemon juice, it is a wonderful protein-rich salad dressing; stirred into chicken broth, it makes a new, fresh-flavored, creamy chicken soup, and it is the basis for an ideal chilled soup in hot weather. You will find recipes for making yogurt at home and for many ways to use it in your Cosmetic Diet.

If you have not yet cultivated a taste for yogurt, I urge you to treat yourself to this exquisite beauty-rich food, as old as the Bible and as fresh as the newly made batch in your refrigerator.

Part Three

---◦❦◦---

YOUR HIGH ROAD

TO BEAUTY

CHAPTER 8

Contours of Beauty: Your Figure

Look into your mirror, Eve. Not your hand mirror, this time, nor the mirror on your dressing table which shows you only your head and shoulders. Look at yourself full length in your mirror on the wall.

What does it say this time? Or perhaps I should ask, do you ever really see yourself as a whole, from head to foot, from the back, from the side, walking, sitting, moving about as well as standing still?

In homes of the elegant era, before the first World War, there was usually a pier glass in the drawing room, as tall as the two tall windows between which it stood. In it a woman could see herself walking forward from the far end of the room. Looking over her shoulder, she could see herself walking away. She could see how she looked in motion, from the flowers on her hat to the trailing hem of her skirt. She taught her growing daughters to watch themselves in that mirror as they walked, sat down, stood up.

In her boudoir she had another mirror, in a frame that rested on the floor so that she could tilt it to any angle. She could see herself in it from top to toe, and not merely standing still, but moving about.

Why do I talk to you of that elegant woman of the Edwardian era? Because I am astonished at the unaware, the *unprideful* way in which so many women carry themselves.

This is true of the pretty and the plain, of the slim, and even more so of the plump. It is true of women of all ages, even of young girls. It is sad to see them, with their youthful resilient bodies, already fixed in ugly distortions which will trouble them the rest of their lives.

I see them teetering along on their insecure heels, waddling, ducklike, with silly, short steps in their too-narrow skirts. I see swaybacks, slopeshoulders, heads thrust forward when they should be carried high and proudly.

Many of these women struggle with one reducing diet after another, when actually they need not reduce at all. Their bulging buttocks, protruding abdomens, and drooping bosoms would automatically go back in place if once the posture were adjusted. All they need is to stand and walk as their bodies were built to do, and they will free themselves for all time from these disfiguring faults.

SEE YOURSELF AS OTHERS SEE YOU

All these young girls and grown women want to be beautiful. No one, it seems, has told them that age-old truth: that a woman who *carries* herself like a beauty, gracefully, proudly, and with assurance has won more than half the battle of being a beauty. To me there is no greater handicap to beauty than what Southerners so rightly call a hang-dog look, and I often wonder why women of today don't see themselves as others see them.

I am afraid that the art of good carriage and natural movement, which women once cultivated, especially in Europe, has been almost forgotten.

And I fear—in fact, I *know*—that American women do not treat their bodies with enough respect and consideration.

American women give endless care to the outer body. They are, without a doubt, the cleanest and sweetest smelling women anywhere. They try to be slim, although too often, alas, they go about it in the worst possible way. They dress, on the whole, very well compared with women in other lands.

But they do not use their bodies well. They do not feed their bodies adequately. And they take no pride in the posture and smooth coordination, of which the body's wonder-architecture is capable.

You are built for action

In all the world of living things there is nothing quite so remarkable as the human body's structure. It is built to do an enormous variety of things. Think of the ballet dancer, the tight-rope walker, the tennis player. Or, to come closer to home, think of yourself and the many everyday tasks you perform in the course of one day, bending, reaching, lifting, carrying, cooking and cleaning, driving a car, holding a baby.

What makes all these skilled, coordinated movements possible? The body is a structure of bones, put together with more than 200 muscles and a great variety of joints. It is not static like a building, but dynamic, fluid, springy.

The spine, the central support of this wonderful structure, is not a single rigid bone, but a flexible column of bones and it is curved like a spring to absorb the shocks of action. Between these little bones are cushions of rubbery cartilage, the disks. The joints of the body are also cushioned with cartilage, and they are securely bound with tough elastic fibers called ligaments.

Do you see that the whole marvelous mechanism is built not to sit and vegetate, but to move? It even has a little sac of fluid to oil each joint! Can you see now, in your mind's eye, what happens to this beautiful action mechanism when it isn't active?

I wish I could impress you with what all this sitting does to a woman's beauty potential. It leaves flabby and unused the powerful abdominal and thigh muscles. It constricts the circulation that is necessary to keep the bones and muscles of the legs and feet healthy, strong and trim. I am afraid that for all her dieting, the modern woman is doomed to TV bottom unless she takes warning.

Muscles against gravity

One of the mighty forces of life to which we are born on this earth is the law of gravity. From the first step that the baby takes, he begins to cope with gravity, and he will cope with it his whole life long. The human body is made of flexible moving parts, it is top-heavy, and furthermore, it has to balance on two legs. It is especially vulnerable to the downward pull of gravity.

But we are earth children, and our bodies are constructed to deal with earth's gravity. We have a built-in reflex in our muscles, called the stretch reflex, so that every time we move, the muscles that are stretched immediately tighten up to hold us in that position against the pull of gravity.

Gravity tugs at every part, at the organs, the body fluids, the blood. Gravity helps the blood to return to the heart from the head and neck and shoulders. But what brings the blood upward against gravity from the two-thirds of the body below the heart? Your muscles do the work. Yes, they are your heart's greatest assistants. Actually, the two-legged human body has a natural corset of muscles all around the torso, powerful muscles that support the organs in their places. And to return the blood to the heart against gravity, the muscles of the legs and this natural girdle of muscles around the hips and torso literally press the blood upward in the veins each time we stand and walk and move about.

Nothing can do the work of this muscular corset. No corset, girdle or foundation that you can buy can support the organs in their places as does this natural muscular belt. As for helping the blood along the veins in the return journey to the heart, every woman knows that a girdle does just the opposite.

Your muscles have a life-saving, beauty-preserving job to do for you. They can do this, and the bones and their resilient connective tissues can respond, only if they are well-fed and well used.

Poor nutrition and poor posture set up a vicious cycle. Either one can be the starting point. Poor nutrition weakens the muscles and connective tissues so that poor posture results. Poor posture deprives them of the circulation that would bring them the nutrition they vitally need.

CHANGING YOUR BODY IMAGE

Some women keep throughout their lives the swayback of their childhood, with the plump tummy pushed out before. Others still stand with the round-shouldered stoop of the adolescent who was embarrassed by her developing bosom.

Surely, once womanhood is reached, that childhood or adolescent body image can be discarded! I believe that most women who do cling to these unconscious old attitudes of the body are quite unaware that they do, because they never see themselves as a whole.

You may need to lose or gain weight. You may need to change your proportions. We shall talk about both those projects in the following chapters. But the first step in changing your body image is to put your body *architecture* back in order, as it was intended by nature to be.

Be taller, slimmer

There are several points at which you can begin to set the mechanism in order again. It hardly matters which you choose, for once one part is set right, the rest almost automatically falls into place.

Let's begin at the middle, with the lower back and pelvis. This bears the same relation to the rest of your body as the keystone bears to an arch in architecture. It is the pivotal point on which the body's weight is balanced, with the support of the natural girdle of muscles.

To perfect your posture from this midpoint, stand with your back against the wall, your heels a few inches away from it. Now try to flatten the curve of your lower back against the wall. You will probably have to begin by bending your upper body forward a bit. Tilt your hips forward, too, and pull your abdominal muscles in. Pull them in hard, as though you were trying to press them right back against your spine. Straighten up slowly, all the while trying to feel your back against the wall.

Now step away, and see if you can keep that feeling of the straight back and well-supported abdomen, easily balanced on the bony cradle of the pelvis. If you have done it right, you should feel and look taller, your head should feel comfortably balanced on a straight neck, your shoulders should hang loose and comfortably, and your bosom should be high. You have reduced your waistline by several inches because you have pushed your protruding

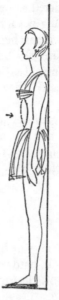

Pull in your abdominal muscles

abdomen back where it belongs and you have tightened and flattened your soft abdominal muscles.

YOU CAN REDUCE INSTANTLY

On my recent Town Hall lecture tour from New York to San Francisco, thousands of ladies were amazed and amused when at the end of my talk I asked for a woman who would like to reduce instantly. Many volunteered and I would pick a nice, plumpish lady and teach her how to straighten the curve in her back. I would put one hand on the lady's back, at the curve, and with the other hand I would help to push back the rounded tummy; then I'd say, "Now walk tall, very tall, push the top of your head, not your chin, into the ceiling," and *voilà*, there was an instant reduction, sometimes of several inches, around the waistline. The audience would applaud noisily as the lady walked across the stage like a professional model.

You, yourself, right where you are, can have a proud and happy posture almost instantaneously. I am not there to help you, but it is so easy! Only follow the directions as I gave them above. Begin by standing against the wall, and follow step by step this simple method of reconstructing your body's architecture of beauty. If you do it before a full-length mirror, you will actually see yourself grow taller and slimmer before your very eyes. It is like waving a magic wand.

BEAUTYFARM POSTURE SECRET

On most Beautyfarms, here and abroad, they spend a great deal of time teaching good posture, and I have seen slouchy, badly postured women leave straighter and taller after two weeks of training. The device which helps to correct bad posture almost instantly is the Beauty Slant, an upholstered, straight board, elevated 15 inches at the foot end, on which you lie and rest your weary bones. The law of gravity does all the work for you. There is a gentle pull all along the spine; exaggerated spinal curves diminish and posture improves, as if by magic.

I first learned about the body slant from Dr. Carl Zukor, the famous physician in Carlsbad. He insisted that all his women patients take the slant position for prolapsed organs, varicose veins and for general health.

But the person who really convinced me of the great value of the Beauty Slant position is one of America's most attractive women, Ann Delafield. I have seen her perform miracles on the Elizabeth Arden Beauty Farm. Miss Delafield laid down the rule that every one of the clients must spend some time on the Beauty Slant before going to bed at night and again the first thing in the morning. In that way, said Ann Delafield, the whole body and especially the inner organs were brought into proper alignment. I assure you that if you adopt this rule you will look and feel better throughout the day.

I have already said in my book, *Look Younger, Live Longer*, that one of the best and most enduring investments any woman can make is a Beauty Slant. I bought the very first one at the Hollywood Elizabeth Arden Salon and presented it to one of the world's loveliest ladies, Greta Garbo. She kept it beside her swimming pool and relaxed on it daily. There are many Beauty Slants on the market now. Try them all and buy the one which feels most comfortable and relaxes you best. An unsteady one made of orange crates is not worth your money; it will not stand up. If you cannot afford a well-constructed Beauty Slant, let your husband make one. Buy a strong board several inches longer than your own height, and elevate one end on legs not more than fifteen inches high. For comfort, pad the board with a thin sheet of foam rubber and cover it with canvas or plastic.

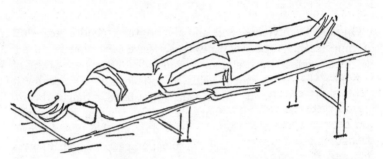

Ann Delafield's Beauty Slant with shoulder brace

BEGIN AT THE TOP

And here is another secret of good posture. This time let's begin at the top. Push the top of your head up as if you were going to push up the ceiling with it. Push and keep pushing. You will feel your neck lengthening, your waist lengthening and slimming, your bosom rising. The abdominal muscles tighten and pull up, the pelvis tips forward, the torso finds its position of balance. And there is no tension, not in the neck muscles, not in the shoulders. Only in the place where tension should be—the powerful muscles of the abdominal wall that should be firm and taut in every upright position of the torso. The only time those muscles can be slack is when you are lying down.

Once you find this natural, *physiological* posture, with your head high, back straight, abdominal muscles firm and strong, your legs will swing easily from the hip joints when you walk, as they are meant to do. When you sit, your torso will not slump down into a weary pathetic figure. It will support itself, as it was built to do. You will prefer a straight-backed chair and you will shun those droopy, big chairs like a poison plague.

When you sit gracefully and proudly on a straight-backed chair, there will be no tension. Good posture is not rigid and tense, but easy and fluid. It is the way in which your body was constructed—to maintain itself *erect* against gravity.

This simple posture exercise will not magically correct your body image overnight. It is a first step, a way of feeling—and seeing, in your long mirror—how you are going to carry yourself.

In order to hold this good functional posture, this beautiful bearing, you will also have to work from the inside and supply your bones and muscles with the strengthening nutrition they need. I invite you to follow my Cosmetic Diet, high in calcium for the bones, high in proteins for the muscles, and high in vitamin C to keep the connective tissue of cartilage, tendons and ligaments resilient and elastic.

And there are two further steps you will want to take to help you become a long-stemmed American Beauty. One of them is to strengthen and exercise your weakened muscles and get them back into healthy elastic tone. And last, but most important, free yourself daily from ugly tensions; don't let it accumulate. Do this, step by step. It is all worked out for you—you will be amazed how enjoyable this can be.

FOOD FOR YOUR ARCHITECTURE OF BEAUTY

The bones are the firm framework of the body, and we think of them as hard and solid, but they are living tissue like every other part of you. It is hard to believe, but 25 or 30 percent of these apparently solid bones is water.

You mothers of the future can lay the foundation for straight and upright bodies by eating scientifically while carrying your babies. Then feed them as Nature intended by nursing them. You mothers are the real beauty chemists of the future. The basic foundation for good bones is laid down, as well we all know, in infancy and childhood, and even before, in the mother's body during pregnancy. The ancient people of the world have long known this. The comparatively primitive people have known it too. For a thousand years or more, Chinese physicians have given a pregnant mother a deer horn, which she scraped into fine powder and added to her food in order to provide her body with extra calcium for her baby's strong bones. The Tibetans give a prized gift of powdered yak bones to a pregnant mother. The Eskimos eat a diet mainly of fish, but they eat it bones and all.

The refined diet of our modern civilization does not give us enough calcium. Dr. Weston A. Price, in his valuable book, *Nutrition and Physical Degeneration,* has shown in figures and photographs how the straight bodies and strong teeth of beautiful primitive peoples have deteriorated *in one generation* of eating overrefined foods.

FEEDING YOUR BONES

We know that a basically good bony structure is built in these early months and years of life. But we tend to forget that the bones continue to renew themselves, that *nothing* alive is final. The real neglect in our way of life is not for prenatal care and childhood, but for adulthood. Adults feel that they have done all their growing, that their bones are fixed and finished for better or worse. The fact is that our bones are scarcely more final than our blood!

Here is what Dr. Martin A. Gumpert says in his fine book, *You Are Younger Than You Think:* "Of the minerals, calcium is often deficient, especially in the American diet. This calcium deficiency often becomes manifest only in advanced age, when the fragility of the bones increases; a symptom of old age that could probably be prevented by a greater calcium storage in earlier years."

Let me say more bluntly what Dr. Gumpert expressed with caution: The trouble that so many adults have in later years with their body framework might well be spared them if their bones had been well nourished through all the years before. When proud, stately, good-looking men and women take on a hang-dog posture, it is a sign to the whole world, not that they are getting old, but that they are failing and have failed to nourish their body structure.

In its daily process of renewal and cell replacement the whole bony structure loses calcium, phosphorus and other essential materials. Day and night, the blood carries away worn-out cells for disposal, and they must be replaced.

And that is why your bones need nourishment every day. Hard as they are, they carry on a constant exchange of these essential materials with the bloodstream. The blood carries away these substances with the worn-out cells, and it must also bring a fresh supply.

It must bring to the bones animal proteins containing the eight essential amino acids that go to make the human proteins of our protoplasm. It must bring the vitamins essential to metabolism and it must bring the minerals that are specific to bone.

Phosphorus, magnesium, and certain other trace elements are needed in comparatively small quantities and are easily available in a good diet. Calcium is the most necessary element, which combines with phosphorus to make the hard substance of bone, calcium phosphate. But calcium is most often short in the diet. Secretary of Agriculture Ezra Taft Benson has warned that American women, especially deprive themselves of needed calcium in their diet.

Dr. Henry C. Sherman of Columbia University has warned us for years that 50 percent of American people are starving for calcium. So I repeat, to keep your architecture strong and straight, you should have at least a pint of milk each day. Cheese, yogurt and all dairy products are, of course, calcium foods par excellence. There are also a few vegetables which contain beauty-giving calcium, especially broccoli, kale, mustard and turnip greens. By all means use these freely.

For the hundreds of thousands of women and their husbands who do not drink their pint of fresh milk daily, I recommend the generous use of inexpensive dried skim milk powder and one of the oldest, but richest of all calcium-rich food, very finely ground bone flour. Some of our better baby foods are already being fortified with this purified and very fine calcium. From this day on, I invite you to include such bone flour for enriching your diet with wonder-working calcium; the fine powder can be taken in your morning fruit juice, it can be used in bread, for fortifying gravies and stews, and it is available even in easy-to-take tablet form. You need never again suffer from a shortage of calcium.

Vitamin D, the "straight leg" vitamin, is also needed for good bone structure. During the summer months we need not worry about this vitamin, especially if we expose ourselves to the sun, but to make sure of a regular supply the year round, it is wise to use a concentrate.

FEEDING THE MUSCLES

If I have convinced you that your bones need nourishment every day, you will not need to be reminded that your muscles also need to be fed, and those important connective tissues that cushion and support the joints and especially the springy spine. For the elasticity of your new body image, for its spring and fluid grace, you will give your muscles the high quality proteins they need, which come chiefly from animal sources: meat, fish, eggs, milk and milk products.

And for the connective tissues, keep up the plentiful daily supply of vitamin C, which doctors today increasingly recognize as valuable in keeping the body structure youthful and resilient. This beauty-nourishing vitamin is not stored in the body. You must have your vitamin C fruits and vegetables or juices every day. Let me remind you again that the Russians cultivate acres and acres of rose bushes, not for their pretty flowers, but for the rose hips, one of the richest sources of C vitamin in all nature!

When you are feeding your new body image these beauty-nourishing foods, you will find it easier and easier to maintain beautiful posture. You will not have to remind yourself to "stand up straight." Your bones and muscles and springy, cushiony connective tissues will automatically do it for you!

GOODBYE FOREVER TO UGLY TENSION

Tension is the next enemy of your new body image. I believe that next to poor nutrition, nothing is so devastating to good looks as the tensions of mind which so quickly express themselves in bodies and faces. And in the pace and drive of our jet age, tension is hard to avoid.

This revelation came to me with great force one day when I was walking along Fifth Avenue at lunch time with a French friend who was visiting New York. The city was at its most beautiful, and up and down the glamorous avenue walked thousands of handsome, well-dressed New Yorkers. Suddenly, to my astonishment and, I confess, annoyance, my French friend exclaimed,

"New York, it is *magnifique,* but the people look so tense and harassed!"

Our beautiful American women—tense and harassed? I looked more closely, and I had to admit that the perceptive Parisienne at my side was quite right. Very few of those well-groomed, well-cared-for women walking down Fifth Avenue did not have that look of tension. You could see it in their faces and even more, in their bearing: chin and neck thrust forward, shoulders held high and rigid instead of loose and free, arms and hands held close and tight against the body instead of swinging in rhythm with their steps.

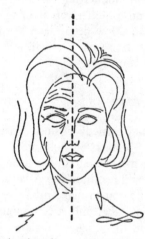

"Tension is ugliness, relaxation is beauty"

You could see tension in their backs as they walked ahead of you, tension in the cramped, jerky action of legs, ankles, and feet. When a professional model or dancer went by in the crowd, you could spot her instantly. The contrast of her free-swinging, *relaxed* bearing made the others even less attractive.

Yes, my French friend was right about those tense American women. So was the famous French painter who said, "Tension is ugliness, relaxation is beauty." Tension writes its ugliness on the face and on the body. Remember that, the next time you find yourself tied in a knot: stop for a moment and relax.

You need not be tense! You need not be imprisoned in tension as in that Iron Maiden of the medieval torture chambers. The first step toward freeing yourself from it is to realize that it is there.

The body has its own healthy way of shaking off tension. For instance, when you have been waiting for a piece of important news, and the news finally comes, what do you do? You give a sigh of relief. Sighing—yes, the deep, deep breath that goes to the bottom of your lungs, expanding your chest all the way, and then a quick expulsion of air in which all the muscles, all the way down to the feet, let go. It is nature's way to snap the tension, to relax you.

Take a cue from your wonderfully wise body. When you feel tension mounting in you, whether you are standing, sitting, walking or lying down, take a few deep, deep breaths, and let them out quickly as you do with a sigh. You will feel the tension let go with each breath that you expel.

SWING-SWAY-SLUMP

Here is my own easy remedy against tension which I have taught to thousands of women on both sides of the Atlantic. It is also never-failing in my own strenuous life in fast cars and jet planes; I have crossed and recrossed the Atlantic in six hours, and without tension. I invite you to make my relaxation secret a part of your daily routine; it takes only a few moments. I call it my Swing-Sway-Slump cure for all ugly tensions. Please try it right *now:*

Stand with your feet comfortably apart, preferably before your big mirror with your window wide open and good fresh air coming in. Let your arms hang loose at your sides; consciously try to let all your body muscles loosen. Now turn and swing your body slowly from side to side, as far as you can comfortably go. Turn to the left, then to the right, letting your arms hang and swing with you like pendulums of their own weight. As you turn to the left, your weight is all on the left foot and your right heel will rise a little off the floor; then you turn to the right, putting all your weight on your right foot and letting your left heel rise. Swing and sway lazily, easily; let go, and when you have the illusion that the window is swinging in the opposite direction each time, you

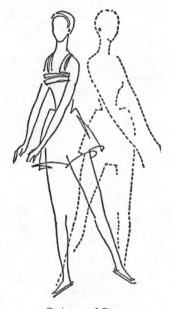

Swing and Sway

are doing the swing-and-sway correctly. Humming or whistling a slow waltz gives my Swing, Sway and Slump drill a pleasant rhythm.

It may take thirty, perhaps fifty swings—hardly more than a minute—but I promise that if you do it correctly, at the end you will have freed yourself of tension from head to toe. Not only your body but your whole face will lose its tension and even your eyes will relax as you swing and sway from side to side.

And here is my very effective 40-second Slump. Besides relaxing you, the Slump gives you an effective one-minute facial, without hands; it is a favorite beautyfarm ritual because it brings the circulation to your face and scalp and relaxes a tense neck. It is a particularly good remedy for tension that comes with long sitting and concentrated work. This is also a stress-and-strain soother for husbands with hectic jobs. It takes less than a minute.

Stand with your feet comfortably apart and slowly, easily bend over from the hips until your head, neck, and arms are hanging loosely. Now, dangling like a rag doll, swing slowly, from side to

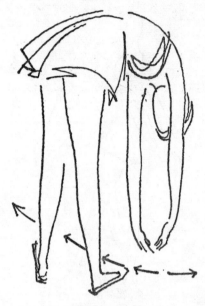

The "Rag Doll" Slump

side, just the way an elephant swings his great head and trunk when he is tied to a chain and bored. As the tightness and tensions drain away, you will find yourself able to hang lower and lower from the waist until your fingers finally touch the floor. But remember, this is not an exercise, so don't force yourself to touch the floor; there is no need to strain or become dizzy. Just hang and swing, back and forth, six, eight or ten times. Then raise your head slowly. Your face is flushed, for incidentally the law of gravity has given you a deep facial—you look pink and glowing. And you will find that your neck, back, shoulders have swung away their tensions. (For those whose blood pressure is above normal, it is best to have the doctor's permission for "Slumps.")

Here is another 60-second counter measure for tension, one that you can perform sitting at your desk, or at your dressing table when you are getting ready to go out and face the world. This is mainly to remove the tension from around your eyes and forehead, but it has brought blessed relaxation, in the midst of work, to thousands of my students. Look into your mirror before you begin. How do you look?

Now close your eyes gently—do not squeeze your lids shut—and cover them with your cupped palms so as to shut out all light, but without pressing against the eyes, without even touching them. Experiment with this until you have shut out the light completely. If your lashes just tickle your palms as you blink, and you still see no daylight, you have the position.

Rest your elbows on the table, breathe slowly and deeply at least fifteen or twenty times and as much longer as you like. When you first closed your eyes and covered them, perhaps you saw lights or colors under your eyelids—that in itself shows that you were tense. But in a little while, as you breathe deeply and the tension leaves, lights and colors fade and you see only restful, velvety black. After a delicious minute of this, cupping the eyes and breathing slowly, open your eyes and look again into your mirror and you will see a more relaxed, unharassed you.

In your campaign to free yourself of tension, look around your home. Where do you sit when you have time to rest and relax? What is your favorite chair? I hope it is not one of those modern, big *sitz* atrocities. A good chair supports your body at the crucial points, the lower back, neck and shoulders, and under the knees. An even better one allows you to put your feet up.

FIRM MUSCLES THE LAZY WAY

I want to give you my seven minute lazy stretching exercises in another chapter; it is a most important subject for beauty seekers. But I cannot leave this discussion of your new proud posture without giving you a wonderful piece of news about how to strengthen those muscles that give your body the proportions of your dreams.

Soft muscles that you have not been using properly in the past will need strengthening. Ordinarily one would have to undertake a regular regime of calisthenics or a particular kind of sport, and practice it faithfully for a long time in order to see the results.

But what if you could strengthen those muscles by only a few seconds of attention to them every day? Would you do it? Now then, here is my good news: *you can!* I learned about this in West Germany.

In the Max Planck Institute of Work Physiology in Dortmund,

Dr. Erich A. Mueller after ten years of research discovered something exciting. He found that with one intense muscular contraction, the maximum possible, held for only seconds and performed just once a day, a muscle grows in strength as fast is it can. Repeating an exercise over and over does not make a muscle develop any faster. Think of it: one maximum contraction performed just once a day makes that muscle become 6 percent stronger in one week, 66 percent stronger in eleven weeks. The once-a-day maximum muscle tensing does more than a long series of exercises with less than the maximum.

These quick muscle tensing exercises have become very popular in Germany and England. In America this fast way of exercising was first described by Dr. Arthur H. Steinhaus, professor of physiology at George Williams College in Chicago. It promises to become popular here, too, especially with our younger people who never did like the idea of lengthy exercise sessions. *Reader's Digest* was the first American magazine to popularize muscle tensing. And now I invite you to symmetrize and strengthen any part of your body with just one maximum muscular tension.

To strengthen those abdominal muscles so crucial to your new body image, just do this once a day:

Pull in your stomach as far as possible, more and more, harder and harder, so hard that the muscles begin to quiver. Then let go. And that is all there is to it; the entire exercise takes less than a minute! On some of the modern beautyfarms you are asked to do this one minute tummy tensing just before you jump out of bed in the morning. You'll be amazed how quickly this one minute of tension strengthens muscles, flattens bulges, and takes off inches. Do it faithfully, and in one week your own natural muscular girdle, the best undergarment ever made, will be 6 percent stronger; in eleven weeks your flabby abdominal muscles will be 66 percent stronger! With that steadily strengthening support, even if you have always hated strenuous exercise, you will be on your way to that proud and beautiful posture which is every woman's birthright.

SYMMETRIZE YOUR CONTOUR

After sitting at your desk all day or watching television all evening, get up, stretch, and with all your might, draw the heavy buttock muscles together, as tense and tight as possible, until they become as hard as a sack of cement; then let go, relax. Do this just once, with one maximum contraction each and every day, and soon you will be free of a flabby, overgenerous derrière.

You can strengthen and symmetrize any part of your body that may have become heavy and out of proportion. Calves, thighs, arms, chest and neck muscles respond equally well if you will give each part its single daily maximum contraction. One only is necessary; two or three contractions will do no more than just one maximum one; the German doctor is emphatic about this. But—and here is the most important point—do your muscle tensing and symmetrizing faithfully, once every day.

I believe many of the present day electric exercise devices are built upon this muscle-tensing principle, but no gadget can do for you what your own muscles—under the direction of your own free will—can do.

Is anyone too busy to invest one minute a day in a new figure?

CHAPTER 9

These Pains Can Be Pleasure:

Reducing

HOW TO MAKE REDUCING A PLEASURE

"Please, Gayelord, not *another* reducing diet. Why, every woman today knows that when she eats too much rich food and doesn't move about enough, she puts on weight and if she wants to reduce, all she has to do is move about more and eat less. You taught me that in Paris in 1938, and look at me!"

This is what the very attractive Mrs. Kingman Douglass, known to millions as Adele Astaire, said to me at her Manhattan dinner party. Adele, who sparkles with vitality, was right. In a few words she summed up what is probably the shortest solution to the reducing problem: move about more, and eat a little less. There you have it. Confucius could not have expressed it more concisely.

A few years ago I wrote an entire book about reducing, *New Guide to Intelligent Reducing*. I did many years of research on that book. I explained the reasons why people overeat, their physical and emotional problems. I gave recipes galore, diets and all sorts of menus, worked to perfection. If you have a reducing problem and want to solve it for a lifetime, I invite you to read that book. You will find it now among the Avon paperback books.

But there is one thing wrong with all reducing diets and books of the past, including mine, and that is what Adele Astaire meant when she said: "Not *another* reducing diet!" Women the world over have developed a deep hatred for all prescribed diets and the pains associated with reducing; the chores of diet and exercise are the greatest obstacles on the beauty road. Why, you ask? Let me remind you of what Sigmund Freud said: "The most powerful urge is to seek pleasure and avoid pain." He called it the pleasure-pain principle. That is a biological and psychological truth. Dieters and also doctors, nutritionists and dieticians of today need to remember that pleasure-pain is the most basic motivation of all and unless we can turn the pains of reducing into pleasure, the best planned diets are of no avail.

When Adele Astaire said I had taught her how to stay slim, she was referring to the very first lecture I gave in Paris. Lady Mendl arranged it for me in her Avenue D'Iena salon, and invited only her closest friends. Before me sat the Duchess of Windsor, Lady Diana Duff Cooper, Princess Aspasia of Greece, the Princess Karputhala of India, Lady Cavendish (Adele Astaire), Lady Carnarvon (Tilly Losch), the beautiful Ambassadress Madame de Saint Hardouin and Mrs. Harrison Williams. I had addressed audiences of thousands but they were mostly Mrs. Smiths and Mrs. Browns. Here were women with position, looks, worldly goods—what could I tell them? It was one of the most difficult lectures I ever gave. Lady Mendl had warned me not to talk too long, so I discussed my Eat and Grow Beautiful plan, with special emphasis on how to *stay* slim, since not one of those glamorous women was overweight and that was twenty-two years ago. And as Adele Astaire reminded me, "Since that day, not one of us has put on an extra pound. You taught us, that day. We don't diet. We just eat smartly."

I learned a memorable lesson another time while addressing the Women's Club in Casablanca, Morroco. During the question period a French woman dressed all in black stood up and said: "Monsieur, some years back my husband and I lived in New York. You had then what is called Prohibition, but never in our lives did my husband and I see so much drunkenness. Now, Monsieur, you come along and forbid us to eat or at least you want to regiment our eating. Don't you know that forbidden fruit is sweetest?"

There was a real stickler. In my best French I struggled to tell the lady that I did not forbid them to eat; I could have given her other answers, but to this day I remember her phrase, "regimented eating," and that is what most diets are.

WHY DIETS FAIL

Let us be absolutely realistic. Every month, hard-working beauty editors beat the bushes for a new diet and exercise regime to take off pounds and inches. How many of them have you tried? How many have been successful for you? And how long has it taken you to get back to your old weight and measurements?

Beauty institutes do a guaranteed job of slimming thousands of women every year. They ask a good price for what they do, and they deliver what they promise. Women do emerge slimmer! Some, I believe, do manage to keep the new figure they have paid for. But I also know that most of the clients of these beauty institutes slip back into their former body contours before very long.

Quick reducing schemes are all deceptive. They often show sensational results, but they do not change the basic pattern. And so the quick miracle is a mirage. It cannot last.

LOSE IT THE SAME WAY YOU GAINED IT

No healthy person gains weight overnight. It is the extra, unnoticed bit of gravy or cream in the coffee, balanced against the energy expended, that puts on perhaps five, perhaps ten pounds in a year or two or three. Sometimes one begins eating a little more, sometimes one eats the same as ever but spends more time sitting at work or riding in cars or watching television.

As Adele Astaire said, eating a little less or expending a little more energy will take off weight. A combination of the two is most successful. Adjusting your food intake to the way you actually live will reduce you slowly but surely to your proper weight and what is more important, it will keep you there!

This seems difficult because it is very slow, as slow as gaining weight was in the first place. And reducers are always in a hurry!

I think it is natural to want to see results. But we must also be sensible in our method of achieving them, otherwise it just will not work.

It probably has taken you two or three years to gain those ten or fifteen pounds, but you are not going to work for two or three years—or even one year—to lose them, and I can't blame you.

Yet neither can you expect to lose them, and lose them permanently, in a few days.

Every time you try one of those quick methods and fail, you lose not your weight but your courage and confidence. All that work wasted! All those daily self-denials, those sacrifices of good spirits and good temper! If the overweight is much more than ten pounds, if it is perhaps twenty-five or fifty, the disappointment in quick reducing, in gimmicks and gadgets and drugs, is a real morale-destroyer.

THE SIMPLE ARITHMETIC OF WEIGHT-LOSING

Let us look squarely at the mathematical facts of gaining and losing. The food that you take into your body each day is fuel. Your body uses up as much as it needs for the day's activities. What it does not use, it stores.

The body has three levels of storage. A certain amount it keeps in circulation as glucose—blood sugar—for immediate use. The next level of storage is in the form of body starch, called glycogen, and it is stored in the liver.

The third, the long-term fuel storage form, is fat. This is the most compact form of stored energy. Any food that you eat in excess of your body's needs (yes, even protein!) eventually ends up as stored energy in the form of fat.

These are the mathematical facts. There are no other explanations, no alibis. And don't blame your glands!

Women have a tendency to retain fluid in the body tissues, and this adds both weight and inches. These pounds and inches are the first to come off when you begin a reducing regime, and that is why the results of a quick-reducing program seem so gratifying. But the moment the program ends, and you return to your normal eating and activity, the fluid seeps back into the tissues and there you are, right where you started.

In most of these quick reducing schemes you do not make a dent in your body's fat. All you do is lose water. Test it and see: drink a glass or two of water and weigh yourself. You will find you have gained a pound!

The biggest handicap is that you try to lose weight without ever knowing HOW you have gained it. You feel guilty, dissatisfied with yourself, obsessed with the question of just what to eat. But you have no real guide to how you can achieve your best contours *permanently*, until you know how you gained weight in the first place.

Let us check up a little. Compare your weight today with your best weight since you reached young womanhood, let us say in your twenties. What did you weigh on your wedding day? What size was your wedding dress?

Now consider: What has changed in your way of life since then? Are you eating more? Or are you using your body less?

Perhaps you have changed dwellings during these years. Have you, like so many, moved from a two-story into a ranch-type house with no stairs, or into an apartment?

One woman tells me that she has been able to trace her gradual gain in weight from the time her children started to school. Another, from the time she went back to a job, at which she sits all day. Still another, from the time she moved six blocks nearer to the bus stop.

And many women, searching for the cause with real honesty, tell me that they began to gain weight when the family acquired its first television set, or its second car! Or from the time when their circle of friends expanded and they began "cocktailing" every weekend!

And then there are people who eat more out of loneliness, boredom, anxiety. Diet alone will not overcome this kind of eating. You need to find new interests and goals. Some very overweight people have benefited by psychiatric help or hypnosis under a competent doctor's care.

One worthwhile new goal is making yourself over into the woman you were meant to be. I can promise you, a lovelier you will not be so lonely, or so bored, or even so anxious. You must break the vicious circle somewhere. Why not break it with a program for your new slim body. And remember, the cause of your own particular weight gain; you can lose the same way you gained, safely, easily, and permanently. You can lose one pound per week. In ten weeks you can lose ten pounds. In a year you can lose fifty pounds.

You can do it without tears. You can do it with pleasure.

Short, shortcut to reducing

Here is the shortest shortcut to reducing, and I promise you this one will not fail you.

> EAT ALL THE GOOD FOODS
> CHEW TWICE AS LONG.
> ENJOY TWICE THE PLEASURE
> AND YOU WILL NEED TO EAT
> ONLY HALF AS MUCH.

It sounds too simple to be true. It is the simplest possible rule to follow. And it works, for reasons which are not quite so simple. If you could follow your natural appetite, and if your foods, like those of the Hunza, came to you directly from the fields, it would be very simple: you would eat only what your body needs and you would never weigh one extra ounce. I am really more concerned with *what* you eat, rather than how much. If your foods were truly full of their natural nourishment, you would never overeat.

You can fool your stomach, but not your brain. In the hypothalamus, that part of your brain that controls your appetites, the signals get all mixed up.

ABSENT-MINDED EATING

We do not eat only to appease hunger. We eat for satisfaction and pleasure. But most of the time we miss the pleasure. We eat absent-mindedly, without knowing what we are eating, without enjoying the pleasure of eating and tasting. And so we keep on eating, still trying to satisfy that psychological appetite.

A woman friend told me how exasperated she was one evening, when her husband had brought home as a special treat some English Cheddar cheese of which she is very fond. She had been looking forward to taking a nibble of it as a midnight snack. And so she did. But as she popped the tasty cheese into her mouth her mind was on something else, and suddenly she realized that she had chewed it up quickly and swallowed, and she had not tasted it at all!

I remember in the old days how Dr. Fletcher taught his followers to "Fletcherize" everything they took into their mouths. At the "Nut and Berry Club," as we used to call their eating place, the people sat chewing like cows—they even chewed water!

Often a good and wise idea becomes laughable when it is followed to excess. I believe that basically there was a good idea behind "Fletcherizing."

Our teeth, our jaws, our facial muscles all were made for chewing, and they benefit from chewing. So does the digestion. But what benefits most of all is the mind. When you chew twice as long, you really taste your food twice as long. You enjoy it. That appetite control in the hypothalamus is really satisfied. And so you will not have the urge to eat more than your body can use. You will no longer need to diet, you can throw away all reducing books, including mine, because your psychological appetite, as well as your physical appetite, will be appeased. That, I believe, is the real secret to most reducing problems.

The French wisely take time at their meals, even though they often do not eat as much as we Americans. If ever you have seen a typical French family eat, you know what I mean by pleasure.

Carl Sandburg, earthy and outspoken American poet, came to New York recently for the opening of his play, and was interviewed by my friend Martha Deane on her radio program. Among many interesting things he said was: "People eat too fast, they don't take time to appreciate their food."

RE-EDUCATE YOUR STOMACH

Let me give you a picture of what happens when a small person —a woman of average size—has a stomach that can hold a quart of food. Yes, just one quart. A large person, a six-foot-three man like myself, has a stomach capacity of one and one-half quarts. Those are normal capacities. But a habitual overeater, a real "fresser" as they say in German, or a "gourmand" in French, can stretch his stomach to hold as much as six quarts! And once he has stretched it to that size, it will clamor for that quantity of food—unless he disciplines it and trains it back to normal.

You do not have a six-quart stomach. Far from it. But you can easily stretch your stomach by absent-minded eating, or empty eating, to a size large enough to accommodate food for a six-foot frame. Unless you are a six-footer, and broad in proportion, you do not need all that food; you cannot possibly use it all up. But your thrifty body will not waste it. Your digestive system will process it, your liver will convert it, and your body will store it away as fat.

SEVEN STEPS TO SMART EATING

The celebrated beauties who came to my lecture twenty-two years ago in Paris have not dieted and have not gained weight. They have only eaten smartly. You can do as well as they. Here are seven steps to unregimented pleasurable eating. See how simple they are:

1. *Chew*, slowly, pleasantly. The longer you chew, the less you will eat, as thousands of my students have proven.
2. *Enjoy* and appreciate every bite consciously. No more absent-minded eating.
3. *See* what you eat. We eat with our eyes, too! No TV dinners in the dark.
4. *Taste* what you eat. Satisfy your need for pleasure in eating.
5. *Refuse* to eat anything that does not satisfy your body's needs. No more empty, foodless foods.
6. *Take time* to eat. Satisfy your psychological need for unhurried pleasure in food.
7. *Eat only* for eating's sake. Find other remedies for boredom, tenseness, and emotions. Thousands have done it.

If you satisfy your physical appetite with truly nutritious foods only, and your psychological appetite with the fullest pleasure in eating, you will lose your extra weight and never have a weight problem again. Please remember: chew twice as long, have twice the pleasure and eat half the quantity.

FINDING YOUR IDEAL WEIGHT

Try on your wedding dress; that is the quickest way to see how much weight you have gained since your honeymoon days. If your Adam makes fun of you, then let him try on his wedding suit so you can both laugh.

Most people are at their best weight between the ages of twenty-five and twenty-eight. After thirty, with the general lack of movement and exercise, weight seems to pile on gradually.

Here are the brand new weights for both women and men. They have been painstakingly tabulated by the Society of Actuaries, an organization of experts, after studying five million policy holders. The Metropolitan Life Insurance Company has prepared these charts which I call "Ideal Weights for Ladies and Gentlemen of 25 Years and Over." Compare your weight with these new figures according to your height and the size of your body frame. If you have difficulty ascertaining whether you are small, medium or large-boned, let your doctor help you.

Remember then that your ideal weight should be figured out according to these new findings:

IDEAL WEIGHT FOR EVE				IDEAL WEIGHT FOR ADAM		
	Small Frame	Medium Frame	Large Frame		Small Frame	Medium Frame	Large Frame
4'10"	92-98	96-107	104-119	5'2"	112-120	118-129	126-141
5'0"	96-104	101-113	109-125	5'4"	118-126	124-136	132-148
5'2"	102-110	107-119	115-131	5'6"	124-133	130-143	138-156
5'4"	108-116	113-126	121-138	5'8"	132-141	138-152	147-166
5'6"	114-123	120-135	129-146	5'10"	140-150	146-160	155-174
5'8"	122-131	128-143	137-154	6'0"	148-158	154-170	164-184
5'10"	130-140	136-151	145-163	6'2"	156-167	162-180	173-194
6'0"	138-148	144-159	153-173	6'4"	164-175	172-190	182-204

CHAPTER 10

The Quick and Happy Way to Exercise

Dr. Jean Mayer of Harvard says, "Combatting overweight by diet alone is like fighting with one hand behind your back. Exercise is the other fist that enables us to deal the knockout blow."

Now we come to the question of that second, knockout punch.

I have been teaching for years that you cannot force the body to exercise on a diet of foodless foods. If it is given the high vitality foods that it needs, it will not need to be pushed. It will demand movement and activity. To the well-nourished body, exercise becomes pleasure.

You need not take my word for this. If you have ever embarked on an exercise regime without looking first to the proper nutrition of your body, you know how hard it was to keep going.

Getting yourself to exercise became more and more like pushing a rock uphill. Perhaps your exercise program just dwindled away. Perhaps it was interrupted by some event—welcome excuse!—and you never went back to it.

This is contrary to all the arguments of the people who urge you to exercise. They say that you will not want to stop exercising because it will make you feel so good!

Or—they tell you—you will see the pounds and inches melt away so fast that you will be encouraged to continue.

You already know that is not so. The pounds do not melt away with exercise. Those attractive exercises that you see pictured in your favorite magazine, modeled always by a lovely slender girl, will not take off an ounce. The diet that goes with them is the reducer although, alas, not a permanent one.

The exercises do something else: They change measurements. They re-proportion you. And that is the essential second step in your program for beauty of contours.

But even this cannot be accomplished by exercises in a short time. The body is not clay. It is living tissue. Remodeling it by exercise, like remodeling it by diet, takes time. Exercise, in whatever form, must become a part of your daily life.

And you will not make it a part of your life until it is transformed from a pain to a pleasure!

REDISCOVER YOUR FAVORITE SPORT

If you have a favorite sport, one that you have allowed to slip out of your life in recent years, go back to it. You are fortunate to possess an active skill on which you can draw; it is like money in an old savings account that you had forgotten about. Do not be discouraged if your skill has become a bit rusty and your muscles protest at first. No one ever forgets how to swim, dance, ski, bicycle, ice-skate, play tennis, or swing a golf club. Your body remembers; only give it a chance, and start slowly!

And give it the energy of your high vitality diet to draw on. You will soon feel again the exhilaration you used to enjoy. Even if you are not and perhaps never have been a champion, what of it? The joy of using your body will keep you happy at it.

Swimming is, as you know, the perfect contour-designer, especially for a woman's body. If you are at all skilled in the water, I urge you to seek out a pool in your locality and begin to swim regularly, all year 'round.

But I do mean swim. Just dunking yourself in the water will be fun, but not really enough fun, and it will do nothing for your figure although it will do a little something for your circulation and general feeling of wellbeing. For real enjoyment, swim your one, two, or three steady laps around the pool. Speed is not important. What smooths your contours is the steady distance stroke.

And let me give you a tip. The old-fashioned breast stroke is far more effective for feminine contours than the stylish, fast-moving crawl. For those vital points of beauty, the throat, bosom, and hips, the breast stroke's upraised chin and extended throat, the spreading arm movement and the frog kick are specific for just those areas that may otherwise elude your best efforts at contour-designing.

Swim, ride, dance—enjoy whatever you like, but *enjoy* it.

GIVE YOURSELF SEVEN MINUTES A DAY

Now here is some more cheerful news about exercise: it does not have to be a long, complicated, strenuous routine. All the women—and men, too—who have told me how they successfully made daily exercise a part of their lives have confirmed my own experience. A few well-chosen, basic, *simple* exercises make the best routine. They can be gone through in a few minutes as part of the getting up, bathing, and dressing ritual that begins your day.

I have studied countless exercise routines, American, European and Oriental, for every country has its favorites. The best ones have been developed out of natural body movements and do not demand a contortionist's or an acrobat's abilities. Let me give you here my seven basic exercises. You can do them well and thoroughly in no more than seven minutes of your day, and they will keep you trim and fit all your life. Remember, we not only exercise to keep slim; we exercise because it helps us to feel so much better and it keeps our "instrument" in tune:

1. Stretch: Rise up on your toes, arms up, with your hands try to touch the ceiling. Drop arms. Relax. Do ten times.
2. Bend: Down, down, from the waist, hands reaching for the floor. Stretch, stretch, until you can touch the floor with the palms of your hands. The best vitalizing and backache exercise. Do ten times.
3. Torso stretch and twist: With arms outstretched to the sides, reach to the left, to the right; twist at the waist and reach backward to the left to the right. A wonderful and easy twist for keeping waistlines. Back and forth. Do ten times.

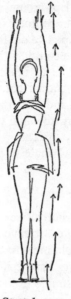

Stretch . . .

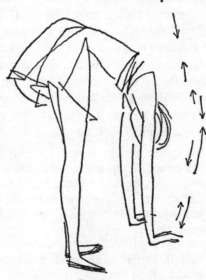

Bend . . .

4. Hip roll: With hands on hips, rotate the middle, holding shoulders still, first to the left, then to the right. Do ten times slowly in each direction.
5. Bicycle: For beautiful legs, lie on the floor on your back, legs up, pedal slowly and rhythmically. The more you breathe the better it feels. Do for two minutes and relax.
6. Tummy lift: This is also good for your Adam. Pull your abdominal muscles in, hard, harder. Hold tight for about thirty seconds or until muscles quiver, then relax. Do just once a day, but regularly.
7. Shoulder shrug: Important for neck, face and scalp. Lift the shoulders to the ears and hold for ten seconds. Relax and repeat ten times.

Now shake yourself all over, take a few deep breaths, and off to your shower or tub. You have done your muscle work for the day. Any other exercise, sport or physical work you do will be so much gravy. Try and make these easy and lazy twists and stretches a daily habit.

Every one of these seven exercises has its particular as well as

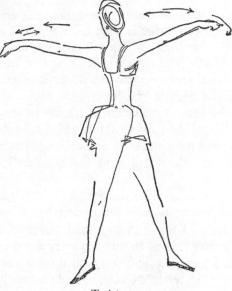

Twist . . .

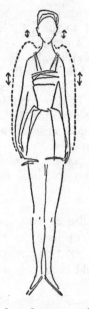

The shoulder shrug loosens neck and scalp

its general value for your beauty. The tummy lift explains itself; you can reduce several inches in just a few weeks, but you must do it regularly. The bicycling and hip roll take care of circulation in legs and the middle. The stretches, bends and twists do wonders in loosening spinal and torso tensions. Those large muscles across your back and ribs contract by reflex, without your conscious effort, and in your sedentary life they are in tension most of the time. The same is true of the shoulder shrug, which loosens tensions in the neck, face and scalp and creates revitalizing circulation to the brain; it also strengthens and firms the muscles that hold the bosom high.

Lively music helps to make exercise fun. I have made a record for myself and I must say it is much more fun to exercise with good snappy music. I urge you to try this easiest of routines for just two weeks; less than seven minutes a day is not much out of your busy life. I promise you, if you do it for two weeks, you will never give it up. The results are amazing and you will have learned to transform pain into sheer pleasure.

FIGURES BY TERRY HUNT

More beautiful women enter the door at 50 North La Cienega Boulevard in Hollywood than any other door in the world. For more than twenty-five years Terry Hunt has conditioned the loveliest stars who came to Hollywood. His scientific methods of strengthening weak parts of the female body have accomplished wonders. Terry Hunt is proud of his work and will not accept a client unless she agrees to cooperate and carry out instructions fully.

Terry Hunt's methods are based upon the solid foundation of health, not via a lot of electric gadgets, but with exercise and sound nutrition. I wish there were Terry Hunt studios in all our big cities to help my students, and not just in Hollywood alone.

One of the greatest beauty assets for a Hollywood star is a high and beautiful bustline, and Terry Hunt has developed what I consider the most effective as well as simplest method for achieving and keeping a beautiful bosom. Here are the simple movements. With these, no matter where you live, you can achieve what every woman desires and every man admires—a high bustline:

1. To strengthen and fill out the pectoral muscles which support the delicate tissues of the breast, you must strengthen the arm and shoulder muscles. You can start these simple movements by extending your arms and closing your fists tightly. But much speedier results, which have amazed everybody, are obtained when you hold a small weight—a book or a bottle—in each hand or, as they do in the Terry Hunt Studio, a one pound dumbbell. Now raise your arms up to shoulder height, then push them forward and backward ten times. This is easy if you breathe in as you push your arms back and breathe out as you push the arms forward.

2. Next do the same thing with your arms at shoulder level: push your arms sideways, back and forth ten times. Breathe in as you extend arms, breathe out as you push arms away from the body.

3. This is most important and effective: push your arms straight out in front of you—straight and stiff and hold for two seconds, then with the arms still straight and stiff, push them right up toward the ceiling. Remember to breathe in as you pull toward the body and push out as you push away from the body. So few women

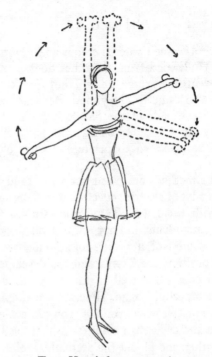

Terry Hunt's beauty exercise

know that breathing correctly makes exercises half as difficult and twice as efficient.

I know of no simpler, easier and less expensive way to achieve the beautiful bustline than these three exercises. Many of the high-bosomed movie stars you watch on the screen have made this simple routine part of their beauty plan. If you will do it conscientiously, Terry Hunt promises it will work every time!!

GIVE DUMBBELLS A LIFT AND THEY'LL DO THE SAME FOR YOU!

That is what the lovely Lydia Lane of Los Angeles printed in her famous beauty column. She tells the story of a matron who cut an unusually neat figure in a sweater. When asked about the transformation, this is what she said: "I received a gift box of dumbbells with instructions; so I started to exercise a few minutes every morning and after awhile I found my brassieres were getting too tight."

Lydia Lane also told of a young mother who worked with dumb-bells and got her figure back in no time.

If you are really serious about achieving and keeping a youthful bustline, I suggest you invest in a pair of one- or two-pound dumb-bells.

DERRIERES AWAY

Firming and tensing the buttocks muscles, as they teach at the Max Planck Institute in Germany, is excellent and easy to follow, but if your "sitz" has gotten completely out of hand, so that it looks as if you are wearing a bustle, and you want to get speedy results, here is where rocking and rolling can do wonders for you.

Sit on the floor; grasp your legs firmly and rock and roll, back and forth. Do this five minutes to begin with and increase to ten minutes. You will be amazed how quickly the bustle disappears.

ACTIVE REST

Your body needs exercise and it also needs rest. Fifteen minutes flat on your back is a marvelous refresher between daytime and evening. But there is a much more effective one, and that is to lie, not flat, but with your feet tilted higher than your head. I have already told you about the Beauty Slant board.

WALKING FOR BEAUTY

Now let me introduce you to a distinguished and rapidly grow-ing society: the walkers. They are anonymous, unorganized, with-out a constitution or bylaws. Some have a favorite daily walk; some will walk anywhere, any time. Your true walker will auto-matically find walking opportunities wherever he or she may be.

Most people will do almost anything to avoid walking, but there are exceptions—and they are exceptional people. Greta Garbo for years walked on the beaches and in the hills of Hollywood; it was the thing which kept her going during her strenuous Hollywood days. Lynn Fontanne, one of the most enduringly beautiful women, walks over the rolling hills on her Wisconsin farm. Marlene Dietrich, famous for her young legs, is a walker; even in New York she takes long walks in the park, sometimes with her grandchildren. Ingrid Bergman is another woman who walks whether she is in Hollywood, Rome, or Paris, often with her children. I could go on endlessly with this list; most glamorous women I know are walkers; they have made walking a pleasant habit and part of their busy lives for which they always find the time. And notice how each of them has developed an unforgettable and graceful walk. Each one's walk has become her own world-famous trade mark.

BE SOCIABLE, TAKE A WALK!

Most walkers are sociable people who would like company if they could find it. A few years ago I discovered that a walking companion is not easy to find. Most of my friends would gladly come to my dinners, adorn my parties, drink any number of cocktails, soft or hard, and stay up until any hour, but few would go walking with me. I began to think that walking, like dieting, is a solo performance.

Then, one season in Paris, I made a contrary discovery. It was a particularly busy season. The popular magazine, *Paris-Match* had given my work so much publicity that it seemed as though everyone wanted an appointment with me. I was beginning to feel like a prisoner behind my desk at No. 4, Rue Faubourg Saint Honoré, when an idea struck me. The Bois de Boulogne was not far; I began asking my friends to come and walk in the park with me.

They were surprised, to put it mildly, but they were too polite to refuse. And I discovered some expert walkers among my friends, and converted some to the society. Maurice Chevalier needed no introduction to walking; we took long walks down the Champs Elysée to the park. King Peter and Queen Alexandra were also confirmed walkers; we walked for miles in the woods of Versailles. Lovely Martine Carol, who had helped me sign autographs for the enthusiastic fans, confessed that she loved walking in the Bois. When she got home she felt wonderfully relaxed and her skin, as she put it, was "blooming."

We need more walks

Perhaps you think I'm going overboard about walking, but I'm not. Walking preserves health and lengthens life. A New York physician said bluntly that half the patients in his waiting room could cure themselves of what ailed them if they would spend an hour walking every day. Did you hear that? Walking cures tensions, insomnia, chronic fatigue, and a host of minor physical and mental complaints that drag down the spirit and body and take the joy out of living. Walking—free striding, free-swinging, rhythmic, unhurried and unharried walking—is the perfect aid to digestion, elimination, circulation, relaxation of mind, body and spirit. Yes, spirit!

The next time you feel low, go out for a walk. Put on your most comfortable shoes (I hope you own a pair of comfortable ones) and your freest skirt. Walk with your head up, take long steps, let your arms swing freely and easily, and deepen your breathing. Keep a good rhythm, not necessarily fast but steady. See how your mood changes, how the dark color of your thoughts becomes gradually brighter. Your low spirits will not accompany you very far on a good walk. Psychologists remind us again and again that the mind cannot remain depressed when the body is in motion.

Believe me, walking does do all this for you, and furthermore it is a very special pleasure. Why do you suppose so many intelligent, gifted people, who could choose any recreation they like, enjoy walking?

There are signs of a renaissance of walking in this country. The doctors are prescribing it. More and more men and women, who want to live well and long, are taking to walking. Several cities have given the streets back to the walkers, by closing off their shopping centers to cars and putting in gardens with paths. If there are enough of you demanding places to walk, they will do the same in all our cities.

In some suburbs there are bridle paths and bicycle paths. Perhaps we shall soon see footpaths as well.

CHAPTER 11

Beauty's Sheath: Your Skin

If you could have one magic gift of beauty, only one, which would you choose?

I am sure I have asked at least 100,000 women this question. And 99,000 of them have answered that the one gift they most long for is a beautiful skin.

A beautiful skin can set a woman apart. It can compensate for many imperfections. It is so pleasing to the beholder that our language is full of poetic compliments for it: it is silken or velvety, smooth as ivory, white as alabaster, soft as rose petals, delicious as peaches and cream.

I can sympathize with the feeling a woman has about her skin. In a very real sense, this sheath that covers her body is the living garment of her person. It is her modesty, her virtue, her sex. It is the outer representation of her inner self.

Women are intuitively aware of this, and it is true. It is not only a psychological and an esthetic truth. It is a biological fact.

The skin reflects the inner state of mind and body like a mirror. The popular surgeon-novelist, Dr. Frank G. Slaughter, once said that it was impossible to put "beautiful skins on unhappy people." It is equally impossible to think that you can grow a lovely skin on an ill-nourished, ill-functioning body.

You can have a beautiful skin

But the most marvelous thing about a beautiful skin is that you can have it. If you do not like the skin you have today, change it— the skin you see tomorrow will already begin to be a new one, and you can begin today to make it a more beautiful one. You can have the clear, glowing skin of your desire, and you can have it for all your long life.

There are many sensible, rational women who throw common sense to the winds when it comes to the skin. They are willing to try almost any cosmetic, in the belief that the skin can be nourished to beauty from the outside.

No, I am not trying to part you from your favorite cosmetics. I do not want you to sweep those jars and bottles from your dressing table. Cosmetic preparations, well formulated with first class ingredients and fragrances, have a definite value in the care of your skin.

But at this point let us be very clear about what they can and cannot do. Your creams, lotions, and oils cleanse, soften, and protect your skin. This is very important.

Even more important is the fact that they can nourish your psyche. They make you *feel* beautiful, and that is a big step toward *being* beautiful. But cosmetics can in no way feed your skin. That wonderful living sheath needs proteins, vitamins, and minerals in ample quantities, such as you will find in the Cosmetic Diet.

Your skin is a living organ

Your skin is not just an inert covering like the glove you put on your hand. It is a living organ, as truly as your lungs or kidneys.

As an organ the skin has two main functions. It is first of all the body's protective covering, its shield against the outer environment. And secondly, it is the body's principal mechanism for maintaining that steady temperature of 98.6 degrees Fahrenheit in which all our cells and body systems are adapted to function. If the skin fails in this task, the body becomes gravely ill. In health and in illness, the skin is one of the hardest working of the body's organs.

Think of it, the skin covering your body weighs about seven

pounds. It has an area of about nineteen square feet. It is made up of living, busily working cells, and every inch of it is supplied with delicate, responsive nerves that keep your body and mind informed about your environment, whether it is hot or cold, wet or dry, soft or hard, agreeable or disagreeable.

This outer covering of your body looks fragile, but actually it is tough and amazingly resistant. It can withstand much punishment from nature. It heals and renews itself, day in and day out. It makes spectacular recoveries from disease and accident.

Your skin is your body's protection against dirt and foreign invaders of every kind. It is a barrier to the billions of germs and viruses in the air and on every surface that we touch. It lets none of these pass into the body; at worst, they may penetrate into the outer layers or pores of the skin itself and set up local infection there, but the skin must be wounded or damaged before it will let anything get into even its own deeper layers. But remember that this same barrier keeps out creams and lotions with which you may be attempting to feed the skin itself.

HOW YOUR SKIN IS NOURISHED

Always remember that the skin needs nourishment and that nourishment comes only from within. I have been teaching this principle of Eat and Grow Beautiful in many languages for many years, and each year science adds some new confirmation of its truth. There is no part of the body that can thrive without good nutrition, and there is no part of the body that derives more glowing beauty from good nutrition than the skin.

Let me tell you how remarkably your skin is made, so that you will carry a picture of it in your mind. It is thin on some parts of the body and thicker on others, as on the palms and soles, but even where it is only one thirty-second of an inch in depth, it is made up of four separate layers.

The outer layer of cells, the epidermis, is the one you see. This layer is constantly flaking and rubbing off. But that need not worry you, for it is forever being renewed from underneath. Under it is always a fresh layer, growing from the buds of living cells below. Interlaced through these growing layers, are the capillaries of the skin's own circulatory system. These tiny blood vessels are of a special design, unlike capillaries elsewhere in the body. They are shaped like hairpin loops, each one curving up and down again, carrying the nutritious beautystream to the cells in every layer of your skin.

And so the skin that you see in your mirror is being newly made every day, *every hour*, by the growing layer of skin cells below. Those cells, which you do not see, can make a finer, healthier, more beautiful skin for you, only if you give them the materials to work with. Those materials can come only through the blood, flowing up and down the tiny capillary loops, in and out among the cell layers of your skin. Your blood, laden with its life-giving freight, is your skin's true beautystream. Your skin can become beautiful, and remain beautiful, in proportion to the quality and quantity of nutritive elements that the blood brings to it.

New skin for old

What are these life-giving, beauty-giving elements?

First, our old friends, the proteins, building blocks out of which new cells are made. And these must be the whole, complete proteins, containing all the essential amino acids for the healthy new protoplasm.

Then, the full list of essential minerals, especially iron which gives your blood its power to carry a full load of oxygen. Your skin cells need a constant supply of oxygen so that the well-oxygenated, rosy red blood, flowing through those capillaries close to the surface can give your skin its live, glowing radiance.

Finally come the vitamins: vitamin A to preserve smooth texture and avoid drying and roughness; all the members of the B family of vitamins, to keep the skin youthful and firm, to prevent excessive oiliness, to keep the color clear and free from ugly pigmentation; and vitamin C for elasticity and also for resistance to infection.

None of these can be fed to the skin from the outside, out of jars. These are nature's own foundation, supplied from within to the growing layers for a healthy and beautiful complexion. See how simple and familiar they are, these ingredients of nature's cosmetic formula!

There is nothing exotic, nothing that you need to seek in

Cleopatra's ancient beauty secrets, nor even in a beehive! This is the real magic, the magic of your own body chemistry which can take these commonplace, *natural* ingredients and transform them into healthy, beautiful new skin to replace the old.

SCANDINAVIAN COMPLEXION SECRET

On my lecture tours, where do you suppose I have found the most radiant and glowing complexions? In Holland, Denmark, Sweden and Norway, those lands where women cherish their fresh supplies of milk and cheese, of greens from their gardens and fish from the seas that lap those shores on nearly every side. In Hollywood it is no secret that the Scandinavian actresses have the most radiant skin and require the least makeup before the cameras. The high protein, vitamin, and mineral content of their diet, from childhood on, is one of the secrets of the fresh wholesome beauty of the Scandinavian complexion.

And we must remember, too, that the fish and seafood, which the Scandinavians eat so plentifully, are rich in iodine, essential to the thyroid gland, for when the thyroid is functioning inadequately, the skin can become coarse, thickened, and dry.

Skin specialists have been paying increasing attention to the role of vitamin A in skin health. Dr. Erno Laszlo, the famous New York skin specialist, who treats a glittering list of beautiful and celebrated women, insists on a high intake of vitamin A, especially for dry skin. I have reports from women the world over who found vitamin A a benefaction for dry, rough, lifeless-looking skin. Since there is a possibility of overdosage with this vitamin when it is taken in other forms than food, your physician should prescribe and supervise any special vitamin A therapy of more than 50,000 International Units a day.

Skin blemished with blackheads and white heads, and with that affliction of many adolescents, *acne vulgaris*, is often the result of vitamin A deficiency. In severe cases, doctors administer high doses of vitamin A, not in oil, but in water-soluble capsules. They also insist on cutting down on animal fats, chocolates, pastries and sweets of all kinds. Remember that your skin may only be advertising to the world that you are far too fond of sweets and pastries!

B VITAMINS AND THE SKIN

It may surprise you that the B vitamins are specific skin vitamins. All the B group play a part in keeping the skin youthful. Vitamin B-2, riboflavin, when liberally added to the diet has been known to help clear those disfiguring brown blemishes, the so-called "liver spots."

Long ago I began to teach the value of food yeast as one of the most potent natural sources of the B complex vitamins. Countless women have discovered that just one or two tablespoons of this wholesome food, added every day to fruit or vegetable juices, brought a new, alive beauty to the skin.

You need never worry about taking too much of the B vitamins; there is no such thing as an overdose, whether taken in natural foods or as a food supplement in capsules. A deficiency is not easy to discover, and it is better to be sure. Among the symptoms of B deficiency are dryness, redness, or pigmented irritations of the skin.

One of this country's most celebrated internists, Dr. Harold Thomas Hyman, who was for many years professor of pharmacology at Columbia University, writes in his book for physicians, *Treatment in Internal Medicine*, on dealing with severe deficiencies:

"It is wise to provide the patient with blanket coverage of the entire B spectrum, particularly since there are no known risks attendant on overdoses of whole vitamin B complex or of its constituent parts."

SKIN BEAUTY FROM THE OUTSIDE

I have referred many times to the brilliant results of correcting skin conditions with unsaturated fatty acids and the remarkable effect they have on fine lines and wrinkles. These fatty acids, which are found in all vegetable oils, were used both internally and externally, with excellent results.

Is there a contradiction here? I have been telling you throughout these pages that the way to skin beauty is from the *inside*. Now I recommend that certain substances are good to put on your skin from the outside.

I want you to think of your skin in a way that might never occur to you: from the inside, as part of the wonderful interweaving of all the parts of the body. I want you to think of your skin as dependent upon the same healthful nutrition as every other part of your body, with some special nutrients that are specifically valuable for your skin. First, you must feed it from the inside.

Second comes protection from the outside. Your skin is your body's shelter. Like the outer walls of your home, your skin is directly exposed to the physical environment. It lives in heat and cold, in wet and dry climates. It copes with sharp changes of temperature, with too little sunshine or too much, with wind, soot, industrial fumes, fog and smog, dust and smoke. Your skin lives an outer as well as an inner life.

Wind and water can wear away stone, and the sun can peel and crack a painted wall or a leather chair. The skin is living tissue, and it can defend itself against the elements far better than these inert substances. But the environment takes its toll all the same. Too much sun makes the skin lined and leathery, too much cold and wind cracks and roughens it, and too much water makes it first puffy and then wrinkled.

DRYNESS, THE SKIN'S ENEMY NUMBER ONE

Even when we protect our skin from the harshest environment, as most of us are ordinarily able to do, there is one continuous threat to its outer surface of cells. That is dryness. More women complain of dry skin than of any other skin condition.

The skin has its own protective mechanism against drying. All over its surface are millions of tiny glands, the sebaceous or oil glands. There are more oil glands in the face and scalp, fewer on the throat and fewest on the hands. These tiny glands spread a thin invisible coating of natural oil that helps to protect the skin against losing its moisture too rapidly.

To living tissue, moisture is even more vital than food. A man can go without food for many days and survive; he will perish of thirst long before he starves. What is true of the body as a whole is also true of each cell. It must have water in order to carry on its life processes.

Your skin is exposed to sun and wind outdoors, and even more to the dry warm air of our winter heating systems. It is constantly losing moisture, in spite of its self-oiling system of sebaceous glands.

THE PROTECTION OF NATURAL OILS

People of the ancient world, 3000 years ago, used to oil their bodies. So did our own American Indians; they rubbed their bodies from top to toe with bear grease. The first Europeans who came to these shores were apparently not too repelled by the odor of this primitive cosmetic to observe its advantages. They wrote home that this was a good way to protect the skin against insects and dirt and also to keep it from becoming chapped in cold weather. Some historians give credit to the Indians for the revival of cold cream, which had been forgotten since Roman times. The Romans made their cold cream out of the natural organic oils, which were the only oils they knew. Only in the last century were these, unfortunately, replaced by mineral oils, which are drying to the skin.

We can learn wisdom from the ancients, and from the peoples who lived close to nature, like our own Indians. Today we are very insistent on keeping the skin clean; Americans definitely believe that cleanliness is next to godliness. Yet, each time you scrub, you wash off not only dirt and germs, but also the natural oils that protect your skin. Soap, even the gentlest, dissolves these oils away. Detergents do it even more thoroughly.

There are some dermatologists who believe we use too much soap on our bodies. They urge that we should rub and scrub the skin more to keep up its circulation and clear the pores of waste. They do not recommend daily soapings which wash away all the natural protective oils.

The wise old Greeks did not use soap. They did not have it. The Romans learned the art of soap-making from barbarian tribes they conquered in central Europe. The Greeks, who always gave their bodies loving care, cleansed the skin by oiling it with their own sweet oils, then scraped off the oil together with the scruff of dead cells. They had a special toilet tool for the purpose, a scraper, which the Romans also used in their famous baths. After all the excess oil was scraped away, a thin film remained on the body or was absorbed into the outermost layer of the skin, and this helped to conserve the skin's own moisture and keep the surface supple and smooth.

And this is the true value of our fine creams, oils and lotions today. They cannot nourish the skin, because the skin cannot absorb nourishment from the outside. But like the fine oils that Cleopatra and beautiful Helen of Troy rubbed on their bodies and then wiped or scraped away, the creams and lotions first cleanse and smooth the skin and then protect it from drying.

SKIN BEAUTY IN THE SUN

You might take another hint from the beauties of antiquity and from those of not so long ago. They protected their skins from the sun. Cleopatra even whitened hers with chalk.

Today our standard of beauty does not exclude a healthy, golden tan—far from it! We also know that in the sun the skin manufactures vitamin D for the whole body, and that water, air, and sunshine and the healthy exercise of the body out of doors are nature's best and finest beautifying agents.

But unless you want your skin to become tough and leathery and aged, do not overdo the sunbathing. Southern women, even today, protect their skins from too much sun. The erring sisters are usually Northerners, escapees from bleak winter, who try to soak up enough sunshine in a few weeks of a southern vacation to last for months of sunless weather at home. Some California women, too, carry their sun worship to an extreme.

English women are famous for their lovely complexions. So are many chic San Franciscans. In London and in San Francisco the moist air is an ally of women in keeping the skin beautiful. By contrast, an Arab scholar a thousand years ago observed that women who lived in the desert had withered, wrinkled faces before they were thirty.

So be wise. Take your sun, but take it in safe doses, gradually, and know when your skin has had enough. Too dark a tan is unattractive, but a sunburn is unforgivable. Sunburn, like any other kind of burn, destroys skin cells. It is an actual wound to the body.

SOPHISTICATED SUNBATHING

No woman in her right mind would court a sunburn, but there are some situations in which you may not realize the intensity of the sun's rays. Be especially cautious in the mountains, at the seashore, and wherever there is a reflecting surface such as snow, beach, water, or light-colored surroundings, for then you are getting a double exposure, twice the sunlight in half the time. When you sunbathe, move about, change your position frequently, and never, never go to sleep.

One of the sun's benefits to your skin is that it draws the blood to the surface cells, a skin exercise that takes place without your having to do a thing, like massage. But for the same reason, be careful not to sunbathe for an hour or more after eating, any more than you would engage in strenuous exercise, because the sun, like exercise, draws the blood away from your digestive organs.

When you sunbathe it is always wise to give your skin the protection of a light natural oil cover. Swiss mountaineers use a combination of oil and quinine to prevent burning in the brilliant sun of their snowcapped heights.

Today the chemists have developed many kinds of protective oils and creams that filter some of the sun's rays. They are helpful to the fair-skinned, and for those features such as the nose and forehead which may get more than their share of the sun.

In Sicily if you want to sunbathe, your Sicilian friends will hand you a cup filled half with olive oil and half with vinegar. It is an old recipe, and as good as any suntan lotion you can buy. The oil intensifies the sun's rays and helps you to tan more quickly, while the vinegar protects your skin against burning. Lotions are helpful, but our best protection against overdoing is to use your watch and time your exposure. Then you can be certain of getting just the right amount that will bring a golden glow of vitality to your skin, along with the golden tan that is the most becoming cosmetic for your good looks.

OUTSIDE SKIN CARE, FOR BUSY WOMEN

A well-nourished skin is warm and glowing. It has its own built-in defenses, as well as its own outside acid mantle to protect itself against the elements and external irritations. Here are just three steps you can take to keep your skin glowing and alive at all times:

1. Cleanse it painstakingly each night so that it can breathe while you sleep.

2. After every washing, protect your skin's acid mantle by applying a mildly acid lotion, such as Cosmetic Vinegar.

3. Oil or cream your skin with fresh clean vegetable oils or your favorite creams. These help to keep your skin soft and smooth.

CHAPTER 12

Beauty's Facade: Your Face

A new face is a new future. It opens doors to you, and it opens people's hearts to you too. When you think of your beauty potential, you look for your most important potential in your face.

It is said of the great Leonardo da Vinci that when he painted his portraits they became so real and alive that he would actually speak to them. That, I believe, is because Leonardo was also a student of anatomy; he was one of the first great painters to understand that the most important quality of a truly beautiful face is harmony, the harmony of bones and muscles underlying the skin.

To this day, in Hollywood, in Paris, in Cine Citta in Rome, or wherever moving pictures are made, makeup artists try to transform their movie stars into oval beauties, with da Vinci's classic proportions.

They divide a star's face into three equal parts: first the forehead from hairline to eyebrows; second, from eyebrows to the base of the nose; third, from the base of the nose to the tip of the chin. These proportions, within a perfect oval, are the measurements of a classically beautiful face.

You can measure your own face right now, but before you do, let me caution you not to be discouraged if you find that you do not have the oval face with its classic proportions. Very, very few women do, even among the movie stars. And here is where the *trompe l'oeil*, the art of illusion comes in. The makeup artists apply color, lights and shadows and shape the hairdo to transform the face into a perfect oval with its three equal divisions. And the camera men with their lighting and camera angles complete the transformation.

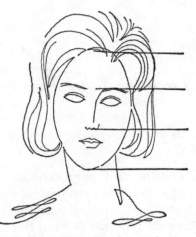

The classic beauty of a Leonardo face

Leonardo did the same. His models may or may not have been perfect beauties—it made no great difference, for the master painter transformed them as he painted, with color, lights, and shadows.

Could you do the same with your face? You can do a great deal with makeup to improve the shape and proportions of your face, and later in this chapter I will give you these secrets.

But remember that the great secret of Leonardo's beauties was within. It was anatomy, that inner structure of bones and muscles that gave them the classic proportions. And remember too, that he painted them as though they were living, *speaking* faces. He gave them the expression of beauty.

And so we have three points: bones, muscles, expression. Let us see now, what you can do with these three.

ARCHITECTURE OF A LOVELY FACE

First are the bones, the architecture of a lovely face. You have heard of women whose faces seem to grow more beautiful with age. Usually this is a matter of the bones which give the face its architecture, and usually the bones that make the difference are the cheekbones. High cheekbones automatically accent the facial structure; they deepen the setting of the eyes and accentuate the curve of the cheek. My friends Lynn Fontanne and Ann Astaire (mother of Adele and Fred) are examples of this indestructible beauty of the bony structure. Some of the new Italian beauties also have this fortunate bone structure.

But this perfect architecture of the face is so rare that if you do not have it, you are no worse off than most of the great women whose names are remembered since the beginning of history!

So it seems that perfect bone structure is not essential. It is the muscles which cover the bone structure which are most important. With the muscles of your face you can accomplish wonders of transformation. They can be trained and strengthened like all muscles.

Let me show you how.

YOUR FIFTY-FIVE MAGIC MUSCLES

Take another look in the mirror. Imagine that you have X-ray spectacles and can see into this marvelous structure. In that small space in front of your ears, between the top of your forehead and the tip of your chin, there are no fewer than fifty-five muscles!

There is nothing like this group of muscles anywhere in the body, and it exists only in human faces. It is called the "mimetic musculature," the muscles of expression. They are slender groups of muscle fibers, interwoven with each other so that they work in teams. A few of them move the jaws and lips for eating and talking, and a few open and close the eyes.

But most of the fifty-five muscles of your face have no other function than to express *you!*

Most of these muscles do not connect two bones across a joint, as muscles of the body generally do. These muscles are divided into small slips, separate bundles of muscle fibers, and they are attached to the inner layers of the skin. Where they are attached, there you have a dimple, or a potential line or fold.

These muscles are your diary. They write the story of you and your life on your face. If you dictated your day's thoughts and feelings to a tape recorder each night, you could not have a more faithful record of yourself.

Not every face can be read. Some faces reveal and some conceal the person behind them. Some people have poker faces! But even a poker face shows something of the character of its owner; it shows reticence, reserve, perhaps a suggestion of interesting depth. When I see an elderly person with a skin smooth and unmarked like a china doll, I think, what a superficial character that must be!

Your fifty-five muscles are capable of an infinite variety of expressions. But probably, like most people, you habitually use only a few, in characteristic groupings.

And that is the first thought for you to remember, when you look at your face in the mirror. The particular grouping of facial muscles that you use, in your habitual thinking and feeling, is the characteristic expression that makes or mars your face.

A ONE-MINUTE FACE LIFT

No matter how beautiful a face may be physically, it is the expression that people remember. How many times have you heard someone say, "Yes, she's pretty, but she has such a discontented look!" Or they say she looks "hard," "spoiled," "selfish." And you have also heard them say admiringly of another face, "No, she's not really beautiful, but she has such an expressive face!" And usually they mean that the expressions are so beautifying as to give the face itself an aura of beauty.

Count on it, your emotional climate is registered in your face. If your habit of mind is happy, hopeful, outgoing, then the lines curve upward. If your inner world is habitually sunny then your face will reflect its brightness. But if your spirit lives most of the time in a world of anxiety and tension, that is what people will read in your face.

Luckily, when the inner climate improves, it is unbelievable how quickly these wonderful muscles respond. A distinguished British psychiatrist once kept a record of the facial expressions of his

patients suffering from depression. He found that when the patient
was on the way to recovery, even the most fixed expression
changed—those seemingly permanent lines magically disappeared!

Many women who think they need a face lift really need only
a change of emotional climate. Lift the spirit and you lift the face!
Yes, you can give yourself a mental facial lift. Right now, look into
your mirror and smile—see the corners of your mouth go up!

NUTRITIONAL FACE LIFT

I have said that your first thought, when you see your face with
your X-ray spectacles, should be that your habits of thinking and
feeling make or mar your face through those fifty-five magic
muscles.

Now here is your second thought: those muscles are very fine
and slender, but they are also very strong. Or rather, they are
capable of great strength, *if you make them so.*

In this way they are no different from muscles anywhere else
in your body. If they are well fed they will be firm and shapely.
They will hold the youthful contours of your face just as your body
muscles hold the youthful body contours. But if you let them become slack and flabby with poor nutrition and poor circulation they
will literally let your face down.

Plastic surgeons have told me that they will not work on a patient until she builds herself up. They can repair and reconstruct a
face to perfection, but without firm, well-nourished tissues all their
skills are wasted. In a little while weak face muscles will fall again.

And even more damaging to the facial contours is the vicious
cycle many women get into, of overweight and drastic reducing.
With overweight the muscles and tissues become soft and loaded
with shapeless fat, which stretches the skin and entirely destroys the
design of the face. Then with a quick-reducing diet, all at once the
fat is removed, and the whole face falls! Women are shocked at the
haggard look their severe reducing gives them, but they should not
be surprised. When the muscles lose their healthy firm tone, when
they are starved of good proteins, vitamins, and minerals, then
there is nothing but fat and bloat which destroys the most finely
chiseled contours.

A London plastic surgeon told me that the biggest job these

specialists have today is to redo the faces of people who have reduced too fast. Especially in the second half of life, when the muscle and skin tissues are not so quick to regain their elasticity, slow reducing, with lots of protein foods, is essential.

It is even better not to have to reduce at all, but to keep one's natural contours for life. If the candy-chewing, pastry-eating, soda-pop-drinking ladies only knew what they are doing to their facial muscles, and through those muscles to their facial contours, they would lose no time in changing to the high-protein, high-vitamin, high-mineral Cosmetic Diet!

THE SAUNA BATH FOR A GLOWING COMPLEXION

Once you have begun to supply beauty for your face from within by way of the Cosmetic Diet, your next step is to bring that beauty-giving, muscle-strengthening nutrition to the face. And by this I mean that you must bring the circulation, your beautystream, to those hungry facial muscles and skin cells.

When the eminent New York skin specialist, Dr. Erno Laszlo, treats his famous clients, his first step is to cleanse the face as a plastic surgeon would, antiseptically clean. No Fifth Avenue beauty salon can compete with the thoroughness of the scientific treatments given at the Laszlo Institute in New York. The list of clients reads like an international Who's Who; among them are several queens, both real and motion picture royalty. When these fortunate ladies emerge after a Laszlo treatment, their complexions glow with the inner radiance of the beautystream shining through the vitalized skin. Dr. Laszlo and his assistants stress individual beauty and each client receives a full hour of relaxing treatment according to her specific needs. Each client is considered a masterpiece and is treated as such. Dr. Laszlo puts his emphasis on a healthy, glowing and clear complexion, rather than on the accoutrements of makeup. Unfortunately, only the lucky few can afford such luxurious treatments to keep them attractive for a life time.

For ever so many years I have looked for a simple treatment which my students everywhere could adopt at home. I believe I found it two years ago. I first learned about it in Finland, the home of the *sauna* bath. Then reports came of how the Japanese cleanse and purify the skin until it shines. Gradually the sauna bath idea gained in popularity in Europe and finally it has come to Hollywood. Some of our movie stars installed their own private sauna baths in their homes.

Most sauna equipment comes from Europe. It is expensive and requires space. But I discovered a small device in Switzerland for a facial sauna bath. I have never seen a simpler and more effective home treatment for cleansing and stimulating the face to a glow. The advantage of this device is that you can give yourself a "glow treatment" when you are fully dressed and without disturbing the hair (see illustration).

But even without this device, you can begin at once to give your face a fragrant sauna bath. All the equipment you need is a two-quart cooking pot; fill it with ordinary water and when it boils, add a heaping tablespoonful of your favorite fresh herbs (if no fresh herbs are available, add a tablespoonful of Swiss Kriss herbs, available at your drugstore).

Now you are ready for a treatment. Take the steaming utensil

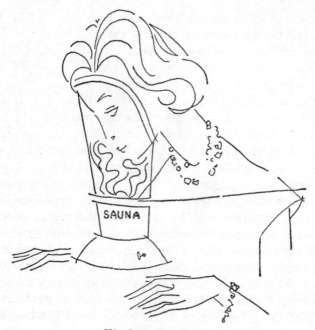

The Swiss facial sauna

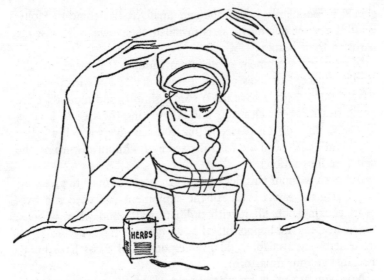

The do-it-yourself sauna

to a table and with a big bath towel, cover both your head and the pot so that the steam does not escape at the sides, but rises straight up into your face. The pleasant herbalized steam penetrates deeply and cleanses every pore as you never thought possible before. The pearls of perspiration coming from the open pores loosen up the accumulated makeup, rancid oils and every bit of dirt. It does all this in just a few minutes. Then close the pores with cold, even ice, water, but do not put ice itself on the face. The herbalized steam is made up of the softest distilled water, as soft as rain, and makes the skin unbelievably soft. The roses that bloom into your cheeks are your own, brought about by your own rushing beautystream. Best of all, the stimulating home sauna facial brings the sparkling beautystream with its nutrition to those facial muscles.

I cannot recommend this simple sauna facial bath enough. I suggest that you take three or more in succession or until your skin is really glowing and clean. Treat your face to your first sauna facial bath right now. Gradually increase your steaming from three minutes on the first day to five minutes on the third day. After that, all you need is one weekly sauna facial bath to keep your skin clear, smooth and in the pink. I urge you to make this a weekly habit. The simple ritual takes only a few minutes of your busy life.

I also suggest that you let your face breathe freely without any sort of makeup occasionally; it will do wonders. Whenever I see a really fine flawless complexion, it usually belongs to a lady who spends more time on *waking up* her face than on *making up*. A healthy, glowing complexion actually needs very little makeup. Remember, we can not stop the march of time, but you don't have to show the mark of time on your face.

HORMONES FOR THE SKIN

Many women have asked me about hormone creams. I have pointed out that we cannot feed the skin proteins, vitamins, or minerals from the outside. But apparently the hormones, which are produced by the body glands, do have a beneficial effect when applied from the outside.

The noted endocrinologist Dr. M. A. Goldzieher reported on this to a meeting of the Society of Cosmetic Chemists. He was able to show by means of slides that estrogenic, that is, female hormones, are effective in revitalizing the skin cells from the outside. Studies made at Yale University also revealed that these hormones have an effect in keeping the skin of older women youthful as long as they continue to be applied. Dr. Goldzieher believes that the application can help to prevent aging if it is begun before skin changes actually occur. The hormones are reported to cause no ill effects if they are used in a concentration of no higher than 10,000 unit per ounce of base. The effective concentration is between 7,500 and 10,000 units per ounce.

If you think a "hormonized" cream or oil may be of benefit for your type of skin, do not hesitate to ask your doctor. One New York dermatologist gives his patients a prescription for a small vial containing a hormonal preparation which they can then mix into their favorite facial oil or cream.

A NEW FACE IN THIRTY DAYS

If you are not satisfied with your face, make yourself a new one. You can do it in a month if you are willing to work at it.

1. Give yourself a mental face lift. Remember, when you lift your spirits you lift your face.

2. Give yourself a nutritional face lift. Feed those magic muscles the vitamins, minerals, and especially the complete proteins from animal sources, the meats, fish, milk and eggs that can restore their strength and firmness.

3. If you have excess weight, redesign your face by losing weight slowly and wisely, at the same time as you nourish the muscle fibers back to firmness.

4. Use water, that best of nature's beauty aids for the face. I have already described for you the sauna facial. A new kind of hydrotherapy I recently discovered in Paris makes use only of cold water to stimulate the circulation to the facial muscles. It is a hose that attaches to the cold water faucet in your bathroom basin, and at the other end is a small needle-shower head in what looks like a giant rubber eyecup which fits the contours of the face. You turn on the cold water, apply this prickling, stimulating shower to the three vital areas of the face: the throat, the chin, the eyes. This brings the blood stream to the three most important parts of the face and has a wonderfully tightening and rejuvenating effect. This Hydro Face Molder is used by many French women to "lift" tired faces. Fortunately this device is now imported to America by Madame Ellene, formerly of Vienna, now in New York City.

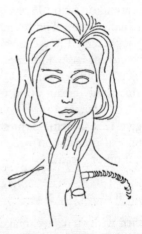

Madame Ellene's Hydro Face Molder

5. And finally, exercise those facial muscles; strengthen them with use, just as you strengthen the muscles of arms, legs, and torso. We all use only a fraction of the fifty-five muscles. It is the ones we do not use that are in danger of becoming soft and letting down the entire facial structure.

THREE FACE-LIFTING GYMNASTICS

1. Your Neck and Chin: Sit in front of your mirror. Look at your face honestly, open-mindedly, or as one student expressed it, "I look at myself as my dearest enemy would." What do you see?

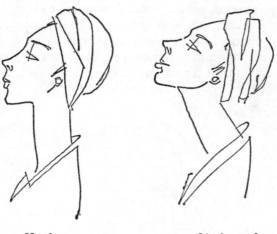

Head up . . .   *. . . chin forward*

A too-full face, perhaps with jowls along the once piquant jawline, perhaps a double chin. Push your head back. Straighten your posture. Sit tall. No doubt, these defects become less noticeable when your neck is in proper alignment. Remember, a hang-dog posture makes everything fall.

And here is good news: you can get rid of heavy jowls and that extra chin with this new gymnastic recommended by the famous German dermatologist, Dr. Hans Weyhbrecht in Stuttgart. Cream or oil the face and throat. Sit high and straight in front of a mirror. Push your chin forward as far as it will go. Now push your lower lip forward à la Maurice Chevalier. Stay in this position and turn your head slowly to the left, then slowly to the right. This brings all the weakened muscles of the throat and jaw into play. The more you push forward with your lip and the more you tighten and exercise these muscles, the sooner you will establish a firm throat and neck line. Do it daily, twelve times left and twelve times right. This takes only one minute.

2. Your Mouth: How does your mouth look in your mirror? I hope the corners go up and not down. If your mouth droops, investigate your upper teeth. If some are missing, have them replaced at once. Nothing can give you such an unhappy look as missing teeth. If your teeth are in order and the corners of the mouth are down, then perhaps your spirits need lifting as well.

Disappointments, sadness, constant worry all register, especially around the mouth. All of us have our share of disappointments, but why advertise it? A brave woman is never defeated. Take out your lipstick and paint your mouth so the corners look as if they were turning up. In the meantime, cheer up! Remember, if you do your best each day you can also expect the best.

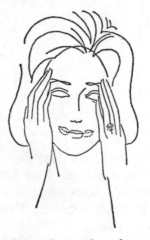

Left and up, right and up

Now this is how you can pull up the corners of your mouth so that they will stay up: Put both hands on your cheeks, hold the cheek muscles tight, and now draw your mouth as far to the right as it will go, then as far to the left. Be sure to hold your cheek muscles tight. Just exercising and pulling the mouth left and right will do you no good. It is the muscular left and right pull, against the cheeks you are holding with both hands, which can do wonders for weakened muscles around the mouth. Do this twelve times toward the left and twelve times toward the right. Dr. Rudolf Drobil, the well-known Viennese physician, teaches the beautiful Viennese scientific face lifting via exercise and insists that unless you give your facial muscles resistance, facial gymnastics are a waste of time. Dr. Drobil in his book, *Gesichts-Gymnastik,* says that women before considering plastic surgery should first strengthen their facial musculature via his face gymnastics; then the face-lift will be twice as lasting.

3. Let the law of gravity lift you: If you are too busy or just too lazy to do these three-minute facial gymnastics, do as Ann Delafield taught thousands of women in the New York Success School: Lie down on your Beauty Slant board and let the law of gravity pull your muscles upward and flood their cells with your own nourishing, reviving beautystream while you rest. The shoulder braces keep the shoulders flat as gravity pulls the neck straight and slender and you can actually feel it lifting your cheeks as it coaxes more blood to them.

A NEW FACE IN THREE HOURS

There are cases that only plastic surgery can help. If there is something about your face that really troubles you, a scar or an ugly feature or if deep lines and sagging muscles make you look older than your years, consider having it corrected surgically. This is an art and a science that has developed fabulously since the end of World War II, as has all surgery. Today it is no longer frivolous or vain to have plastic surgery when it is needed.

In Moscow I went to visit the Medical Cosmetics Institute on Gorki Street. There scars are removed, ears and lips are corrected; a nose is shortened and straightened for 600 rubles.

In Tokyo, at the Jujin Institute, Japanese girls have eyelid surgery to make their eyes look wider and rounder, more like those of the American movie stars they adore. The cost: $8.33. For $13.88 one can have bags under the eyes removed.

But the center of this work is the United States and England.

A good plastic operation is still expensive, but in New York City there is already a clinic headed by the distinguished Dr. Herbert Conway at New York Hospital, and I am sure that similar clinics will soon spring up all over the world for those who need this work done and cannot invest a large sum of money.

If you have a really troubling facial problem, and want to consider plastic surgery, this is my advice: Take the utmost pains to find the best doctor within your reach. Travel to find him, if necessary. Write to the state medical society at your state capital; you will get from them a list of reputable specialists in your locality. If you live near a large hospital or medical center, ask there for the names of staff surgeons or affiliated surgeons who specialize in plastic surgery. When you have the names of several, find out all you can about them.

For a woman who has to make a living and appear before the public in her middle years, plastic surgery is often a sound solution. This is the advice I have given to women in this situation who have taken all other measures to keep up their energies and good looks, such as intelligent eating, exercise and sufficient rest and relaxation.

Here is one of many cases, one of my New York students, a woman who owned her own dress shop for many years: She was in her fifties when she suffered business reverses, lost her shop and all her capital, and was faced with creating a new future for herself. She looked her age, with bags under her eyes and a sagging jaw line; altogether she made a sad appearance for a woman who must go out and seek employment. Even though she was both capable and experienced in her field and would be an asset to any retail establishment, I knew that no personnel manager would give her the opportunity to prove her abilities. I advised her to investigate plastic surgery before she went looking for a job.

She made doubly sure to perfect her nutrition with extra protein drinks and vitamins. Finally, she entrusted herself to a first-rate plastic surgeon, who performed a three-hour operation, removing the under-eye bags and lifting the cheeks and the drooping mouth. I saw her three days after the operation and she looked amazingly well, with only a little black and blue evidence under the eyes and very fine red lines showing where the face-lift incisions had been made at the ears. Three weeks later, not even I could see the lines. Just four weeks after the operation she found a position as a buyer in one of the large New York department stores without difficulty, and is completely happy with the operation that insured her future livelihood and independence. Needless to say, she realizes that for her skin and muscles to remain firm and her face to keep its attractiveness—as she says, to protect her investment— she needs a high-protein diet and she also fortifies her diet with all the necessary vitamins.

I know many, many instances in which these three operations in particular have worked wonderfully for the women who underwent them: the nose plastic, the face lift, and the eye plastic. Here is what you should know about them:

THE NOSE

This is the most frequent plastic operation, three to one compared with any of the others. Straightening and shortening are the simplest repairs; narrowing can also be done within limits. The operation takes about one hour under local anesthetic, and it is best to remain in the hospital for a day or two. There are no scars because the work is done within the nose and the improvement is permanent.

THE FACE LIFT

This is the second most popular and a blessing to many women— men, too—who need to keep up a youthful appearance. The operation tightens the loose folds of the neck by pulling the skin upward by incision behind the ears, and tightens cheeks and forehead with another incision within the hairline at the temples. It takes about three hours, under either local or general anesthetic, and the hospital stay is about three days; after two to three weeks there is almost no sign that an operation has been performed. The improvement may last five or ten years depending on how well you take care of your health and your skin. The scars are the thinnest possible, and can be covered by the hair.

THE EYES

Disfiguring under-eye bagginess and eyelid wrinkles may not be the result of late hours and over-indulgence; they can be constitutional. Some faces have a tendency to develop a small grape-sized lump of fat under the eyes, and some skins tend to stretch and wrinkle at the lids. These repairs are two separate operations. Each takes about an hour or less under local anesthetic. The hospital stay is one or two days. In a week or ten days the signs of the operation are completely gone. The only scars are thin lines at the eyelid edges and can be successfully concealed by light makeup.

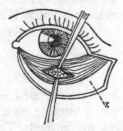

Surgery, not cosmetics, is necessary for removal of eye puffiness caused by a fat deposit

Where there is surgery, there are scars, but the art of the plastic surgeon includes the artful placing and concealment of the scars.

Take your time in deciding whether you want to have plastic surgery and in choosing your doctor. It is not an emergency operation and you can consult several doctors for their advice. The good surgeon is also kind and thoughtful and he will advise you whether you really need the operation and what success you can expect, so that you can feel confident in taking his advice. He will ask you why you feel you need it, and you should tell him your reasons honestly. Plastic surgery as American and English doctors perform it today can do wonders, but you can only expect it to improve your looks, not to solve all your problems. A good plastic surgeon will not exaggerate the results his reconstruction can make in your life. If your expectations are reasonable, and if you do everything in your power to build up your good looks *from within*, then your plastic surgery can give added contentment and renewed self-confidence for many years to come.

CORRECT THESE BEAUTY DEFECTS

Facial hair is not considered a defect to a woman's beauty in some parts of the world, but in this country hair on the upper lip and chin is looked upon as unfeminine and it causes distress to one who has it.

Where there are a few hairs, they can be tweezed, and a thin or downy growth of hair can be bleached with a little peroxide so that it is invisible. A heavier growth should definitely be removed, and nowadays this can be done safely and permanently, without scarring.

Electrolysis for removing superfluous hair has been used by dermatologists since 1875. It should be done by a trained technician. On the skin of the face usually a single needle is recommended rather than multiple needles. Strong hairs may offer resistance and they may have to be removed more than once, but with patience and a skilled operator they can be conquered.

Moles, with or without hair, and especially pigmented moles, should also be removed. For these it is wise to consult a dermatologist. Doctors usually recommend that moles be removed not only for beauty but for health reasons. An excessive growth of hair on the face may be a sign of glandular imbalance; your doctor should check on your glandular functions and consider whether treatment is needed for endocrine deficiencies.

First Wake Up, Then Make Up

Now we come to a phase of beauty in which you are already expert. The cosmetic manufacturers have done a marvelous job of teaching women how to use their cosmetics. After you have worked from the inside and enriched your beautystream with all the beautifying foods, there is no reason why you should not enhance your good points and tone down any weak points you may have.

I had an unforgettable experience with cosmetics in Hollywood some years ago. Lady Mendl cabled me from Paris: "Am very tired and need you badly. Can you take care of me for four weeks." Lady Mendl had helped me and my work so much in Europe that I welcomed an opportunity to be useful to her. She arrived at my home in Beverly Hills with a secretary, a chauffeur, a Rolls Royce, a maid and two dogs.

Sunrise Hill was turned into a private beautyfarm for Lady Mendl who weighed less than a hundred pounds at the time. My whole staff was at her disposal, including my cook, Anna Lee, whom I had trained to cook beauty-full foods. We called in the best doctor to make sure that there was nothing wrong physically. There was a masseuse for body massage; a chiropractor to adjust Lady Mendl's feet (which had begun to give her trouble); every day a woman from the Frances Fox salon came to brush her hair for one hour and at five each evening came the best hairdresser. I taught Lady Mendl to relax; she swam in my pool, she took air and sun baths and the cook outdid herself trying to put some weight on Elsie.

All Hollywood was excited about Lady Mendl leaving her fabulous villa at Versailles and coming to faraway Beverly Hills. Ann Astaire, Mary Pickford, Ann Warner, Hedda Hopper, all her devoted friends were anxious to see the Beloved Elsie, as we called her.

After we had worked day and night with her for about two weeks, Elsie visibly started to bloom; she looked pink and fit and walked once more like a debutante. Since Elsie always lied about her age (a lady's privilege), we did not know she was then eighty-four! And here is the point of my little story: When I asked her if she felt ready to see her Hollywood friends, she said she was delighted, of course, she never felt better in her life. Then she added wistfully, "But dear Gayelord, what will I do about make-up?"

It was then that I discovered the reason for makeup: even this fabulous woman needed it to bolster her psyche!

We did it in the Grand Hollywood Manner. We consulted the greatest "portraitist" in the United States, Eddie Senz from New York, who restyled her silver hair and gave her a flawless smooth complexion. Most of the brown spots had faded with our good diet, but Elsie said, "I don't want any old lady liver spots," so Eddie covered them beautifully. He highlighted Elsie's eyes and gave a more generous look to her mouth.

The "coming out" party of Elsie Mendl at eighty-four was a great success. Lady Mendl's salon became the place where the world's most interesting people met, but she herself remained the most interesting of all.

It was about that time that I had the unique opportunity to bring two of the world's most extraordinary women together: I introduced Lady Mendl to Greta Garbo. Here were two amazing women, direct opposites, one an out-going extrovert with trunks full of Mainbocher clothes and a suitcase of jewels, the other a complete introvert who shunned people, whose wardrobe consisted of twenty pairs of slacks, twenty-four sweaters, twelve pairs of walking shoes and not even one lipstick. They got along famously. Elsie, with her Eddie Senz complexion and Mainbocher clothes, played mannikin and strutted up and down my living room. Garbo, hilarious with laughter, tried on some of Elsie's dresses and finally asked for a lipstick. We had one made to order, a beautiful cherry red, by Beautymasters of Detroit.

Up to this time Garbo had shunned the use of cosmetics, with one exception: mascara. She felt undressed unless her famous, natural, long, blonde eyelashes were carefully mascara-ed. She used her new lipstick for a few days, decided that she liked it, and has continued to use it ever since. Her extraordinary natural beauty needed no embellishment, but the slight touch of makeup had the same effect on her face as a perfect frame has on a lovely picture.

In direct contrast to Garbo, Elsie Mendl delighted in every conceivable artifice. Even as a young girl, when as Elsie de Wolfe she was a Broadway star under the management of David Belasco, it was never said of Elsie that she was beautiful, but she had a quality which transcended beauty. She had personality, magnetism, charm, intelligence and determination all rolled into one, plus a magic ingredient: taste. Elsie lived in beauty and for beauty. She created beauty for herself and for hundreds of famous people for whom she decorated homes during her career as an interior decorator.

MAKEUP LIFTS THE EGO

We must never underestimate the psychological value of makeup. I remember stories told by our war correspondents overseas, of the women who came out of the bomb shelters, shocked and shaken, only to reach first of all for their lipsticks. In the terrible forest fire that swept Maine some years ago (as Gertrude Mackenzie tells it in her book, *My Love Affair with the State of Maine*) the Red Cross thought of everything that people driven from their houses might need, from baby food to shaving cream. The women, deeply grateful, longed for only one thing more— lipsticks. I hope the Red Cross has added lipsticks to its disaster list since then. The Red Cross understands the value of morale.

It shocks me to see women take out their cosmetic kits and fix their faces in public, even combing out their hair in a restaurant. I remember when little girls were taught that they must never never touch their hair at the table, and in nice houses to this day the ladies excuse themselves at the end of dinner and come back to the party with their coiffures and faces freshened. It seems to me that a woman would want to guard her makeup secrets and keep a little mystery about her, instead of boldly revealing to everyone how she achieves her effects!

Again I must say, if your beautystream nourishes you well from the inside, your eyes, hair and skin will reflect it and very, very little artifice is needed. Remember, we do not argue against eating, we argue against *over*eating or *over*doing anything. And it is the same with paint, powder and makeup. The inside-outside beauty, to which most of this book is devoted, means first mustering up all the inner resources with the Hi-Vi nutrients for the trillions of cells of the bodyhouse, via the bloodstream.

Perhaps you ask, what then is the difference between the old beauty culture and the new beautyfarm idea? This is my answer in two sentences:

The new Eve first nourishes and wakes up her inner biologic resources. *Then* she uses makeup to highlight her best features.

LET YOUR LIGHT SHINE

In my book, *Look Younger, Live Longer,* I quoted wise old Confucius, who said 2500 years ago, "Everything has beauty, but not everyone sees it."

I believe a woman's makeup can help to bring out her good features so everyone *can* see them, most of all herself. When her mirror tells her she is beautiful, it gives her an added lift and assurance.

THE OUTER YOU

Perhaps the one great secret of success in using makeup is to *underdo,* so that the natural radiance of the skin shows through. If you use a foundation cream to tint your skin, apply it lightly and blend it into the skin so that it looks like a fine veil and never like a mask.

When you make up your eyes, do it with a light touch. Remember that the eyes are your most precious jewels and makeup should enhance them, not overshadow them. Use only a bit of coloring as a frame or background for your jewels. Eye makeup that is heavy and obvious has missed its real purpose. It is like putting a vulgar frame around a noble painting. The eyes of Garbo, which have become world famous, have been given greater depth and mystery by penciling a single delicate line along the roots of the upper eyelashes. Thousands of women have learned to highlight their eyes with the simple Garbo line.

Cleopatra long ago knew the secret of framing her eyes to give them extra dimension and greater depth, and Beautymasters of Detroit have been immensely successful in correlating all makeup around the jewel-like color spectrum of a woman's eyes.

Your mouth

If the eyes are the windows of the soul, you might call the mouth the gateway to your bodyhouse. A generous up-turned mouth tells the mirror that all is well with you and the world. Lovely young creatures in their full development of strength and with the young beautystream reddening their lips, need no external adornment. A young girl can be beautiful with a clean scrubbed look, but women in the midstream of life look better with red full lips.

Lips are meant to be generous and red, not blue or purple. A clear red is most flattering because it is natural; it is the color of the beautystream. Periodically, the cosmetic stylists create unnatural lip colors such as the cadaverous, pasty, purplish colors the Italian beauticians tried to introduce recently; smart women do not accept them and they are quickly forgotten. Stylists must remain humble and go to Mother Nature who created all basic colors for her children.

There are four unforgettable paintings in a London gallery called the "Four Seasons." They represent spring, summer, fall and winter. The faces of the women representing the season in these paintings are made up entirely of the fruits and vegetables of the season. Miss Springtime has a delicious mouth of red cherries and a necklace of ripe, red raspberries. The Flemish artist-painter knew intuitively what every woman should know: follow nature's coloring and not the dictates of fashion, fads and fancies. If your mirror tells you that your mouth is not a happy one, lift your spirits and use your gay, red lipstick to help you create a happy mouth.

YOUR AURA

More than any other people, the French know how to extract the perfumes of exotic flowers and fruits and blend them into mysterious scents. There are dozens of delightful fragrances which you can make a part of your beauty ensemble. There is one to fit your type and personality. You already know some of their popular names: Femme, Miss Dior, Chanel No. 5, Lanvin, Ma Griffe.

American perfumers are also now learning the art of creating fresh scents such as Mary Chess' pure Flower Fragrances, Beautymaster's fragrant Beverly Hills Cologne and many others.

If you are young and full of life, you can use any and all of the perfumes, even the strong musky ones, but if you are in the midstream, it is wiser to stick to the fresh, natural flower scents. You might prefer to make and use your own fragrant concoction of toilet water. Sophisticated women frequently create their own individual combination, putting together half a dozen different perfumes to make their own distinctive scent. They apply this scent directly to the skin, never to the clothes, and this surrounds them with an aura which is theirs and theirs alone. A chic French woman to this day prefers to have her own blend of perfumes, and her cologne, bath oil and even her soap which is made with her individual scent.

YOUR CLOTHES

If you want to stand out among the thousands of well-dressed women in America, according to Ann Hunter, the brilliant American designer now living in Paris, you must *underdress*. Take off ribbons, buttons and furbelows and follow the simple lines of the body and you are always architecturally correct and in style. A smart woman never blindly follows any fashion. She may like something of the Dior look, the Fath look or the Lanvin look, but she aims at all times to create her *own* look, one that makes the most of her good points.

I have often wondered why American designers do not create more specifically American clothes for American women. We are "go" people, working people, always going somewhere and many of the eccentric foreign designs are not for active American women. Now, I am happy to say, two outstanding women have done just such designing for busy American women, giving good basic body lines—as I like to call it, architecturally correct—and at prices American women can afford.

The Duchess of Windsor is one of the best dressed women of all time. The great friend of our mutual friend, Lady Mendl, now designs simple new patterns for dresses and slim-line suits to give you that active American look. In all the years since I first met the Duchess of Windsor in Paris in 1938, I have never seen her over-dressed. She expresses her excellent taste in extremely simple clothes. Now, for you who have dreamed of dressing that new body of yours simply and beautifully, here is your chance to procure the Duchess of Windsor's simple and elegant patterns.

Gloria Swanson is the best example of her own ever-young, ever-vital philosophy. She is a one-woman organization who gets things done. Her attractive and beautifully designed clothes are available from coast to coast. Nobody knows better than Gloria herself that a trim body is the best foundation garment for any dress. What I like best about Gloria Swanson is her devotion to her work. She is not like so many of our cinema stars—pining away and bemoaning their fate. She not only works for her own family and grandchildren, but for all children. Her speech before the Big Brother Club at the Press Club in Washington, D.C., was a classic which every mother should read. She traced many of our juvenile troubles to the bad meals the youngsters get in their homes, and at Saks Fifth Avnue in New York City she had the courage to tell the thousand women who oh'd and ah'd at her face and figure, that they should go home and learn to build better bodies with better food.

MARUSIA MEANS GLAMOR

There are those who scoff at Hollywood styles and it is true that many atrocious fashions came from there, but let us not forget such splendid designers as Irene, or Adrian, who designed beautifully classic clothes for our greatest stars, Garbo among them. There are many good designers in Hollywood today, but there is one remarkable Polish designer who has a fantastic flair for elegant clothes. Her secret is harmonizing line, fabric and color. With these, Marusia performs modern miracles. She has learned never to overdress her glamorous ladies; she tells them: "All I do is put a beautiful frame around a beautiful woman." This, I believe, is Marusia's own secret. In private life, Marusia is the Princess Toumanoff. She is her own best model. She is probably one of Hollywood's busiest designers to glamorous ladies, including the regal queen mother of Egypt and those fair and fabulous Gabor girls, Zsa Zsa and Eva.

CHAPTER 13

Beauty's Jewels: Your Eyes

Your eyes were made to be beautiful. They sparkle like jewels with their own moisture. Whether they are brown or blue, gray or green or hazel, they are the only natural spots of true color in the face. And consider their setting. Could any jeweler do better for his finest gem than that shining white background, that frame of lashes, that shadowy hollow between cheekbone and eyebrow ridge? While above, the eyebrow sweeps up and out in emphasis, final flourish of the artist's brush!

If they never expressed a thought or communicated an emotion, your eyes would still be beautiful. But with all their other beauties, they also happen to be the most eloquent features of the human face, the true spokesmen of your inner self. The eyes speak a language that transcends words.

The wonderful mechanisms of pupil and lens adjust themselves instantly to the constant changes of light and distance. The muscles of the eyeball, six of them for each eye, automatically turn and adjust the eyes together, focussing these twin cameras without any effort on our part.

If they are so sturdy, you may wonder why your eyes sometimes look and feel strained; why they lose their luster, why sometimes they seem smaller than usual and give a look of tension to your face. Remember, of all our senses, we human beings depend most on our vision. Our eyes work constantly except when we sleep. They *need*, and they deserve, the best of care from the inside as well as the outside.

Those six little muscles that move your eyes up and down and from side to side are delicate as silken threads and strong as steel springs. Yet they can become tired, and when they do their fatigue will be reflected in lines of tension not only around your eyes but throughout your face.

The tiny circular muscle that pulls open and draws together like a purse string to widen and narrow your pupil, letting in more or less light, is made of smooth muscle tissue. This is the same kind of tissue that makes up the walls of internal organs such as the stomach and intestines, and it almost never becomes tired. But it can lose its elasticity. So can the lens, made of crystal clear elastic tissue, that bends the light rays as they enter your eye and focusses them on your retina. So can the strong, resilient ligament that holds the lens, and pulls or releases it to change its shape for seeing objects far or near.

But the most dangerous beauty thief of all is poor nutrition. It is a sneak thief because it creeps up so gradually.

Today we know that when some vital element of nutrition is lacking from the diet, the eyes are the first to suffer.

Food for seeing

I have been teaching for many years that of all the body's mechanisms, the eyes most need the entire alphabet of vitamins, minerals, and amino acids, and in the past decade this belief has been confirmed by reports from many ophthalmologists, eye surgeons, and research scientists.

It could not be otherwise. The mechanisms by which we see with our eyes are like the finest, tiniest Swiss watch.

Only these mechanisms do not work mechanically, by means of wheels and springs, like a watch. They are made of living cells and they work *chemically*. For the miraculous chemistry of vision, all the vital nutrients are needed.

Let me give you an example.

You undoubtedly know that vitamin A is important for your vision. But do you know why? It is an interesting story.

At the back of your eyes, lining your eyeball like the thin inner skin that lines an egg shell, is the retina, the film of the eye-camera. It is composed of the very special cells of vision. In each eye there are about 137 million of these seeing cells. They are developed from the same tissue that goes to make brain and nerve cells, but they are specialized to respond to light. They are even further specialized among themselves. Some, which are cone-shaped, do all our seeing in bright light, and they also see colors. Others, which are rod-shaped, are for seeing in dim light.

Each kind of cell reacts to light with its own kind of sensitive chemical substance. The cone-shaped cells have special substances that react only to bright light and to light of different wave lengths for the different colors. There is still a great deal the scientists are trying to solve about the differences among the cone cells.

The rod cells have a substance for dim light called visual purple; the cells themselves make this substance out of a special protein plus vitamin A.

Cats see better in the dark than we do, and some human beings see better than others. But if the body is lacking in vitamin A, then the cells cannot make their visual purple. And one result of this lack, the most apparent one, is the inability to see in dim light—night blindness.

The fighter and bomber pilots who flew night runs in World War II were given heavy doses of vitamin A. Long before that, in my first book on beauty and nutrition, *Manger Pour Être Belle*, I told of the experience of thousands of Belgians in World War I who suffered from a mysterious eye affliction, apparently incurable —until spring came and they began to eat fresh green vegetables and butter and cheese and to drink their good rich milk. And then, miraculously, their eyesight recovered! The explanation was that the enemy had confiscated all their fresh foods, and their apparently incurable eye ailment was nothing else but a serious lack of vitamin A.

But the story of vitamin A and the eyes is a great deal older than our two world wars. Five hundred years before Christ, the wise Greek physician Hippocrates recommended raw liver to his patients who had difficulty in seeing at night. Today we know that liver is a rich source of vitamin A.

THE HUNGRY BEAUTIES

Let us talk about vitamin A again. Your eyes need it not only for seeing in the dark, but for their good looks, whether in the dark or the light. If vitamin A is lacking, the cornea and eye tissues lose moisture and luster. If there is a serious deficiency, actual dry spots appear on the eyeballs, giving a grainy feeling as though there were grains of sand in the eyes. Dark spots may also occur in the field of vision. A still more serious lack can cause softening of the cornea, a grave condition.

The B vitamins cover a whole range of beauty factors. When there is a lack of vitamin B-2 or riboflavin, the eyes become bloodshot, itchy, burning; they water frequently, and they are sensitive to light, the condition called photophobia. When these symptoms appear, the recommendation is not only to take riboflavin, but to increase the whole B group in the diet, just as it occurs in natural foods such as food yeast, wheat germ, liver.

In my classes I have told the story of a famous motion picture star who suffered for years with burning, bloodshot eyes. She blamed the studio lights, and since she was past her fortieth birthday she also blamed her age. She undertook to follow the Cosmetic Diet with the same vigor and persistence that made her one of Americas most distinguished artists. The results surprised even me. After three months her eyes were clear and beautiful as they had not been for years. And because they were no longer sensitive to light, and she could open them wide despite the hot glare of studio lighting, they even photographed larger than before.

The diet that worked this magic was nothing mysterious, simply a diet rich in vitamin A and the entire B complex: green broths, food yeast, liver, milk, all the natural foods that restore health and beauty to hard-working, hungry eyes.

VITAMIN C FOR YOUTHFUL EYES

After vitamin A and the B vitamins, in our vitamin alphabet for eye beauty, comes vitamin C. Here some exciting studies have been made, in connection with the serious condition of cataract, the clouding of the eyes crystalline lens. Several years ago Dr. Donald T. Atkinson of San Antonio, Texas, found that when he persuaded many of his patients, who habitually lived on salt pork, corn meal, and coffee, to add plentiful fresh greens, oranges, and tomatoes to their diet, as well as eggs and other good proteins, the condition improved or the growth of the cataract was arrested.

We do not know just how vitamin C is connected with this serious ailment of the eyes, and anyone suffering with cataract urgently needs the help of an ophthalmologist. But we do know that the eye, and especially its lens, normally contains more vitamin C than any other part of the body except some of the endocrine glands. And we know that in cataract the vitamin C is conspicuously missing from these tissues.

We also know that vitamin C is crucial to the health of the capillary walls in the body generally, and that a lack of it goes hand in hand with aging of the connective tissues. And if healthy eyes keep up such a high level of vitamin C, there must be a reason!

So let us give them this vitamin in maximum, not minimum, amounts. The body does not store it, and you need to replenish the supply every day. With plenty of vitamin C in your diet, so easily supplied with citrus fruits, green peppers, tomatoes and the richest of all foods, the rose hips, you are feeding your eyes what they themselves take in great quantity from the body's supply.

VITAMIN D FOR GOOD VISION

Next in our vitamin alphabet is D. This is the sunshine vitamin which the body must have to absorb calcium and make good bones and teeth. Now here is a curious fact that came out of two separate experimental studies: a lack of vitamin D and calcium produced nearsightedness in puppies, and the addition of vitamin D to the diet of nearsighted children improved their vision or prevented it from getting worse.

Here again the scientist cannot explain exactly how this worked. We do know that a proper balance of calcium in the blood is essential, and that if this balance is disturbed, cramping spasms of muscles, big and small, can occur. Quite possibly, especially in young growing puppies and children, a disturbance in the calcium and vitamin D balance could result in excessive tension of muscles and ligaments, so that the eye fails to accommodate for near vision.

And finally there is good evidence that amblyopia, a general dimming of vision without any apparent defect to account for it, can be a result of general nutritional deficiency. Dr. A. J. Cameron, surgeon at the Royal Eye Hospital in London, found this to be so during the post-war years of austerity diet in England. We can go a step further: in countries of generally poor nutrition, for example India, and in the Soviet Union during the war years, cataracts appeared at a much earlier age than the average in well-fed countries

There is still one more point in this beauty-feeding of the eyes. It is not enough to take the food into your body. It must also be distributed, and this means good circulation of the blood via exercise.

BEAUTY GYMNASTICS FOR THE EYES

We are going to talk about exercise for the hair. It should not surprise you that exercise makes the eyes more beautiful. Good food, remember, creates a good bloodstream, but only exercise can bring that bloodstream where it is needed.

Attached to your eyeballs are those six fine, silk-like little muscles which can be exercised and strengthened like all other muscles of the body. Simple eye drills, which take only a few minutes a day, can greatly improve the looks and function of the eyes. Here are two basic eye gymnastics:

1. Turn your head from side to side as if saying an emphatic "no." Do this ten times.

2. Hold your index finger or a pencil about ten inches away from your eyes. Look at its tip, then into the distance. Do this ten times.

Do these two simple eye drills every day; do them especially when you are using your eyes intensely for close work or for

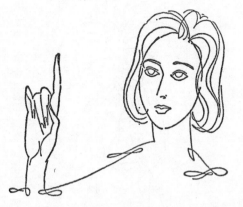

Look at your fingertip, then into the distance

reading, and your eyes will be more beautiful and also serve you better. Here are two additional aids to eye beauty and eye comfort:

EYE RELAXATION

Palming is still the best way to relax tired eyes. This simple method was discovered by Dr. William H. Bates of New York City It is the same as the exercise I recommended for relaxing tensions.

Sit in front of a calendar or a picture. Look at it. Now, gently, close your eyes and cover them with your palms. Be sure not to press on the eyelids. Rest your arms. Relax. Let go. Breathe slowly and deeply 30, 40, 50 times. As you relax your covered eyes will only see restful gray-black, and as you gradually let go of all tension, your eyes will see a deep dark black. Then open your eyes. Look at the calendar or picture again. You will see it more and more clearly the more you relax. Your eyes and your whole face lose their tension whenever you palm. Do it often.

EYE REFRESHER

Plain cold water refreshes your eyes more than anything I know of. The same hydrotherapy device that is described in Chapter 12 for the face is ideal for the eyes. I have used it constantly during the writing of this book. If you do not have this device, wring out

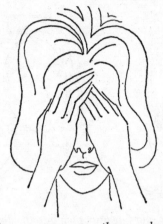

Close your eyes, cover them, and relax

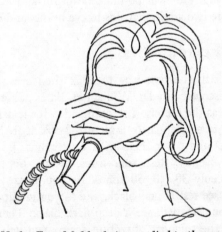

Hydro Face Molder being applied to the eyes

a washcloth in cold water and apply it specifically to the eyes. Do this several times. The cold water stimulates the tissues and tiredness simply disappears.

EYEGLASSES

My students in many lands have made these simple eye drills part of their daily living and many have had remarkable success in keeping their eyes young and attractive. Some have succeeded in keeping their eyesight sharp and keen. I actually have met hundreds of men and women who believe that good nutrition, exercise, and the eye relaxation originated by Dr. William Bates have kept their eyes young and attractive.

Today there are many teachers of the Bates Method of Eye Relaxation. I have met them in Germany, England and Switzerland; Mrs. Margaret D. Corbett of Los Angeles, California, an outstanding teacher of the Bates Method, has helped many of our movie stars to strengthen their eyes. I myself have studied these methods and find them valuable for relaxing the eyes; you have found some of them described in this chapter. We cannot ignore the successes these eye teachers have with their pupils. The only difficulty I see is that eye exercises and eye relaxation require constant practice and application, for which the great majority of human beings are either too lazy or too busy.

So I definitely do not belong to the school that says: "Throw away your glasses." Unless you are willing to work on your eyes constantly and daily, I suggest that you consult the best eye doctor in your city and let him decide, after a thorough examination, whether or not you need glasses. There are few things so damaging to a woman's looks as her straining, squinting effort to see. It is not only detrimental to the eyes, for tissues around the eyes become a mass of fine, squinting lines. Along with the muscles of the eyes, your whole face and even the muscles of your neck and shoulders become tense in the struggle to see.

The decision rests entirely with you and your eye doctor. If you need glasses, wear them boldly and confidently. Today women treat eyeglasses not as a handicap to good looks but as an accessory. You no longer need to change frames and shapes that will make the glasses inconspicuous. Quite the contrary—the bolder the better. Girls with small faces and small features can wear glasses with thick frames and bold colors. The rule used to be "small face, small frames," but chic women everywhere have discovered that the smaller the face the larger and more self-assertive the spectacles can be.

CONTACT LENSES

For actors and actresses and for those before the public, especially if the eyes need help not only for reading but for seeing around the clock, the new types of contact lenses may be a boon. In the past several years there have been improvements that minimize and perhaps eliminate some of the disadvantages of these plastic lenses that fit directly over the eye.

Formerly, contact lenses were fitted to cover the entire front of the eyeball, but today they can be made to fit only the seeing part of the eye. Recently, two Boston specialists, doctors Donald R. Korb and Morton Shaw, found that they could make these tiny lenses with a pinpoint hole through which the cornea can, so to speak, breathe. Through this opening the heat of the cornea can escape and air and fluids can circulate to keep the eye comfortable.

Whether contact lenses are for you is a very personal question. Some swear by them; others still claim they are uncomfortable. Of course, absolute cleanliness is essential for lens wearers to protect against the danger of infection.

OUTSIDE CARE

Very little is needed if you make good nutrition, exercise and relaxation the basis for better-looking eyes. In case your eyes are often exposed to smoke or smog, refresh them with an occasional herbal compress; or an herbal bath; these can be very comforting and soothing. A delightful herbal infusion can be made right in your own kitchen.

PLAY FOR THE EYES

Whether or not you need lenses or glasses, whether you use your eyes little or much, if you want them to keep their beauty, treat them well. Give them good food, good working conditions, rest and relaxation. And give them not only work but play as well.

Muscles thrive on use, as I have said many times. But they do not thrive on being held long in one position. The use that they thrive on is action.

That is what the standard eye exercises are designed to do: they give the muscles of the eye a series of active movements, turning the eyes in all possible positions. Thus each pair of muscles has full opportunity to contract and relax, to tense and stretch.

EYES OF THE MIND

Give your eyes a change of pace, a change of view, a vacation. Do you really use your eyes for seeing in the truest sense?

If you truly see what you are looking at, it is yours forever. If you look well, even at the most familiar faces and places around you, you will see something of interest, something of beauty. Perhaps you will find in the most unexpected place a masterpiece to hang on the walls of your mind, one that will forever enrich the home in which your spirit lives.

I have been lucky in people and places. I have been able to collect many great pictures to hang in my mental picture gallery. I have many happy pictures of Taormina in Sicily. I have pictures of my childhood home in the Black Forest where I was born. I have a portrait of Albert Schweitzer, seated at an organ in his church in Gunzbach. In my memory's collection I have portraits of many dear friends, some of them famous, some whose names are important only to the few like myself who knew them.

These pictures are mine forever. I carry them with me everywhere, and I can look at them whenever I like.

Anyone can collect a gallery of masterpieces for the mind's eye. It does not matter whether you roam the world, or live in one town and on one street all your life. It does not matter whether you ever see new scenes and faces or only the everyday familiar ones. I have known many people who travel far and to glamorous places, and meet interesting people—and yet have not one picture in their mind's collection! They never see what they look at; they have never learned to use their eyes.

And I have known people (so have you) who never stirred more than a mile from the place where they were born, who yet stored interesting pictures of a flower, a bird, the sky, a child's face, sunlight shining through green leaves.

I grant you, it takes more seeing to see the everyday commonplace sights than the new and strange ones. But you will be amazed, if once you begin, to discover how much there is to see, how much that is interesting, funny, and even beautiful, which you have been blindly passing by in your daily, seemingly uninteresting rounds.

Your eyes reflect the living spirit of you. If your spirit is alive and eager to drink in the world around you, your eyes will shine with that eagerness. They will grow wide and beautiful with your appetite for life.

CHAPTER 14

Frame for Beauty: Your Hair

I believe there is no other single feature that can do so much for a woman's looks as a mass of sweet-smelling, shining hair. Also, there is no feminine feature that can glamorize, minimize or balance facial shortcomings as can beautiful hair. In the same way that a good frame brings out and highlights a picture, just so can beautiful hair frame and highlight an almost beautiful face into extraordinary beauty.

The great painters knew this. The Venetian painter Titian always framed his women's faces in masses of copper-tinged hair. There is another secret that Titian used so well. He bestowed on his ladies' hair not only fabulous color, but also texture and luster that have not faded in 400 years.

I have learned that most women at some time worry about their hair, so let me say at once that I believe you can have beautiful hair. The texture, color and luster of your hair are mixed right in your own body cells, a feat so mysterious that biologists to this day do not have all the answers to the puzzle.

YOUR HAIR IS ALIVE

We do know that your hair is a living part of your body; it grows from living roots in the soil of your scalp which is a specialized part of your skin. Your hair draws nourishment from the same beautystream, your blood stream, which nourishes every other part of you. Every single hair has its own tiny muscle at the root which can make it stand up when you are cold or make your hair misbehave when you are nervous. The tiny sensory nerve ends of your hair can telegraph to your brain every whiff of wind that stirs and every change of temperature. Yes, and each hair has its own minute oil gland that lubricates it and keeps it soft and shining. And here is the wonder of wonders: every hair on your head has its own pigment-mixing chemistry which decrees whether you shall be blonde, brunette or a redhead. Like the same wondrous cell chemistry which tints your skin, each hair is equipped with a tiny color factory that manufactures the color of your hair.

And now you ask, and rightly so: how can I provide this inner support for my hair? Where do the texture and body come from? Where does the mysterious color come from? And how can I keep the natural color of my locks? And the answer is: Your hair is nourished from the foods you put into your body. Your particular hair color is inherited, like the tint of your complexion, but its texture, luster and sheen can be maintained only by the foods you eat and by the vitamins and minerals that you provide for the individual color-making factories located in each of your hair follicles.

Perhaps sometimes you regret that you are not a blonde, a redhead or a raven-haired beauty. These extremes of hair color are comparatively rare in the United States and among the mixed peoples of Europe. More people in the western world have brown hair than any of the striking shades, and curiously enough, most of the great artists painted the hair of their beauties in shades of brown, including da Vinci's smiling Mona Lisa and Goya's Duchess of Alba. I would like to emphasize that it is not the *color* of your hair that makes it beautiful, but its texture and luster. I repeat, whatever the color of your hair may be, even if it is already mixed with silver, your hair can be beautiful as long as it has good texture and shines with cleanliness and health.

In my travels I see many women in many lands and I must say that our American women, on the whole, have the best-groomed hair. They tend it most carefully on the outside. But they neglect to care for it from the inside.

HAIR BEAUTY FROM THE INSIDE

If you have hair you "can't do a thing with," nine times out of ten it is not a new permanent nor a new color job you need. Your hair first of all needs more body, and for this it needs feeding from the inside. Contrary to what you may have heard, there is nothing known to scientists which can in any way, shape or form feed your hair from the *outside*. Beautiful hair requires an inside approach. Dr. Irwin Lubowe, the famous dermatologist of New York's Flower-Fifth Avenue Hospital, says: "If the diet is unbalanced, particularly if there is an excessive intake of carbohydrates and animal fats, the sebaceous glands are adversely affected."

Here is an answer to many hair problems. It is well known that we food-rich Americans consume more sugar and sugary drinks, more starches and more saturated animal fats than any other people in the world. Even the most skillful hairdressers cannot create flattering coiffeurs with starved, dry, dank and oily hair.

There is one way to correct a multitude of hair troubles, and that is to start from the inside. Follow the Cosmetic Diet; replace empty starches and sugars, cakes, candies, soda pops and nutritionless cereals with beauty-full foods that will nourish your hair.

Most important for hair are the first class proteins like lean meat, fish, eggs, cottage cheese. Use only whole grains, good breads, fruit juices and honey. Cut to a minimum all animal fats with the exception of butter. But be generous with the golden vegetable oils. You have a wide choice to fit your taste and pocketbook: sunflower oil, sesame oil, soya oil, wheat germ oil, corn oil, olive oil and many others. These oils make tasty salad dressings. Use them singly or mix them in a beautyfarm salad dressing. Cook with these oils and bake with them, and if your hair is especially dry and mousey, take a tablespoonful of oil every day. You will find that these natural golden oils taste sweet and fresh.

EXERCISE FOR THE HAIR

If your hair is excessively oily and dank, it tells the nutritionist that something has gone wrong with the little sebaceous glands in the scalp. That is why, first of all, the animal fats should be cut down and replaced by vegetable oils. Excessively oily hair also shows a lack of "exercise." Brushing is one of the million dollar secrets of healthier and more beautiful hair. But there is a right way to brush it.

I believe that learning how to brush your hair correctly, as they do on beautyfarms, is worth the price of a two week's stay. Out in the open air, the professional hair brushers use an assortment of all kinds of brushes—soft ones, hard ones and very stiff ones, depending upon the sensitivity of the scalp. I strongly recommend that you use natural bristles, rather than the synthetic ones which are often so stiff and sharp that they irritate sensitive scalps.

You can brush life and luster into your hair, provided you are following the Cosmetic Diet; brushing weak and sickly hair is likely to break the hair shaft. Once you have begun to give your hair its needed nourishment, here is the way to brush it: begin with your brush at the scalp; remember that at the root of each hair is a little "oil can," the sebaceous gland that supplies oil to keep each hair soft and glistening. It is also this little "oil can" at the root of each hair which makes your hair easy to manage and arrange, so press the bristles of your nice clean brush against the scalp to exercise and squeeze the little "oil can" and distribute your own natural scalp oil to each single strand of hair. From the root of the hair let your brush carry the oil to the very ends of the hair.

Oily scalps and strawy hair ends tell the biologist that you either eat too much animal fat or are too lazy to brush your hair, or both. In your grandmother's day, girls were taught to give their hair 100 strokes each night. Whether they knew it or not, that was how they distributed their own natural oil to their very long hair, and that is how they kept it shining and sweet-smelling. It is still a good practice.

DON'T SHAMPOO TOO OFTEN

It is folly to wash your hair too often, especially if you use a drying, synthetic shampoo. Brushing your hair and scalp 50 to 100 strokes each night keeps the hair clean so that you will need to wash it only every two weeks. You will also save time and money when you do shampoo if you use a preparation with natural oils and lanolin.

Before shampooing, give your scalp this simple beauty treatment. Take a tablespoon of your nice fresh vegetable oil, the same kind you now use in your food, and massage it into your scalp. Wring out a towel in very hot water, wrap it around your head, and leave it on for five minutes. Then wash with an oil-lanolin base shampoo. Lather and rinse once or twice, depending on how much hair you have.

And now for another million-dollar beauty secret your grandmother already knew: always rinse your hair in a gentle acid solution to get rid of the alkaline curd of shampoos and, what is so very important, to re-establish the protective acid mantle of your scalp. This is easily done by adding a tablespoon or two of Cosmetic Vinegar (see formula, page 353) to your last rinse water. This forgotten beauty secret alone can save you much grief and money. It helps to prevent excessive oiliness, it gives your scalp a chance to defend itself against invaders, and it is one of the finest insurances against troublesome dandruff.

Obviously, there are some scalp and hair conditions which are medical problems and should only be handled by a dermatologist. If you have a problem like an infected scalp, or if your hair comes out in bunches, do not waste your money on tonics and salves, but get the best professional help.

There are also some hair problems which can be caused by poor thyroid function. Some years ago, in our Great Lakes region in the Middle West, the farmers complained that they were having trouble growing wool on their sheep. This is one of the areas in the world where iodine is lacking in the soil; Switzerland is another such area. When the farmers added an iodine ration to their animals' feed, the animals responded with good healthy fleece. Unfortunately, growing hair for human beings is a much more complicated affair, but it is always wise to make use of the iodine-rich foods or at least use salt that has been iodized.

What goes on inside your head, believe it or not, can also affect your hair. Stresses and strains can definitely interfere with the circulation in the scalp and so can constant worry affect the health of your hair. Obviously this is where the art of relaxation comes in and I strongly urge you to make my easy "Swing, Sway and Slump" method a daily habit. It takes only a few minutes. If you tell me you are too busy or too lazy to work off your daily tensions, then I am sincerely sorry for you and suggest that you rearrange your life. In the meantime, at least lie on your Beauty Slant board for ten minutes whenever you have time during the day or especially before going to bed. Remember the straight board helps to put the spine in alignment and the law of gravity does the rest. Lying with your feet higher than your head can remove the tension from your neck, face and scalp and the pink glow is brought to your face and scalp by your own beauty-stream.

DID YOU INHERIT GOOD HAIR?

A famous New York dermatologist tells his patients that the surest way to have a good head of hair is to choose parents with good hair. No doubt he has a point. Heredity has a good deal to do with good hair, but I insist, and I have thousands of students to prove it, that it is not heredity we should blame for many defects. We inherit not only the traits but also the cookbooks and eating habits of our parents.

Think for a moment: how different is your diet today from the way your parents ate? Have you taken advantage of the scientific advances in nutrition that have been made since your mother's day?

Our bad eating habits are more often at fault than our inheritance. Let me give you an example. The Chinese people in general have handsome, thick, black hair as long as they stick to their native diet. They rarely suffer from baldness and their hair keeps its blue-black color until late in life. Inheritance? No doubt, but it is also true that the Chinese cuisine is very high in minerals and many B vitamins. They eat quantities of soya beans and soy sauce and a great variety of vegetables, and their diet is rich in first class proteins as fish and sea food. They also consume quantities of iodine-rich sea greens of all kinds. The Chinese never overcook their vegetables, they never throw away the cooking water, and their cooking fat is golden vegetable oil, rich with the unsaturated fatty acids. You never find hardened fat in a Chinese household.

SICILIANS HAVE GOOD HAIR

The Italian people and especially the people of Sicily, where I spend a good deal of my time in summer, also have thick, black, curly hair and I have many Sicilian women neighbors who still have beautiful black hair at the age of seventy. No doubt inheritance plays a part, but listen to this: The Sicilians practically live on the foods coming from the sea. They eat quantities of clams, oysters and other shellfish fresh out of the ocean, and also quantities of fish, broiled, boiled and roasted over wood fires. They also eat vegetables coming from the sea. I have already spoken of one of their favorites, Spaghetti del Mare, a sea green that looks like spaghetti, which they eat both fresh and dried. And, of course, Sicily also produces some of the finest olive oil in the world. This is their only source of fat, and as with the Chinese, you find no hardened fat in a Sicilian kitchen.

NATURAL HAIR COLOR

The Chinese and Sicilian diets are both rich in B vitamins. I am convinced that the vitamins of the B complex are important for the health, beauty, and even the color of the hair. Scientists have been able to prove in animal experiments that there are three so-called anti-gray hair factors. They are called pantothenic acid, para-amino-benzoic acid, and folic acid. In animal experiments there have been definite successes, but with human beings the results have not been satisfactory. Some of my students have reported that with large amounts of the three anti-gray hair factors taken as part of the Cosmetic Diet, their hair did get darker. Many others found the diet had no effect on the color of their hair but their hair became healthier and more vigorous.

Those, I believe, are the qualities that every woman should strive for: well-nourished, well-brushed, strong hair, regardless of color, is beautiful even if it contains gray or silver. Gray hair can make a very flattering frame around the face. Many young girls have discovered that the Paris fashion of silver streaks and silver tipped hair adds interest and piquancy to their faces. Let me assure you that you need not worry about the silver in your hair. It is no longer a sign of many birthdays.

A CHANGE OF COLOR

Nowadays one out of three women colors or highlights her hair.

Hair coloring is nothing new. In Cleopatra's time, and even before, Egyptian ladies used henna and indigo. Roman matrons, admiring the blond Teutonic slaves brought back by Caesar's legions, bleached their hair with such mixtures as ashes of plants, oils, nutshells and vinegar. Renaissance women were known to mix alum, sulphur and honey to become fair-haired. Powdering hair with gold or silver dust was the vogue among fashionable Americans after the Civil War, and, at the turn of the century, bleaching and dyeing were considered smart by actresses and playgirls. Henna rinses again became popular just before World War I, then were replaced by peroxide bleaching which became so popular in the thirties.

A woman may have many reasons for wanting a different hair color. A shining crowning glory is still a mighty symbol of femininity, and the woman who does not care how her locks look may have deep-seated problems. A New York psychoanalyst, Dr. Harold Green, tells of a patient he had under treatment who did not appear to be responding, when one day she came with a new hair color. "Suddenly I knew she was getting well," said Dr. Green. "At last she was ready to establish a personality, to respond to attention. Vanity in a woman is a sign of mental health."

CHAPTER 15

Gateway to Beauty: Your Mouth

Your mouth is the most mobile, expressive, eloquent feature in your face. It speaks for you even when you do not say a word. Around it your personality sketches itself in smiling upward lines or drooping downward ones, in generous sweetness and warmth, or in cold, tightly pressed tension.

When your lips open to speak or to smile, do they reveal attractive, well-cared-for teeth and gums?

In every real sense, your mouth is the gateway to beauty. It reveals the state of body and spirit, the vitality or lack of it, the intelligent care or the unfortunate neglect. Neglect of a potentially lovely mouth and teeth can bankrupt all your other efforts to create beauty. Makeup, lipstick cannot redeem this asset from the outside. The beauty of the mouth can only be an inside job.

Of all the visible assets of beauty, the teeth are most often the victims of careless nutrition. Some defects are inherited, as we believe. A tendency to caries, or tooth decay, may run in families, but as a nutritionist I thoroughly believe that it is the inherited bad eating habits which are the real culprits when it comes to teeth.

Recently I read of a fascinating experiment that a Swedish dentist, Dr. Alfred Askander carried out with his own children.

He and his wife both had very bad teeth, and he was determined
to give his own children a better start. Incidentally he thought he
might prove that although poor teeth may be inherited, an unfortunate heredity could be corrected. And he did prove just that.
He prescribed finely ground bone meal flour to be added to the
family's food, and he also prescribed that the family should have
a plentiful supply of the little sardines that their Swedish ancestors
used to eat *with the bones*. The result is that this foresighted
father's lucky children have grown up with beautiful, sturdy teeth
which will probably last them all their lives long.

YOUR TEETH, KEYS TO BEAUTY

Your teeth can make or destroy your beauty. They are your
keys to beauty, not only of your face but of your whole person.
Let me tell you why.

Look in your mirror. Smile! A smile lights up the face like the
sun breaking through clouds. Does your smile do that? Or is it
dimmed by teeth that are not white, strong and healthy?

Study the contour of your face, the curve of your cheeks, jawline, chin. Your teeth decide what that contour will be. They are
the architectural framework, the foundation upon which the chin,
the lips and the mouth, the cheeks are dependent. The teeth can
make the lower half of the face beautiful or ugly. They determine
the proportions of the face from brow to jaw. They even influence
the shape of the nose! Many a nose looks too long, not because it
is too long, but because uneven or unfortunately positioned teeth
make the distance from nose to chin too short. Many women
think they need a face-lift, when what they need is repair and
reconstruction of their teeth.

And now look at your eyes, your skin, your figure. If they please
you—if your skin is smooth, your eyes bright, your figure trim—a
good part of the credit must go to your teeth!

It is your teeth that have prepared the food for your good digestion. They have ground it and mixed it and made it ready for the
wonderful chemistry of your digestive system. Your good teeth
have begun the work of turning nutrients into the materials of
beauty. Without strong, healthy teeth, very often the sad results

are indigestion, constipation, and the other digestive ills with all their unfortunate effects on your looks.

For your beauty's sake, have these keys to your beauty looked over and cleaned frequently; take good care of your teeth.

FEED YOUR TEETH

But one truth is unquestioned, and that is that besides the best external care, the health and looks of your teeth depend on good solid nutrition.

The teeth, hard and inert as they seem, are alive. They build themselves and renew themselves with the materials that you give them. Their materials come, as to all other parts of the body, in the blood stream. Like plants, the teeth take their nutrition through their roots. Tiny branches carry these precious molecules of building material through the living core of the tooth, the pulp within its casing of hard enamel, and the cells take what they need for their health.

"If the repair materials supplied to the blood by our daily food is second or third rate, the teeth are rebuilt with shoddy material that deteriorates as surely as a shoddy piece of cloth in a suit deteriorates," says Dr. Fred D. Miller in his very fine book, *Open Door to Health*, a book which I highly recommend to parents.

One of the most widely known facts about the teeth is that they need calcium. The teeth are composed of the hardest substance in the body, calcium phosphate, which is also the hard material of the bones. But here are some curious facts that few people know:

A lack of vitamin A can lead to decay of that hard substance. And a lack of vitamin D means that no matter how rich in calcium your diet may be, the body is unable to absorb and use it, and the badly needed tooth-building material will never get to the teeth at all.

Vitamin C is essential to the production of collagen, the connective tissue that provides the framework for the dentine or bony structure of the teeth. And the bone of your jaw, in which each tooth is implanted, needs its proper supply of calcium and phosphorus like any other bone.

EXERCISE YOUR TEETH

And here is another almost forgotten fact. Your teeth and gums need *exercise*: exercise to strengthen the surrounding tissue and to stimulate the circulation for gums and teeth. This is essential to the health and beauty of all living tissue and your mouth and teeth are no exception.

How does one exercise the teeth? No doubt your dentist told you, when you were still a youngster, how to massage your gums vigorously with your brush, and I hope you still do it conscientiously. Another way to stimulate the circulation of the mouth, gums and teeth is simply to do what your teeth were meant to do: CHEW!

Chewing your food well not only helps your digestion (and your weight: see chapter 9 on reducing). It also brings the blood stream to gums and teeth, and incidentally it brings the cleansing, germ-killing saliva to them as well. By chewing, I mean chewing good solid food like whole grain bread or toast, raw vegetables such as celery and carrot sticks or any of your own favorites.

Perhaps you have seen—and perhaps you have envied—the strong white teeth of primitive men and women. Those people's teeth remained handsome and healthy because they chewed on bones! Emily Post would not have approved. I find that for our more sophisticated ways, any salad with a generous proportion of chopped vegetables is a good substitute. I would also recommend another group of good, nutritious, chewing foods, the various seeds and nuts.

Munching a handful of firm, nutritious seeds not only exercises the teeth but also gives them real nourishment. Try them, all kinds, fresh or lightly toasted: sunflower, pumpkin and other melon seeds, plain or salted.

COSMETIC DENTISTRY

If your teeth are already in trouble, then you cannot chew raw or other solid foods, and the first and best thing for you to do is to find the best dentist in your city.

If you have lost some teeth he can skillfully replace them for you, and if you need a whole denture, a modern dentist can adjust your bite and give you chewing comfort. Cosmetic dentistry has made tremendous advances; today no one needs to know that your teeth are artificial, thanks to a Swiss dentist who introduced new artificial teeth that look transparent and alive.

I am always sad when I see an otherwise lovely face with a bad denture, the teeth evenly divided like so many navy beans. Nothing can make a woman more self-conscious than an obvious or badly fitted denture.

Today, especially in the United States, dentistry has developed splendid solutions to repair the damage done by neglect or inadequate dentistry performed in the past. Teeth may be sturdy and still be unbeautiful if they are crooked, badly spaced, or discolored. I urge you to look into this new kind of dentistry, which combines beautification with skillful engineering that saves teeth for many years and saves your beauty, too.

This is the system of capping the teeth with porcelain jackets lined with platinum alloy. Missing teeth are replaced; broken or injured teeth, badly discolored or misshapen teeth are given a coat of glistening, natural-looking porcelain, shaped to make a beautiful mouth and also to give you a sturdy, comfortable bite.

It is an expensive kind of dentistry. But automobiles and air conditioners and big shiny refrigerators are also expensive. I believe the improvement to your looks, in teeth that truly need this kind of dentistry, is worth more than some highly advertised appliances of modern living. Ask your man whether he would not rather look at a beautiful woman in the parlor than a beautiful refrigerator in the kitchen!

SEE YOUR DENTIST BEFORE YOU ARE BORN!

You young mothers can spare your children many of the tooth agonies you have gone through, by eating intelligently while you are carrying a child. The first months of pregnancy are especially important; during the fourth month the baby teeth are already forming in the gums, and by the time your child is born all twenty of them are there, although he may not show his first tooth until many months afterward. During those first three or four months of pregnancy you yourself can lay the foundation for his good, sturdy

teeth, and by good nutrition for your baby's teeth you also protect
your own.

Lucky babies, born to such wise mothers! And lucky mothers,
too. For wonderful as our American dentists are (and they are
acknowledged to be the best in the world today) there never seem
to be enough of them to repair the damage of tooth decay and
gum disease. It is high time for you smart young mothers to begin
to prevent tooth decay at the very source. Eat correctly while you
are carrying the little rascals! And then, as they grow up with their
handsome strong teeth, they can smile their beautiful smiles and
say, "I saw my dentist before I was born!"

The voice of beauty

Beauty-full foods and beautifying dentistry can transform your
mouth into the gateway to beauty that it should be. But from your
beautiful mouth, what kind of sounds emerge? Your voice is
definitely a part of you.

Perhaps you remember a very funny play about Hollywood
movie-making; "Once In A Lifetime." The regally gowned young
lady floated down a red-carpeted stairway in an aura of grace and
beauty. Then she opened her mouth, and uttered one sentence in
a voice so brassy and shrill that it would have cracked a mirror.
The spell of beauty and mystery was shattered.

I have seen this happen in real life. I have seen good-looking
women, beautifully groomed and gowned, destroy the illusion
they had labored so hard to create, the minute they opened their
mouths.

Did you know you can have wrinkles in your voice, as well as in
your face? Dorothy Uris, speech educator and author of a new
book entitled, *Everybody's Book of Better Speaking*, describes these
"vocal wrinkles." The quavering voice that is usually heard in old
people can come long before the first gray hair. She points out
that American women, with all their care for their appearance, are
shockingly neglectful of their voices.

Your voice is a mirror, but be careful that it does not misrepre-
sent you! It may make you sound older than your years, or like a
retarded child. Worst of all is the whining, complaining, nasal
voice—yet the woman who speaks that way may not be a com-

plainer at all. She simply does not hear herself. Make a record of your voice and listen to yourself. It will tell you the truth about how you sound to others. You may be quite shocked at what you hear.

One of the most attractive speaking voices I know belongs to Jessica Dragonette, a long-time friend and student of mine; many know her as America's "princess of song." She now lectures on singing and speech, and from her I learned some important truths about the voice. Your voice, says Jessica, is as much a part of you as your skin. Your voice is you, showing your depth of feeling or lack of it, your warmth or selfishness. You can improve your voice just as you can improve your skin. Most important, she says, is to put a smile in your voice.

SILENCE IS ALSO BEAUTIFUL

Listening to a lecture by Dr. Spiske, the head physician at Dr. Buchinger's famous clinic in Uberlingen-am-Bodensee, Germany, I learned a new word; he spoke of an ugly disease which is spreading all over the world. He called it *verbalismus*. Talking too much, idle chatter, can become such a waste of life. At times we are all guilty of it, from the housewife who chatters all day and leaves her dishes piled high in her electric kitchen, to the head salesman who can tell endless corny stories. If only we could learn to be silent unless we have something constructive to say, it would be a much more relaxed world to live in, and if ladies with loose tongues would remember to gossip less they would have fewer wrinkles around their mouths.

CHAPTER 16

Beauty in Your Hands

Dr. Charlotte Wolff, the brilliant London psychiatrist, has written an entire book about hands. It is fascinating to learn how much the hands themselves and the way they are used can reveal to the trained observer—more than even the face. We can hide our emotions behind a poker face, but our hands give us away every time.

The hands are always on parade, and their defects cannot be covered by makeup. Also the hands, even more than the face, are constantly exposed to wind, weather and irritants, and in our beauty plan hands also need special attention, both from the inside and from the outside. Whenever I see a woman with a truly beautiful complexion, I usually also find well-cared-for hands. There is nothing surprising about that, since naturally the skin of both face and hands depends upon sound nutrition.

What most women do not realize is that one reason the hands often look older than the face is that the skin of the hands has fewer oil cells than the skin on the face; therefore the skin on the hands dries out much more quickly.

Practically the same nutritional program that I have given for the complexion also helps to keep the hands attractive from the inside, but to counteract the excessive drying effects of detergents and soaps, women must give special outside attention to their hands. First of all, dermatologists tell us that most household tasks could be done with only half as much detergent as women ordinarily use. They also urge women not to neglect entirely the old-fashioned fatty soaps, which are kinder to the hands.

Then, of course, there is one simple, easy outside protection for the hands which is better than many of the fancy lotions. Your grandmother long ago used this simple formula, a combination of rose water and glycerin. Glycerin is the original moisturizer for the skin of the hands. It is hygroscopic, meaning that it has the chemical power to attract moisture from the air.

Another simple remedy, after washing the hands with soap and water, is to help the skin re-establish its normal healthy acid mantle. A few drops of lemon juice massaged into the skin does wonders for hard-working hands; so does a little of any mildly acid lotion, such as Cosmetic Vinegar.

STRONG FINGERNAILS

Most women know today that their fingernails reflect their diet. We must thank the gelatin manufacturers for their campaign persuading women to add more protein to their diet. They have done a splendid job of pointing out the vital connection between food and beauty, especially between protein and the beauty of the nails, but I am amazed to see many women, and a good many physicians, willing to accept such an inadequate protein as gelatin for their beauty magic from within. We know now that we must turn to animal sources for our most complete proteins, that these include all the essential amino acids. But while gelatin is an animal protein, it is not a complete one.

Here is what the *Yearbook of Agriculture 1959*, a United States Government publication, says:

"Gelatin is the only food from an animal source that does not meet the specifications. It contains almost no tryptophane and has very small amounts of threonine, methionine and isoleucine."

If you will look at the list of essential amino acids—by which we mean essential to human metabolism—you will find that these are four of the eight. Gelatin thus ranks as barely more than a fifty percent protein.

Now that we know that the nails need protein, I ask you not to put your faith in gelatin alone, but also to increase your intake of milk, eggs, fish, and lean meat. These contain all the amino acids, the building blocks of new nail tissue, and the results will be quicker and more permanent.

The nails are among the miracles of the human body. Like your hair, they are a specialization of the skin cells, and they are one of the marvels of evolution.

In nature their value is to protect the tips of fingers and toes. To other creatures than man, the nails are quite fearsome weapons, or else they are essential for locomotion. In the cat family and many others they are claws for climbing, and in the grazing animals they have evolved into hard thick hoofs for running over open ground.

On your hands your nails are not only useful but esthetic. Deep under the cuticle, the special cells of the nail bed assemble the materials for the smooth, transparent, firm and yet flexible substance of the nails. You can see part of that growing area, the pale half-moon that adds its own touch of natural beauty to your fingertips.

WHAT YOUR NAILS REVEAL

Nails are peculiarly sensitive to your general body condition. To some extent the sturdiness of nails, like that of teeth and hair, is inherited. But every physician knows that the nails can tell a great deal about his patient's general health. English physicians during the First World War found that they could tell the date of a man's wound with surprising accuracy, just by looking at his nails. Wanda, the famous Hollywood fortune teller at the Assistance League, confided to me that when she tells a film celebrity about a recent illness, she is not guessing, nor does she have to depend upon that mysterious gift we call second sight. She only has to look at her client's nails!

The nails grow slowly, an average of .119 millimeters a day, the merest fraction of an inch. Dr. William Bennett Bean, who kept track of his own nails for ten years and reported his findings in the *Journal of Investigative Dermatology*, found that when he had the mumps his nails stopped growing altogether for the duration of his illness. He also reported that the nails of malnourished children grow much more slowly than those of well-nourished ones.

Those little factories deep in the nail bed need their full supplies of high-quality proteins, and of calcium for the hardness of your nails, as well as all the vitamins and minerals essential to efficient body metabolism. You cannot expect your nail cells to turn out a sound and beautiful product without sound and beauty-full building materials!

Nourish these nail factories well; give them the complete proteins, never less than 75 grams a day; be generous also with the vitamin and mineral-rich foods, especially calcium and the vitamin B complex. Then, and only then, can you expect to have healthy, good-looking nails, clear and transparent, without ridges or scars.

CIRCULATION FOR THE HANDS

A few years ago in Hollywood, a Frenchwoman whose professional name was Juliette opened a salon devoted entirely to the beauty of the hands. This woman had studied anatomy and nutrition and knew what she was talking about. She instructed her clients, among whom were most of the important movie stars, to double their protein intake for sixty to ninety days. She also recommended calcium tablets with vitamin D.

Her final innovation was to begin her hand care with a massage, starting at the elbow, working down toward the nails, kneading and pressing until the fingertips were tingling with increased circulation. Only then would she give her manicure, ending with the application of her famous wax and nail colors.

OUTSIDE HAND CARE

Well-nourished nails are great time-savers; they actually take very little care beyond filing the tips and keeping the cuticle neat. Healthy nails also take and hold nail colors much longer than problem nails. Do your inside beautifying job first: make your nails good and strong with the Cosmetic Diet, and then and then only, spend your money for manicures.

Every woman should know that her nails need an occasional vacation from makeup. On one of the California beautyfarms, nail polish is removed on arrival and stays removed during the entire stay. This gives the nail tissue a chance to breathe. During this time the warm oil treatment is applied, for oil is as good for the nails as it is for the hair. Here is the treatment: simply warm up half a cup of salad oil, the same oil that you use in salad dressings and in cooking, and soak the nails for five minutes in this warm oil bath. Then gently massage oil into the nail roots; wash the hands and finish, as you always should, by rubbing in a few drops of lemon juice or a bit of Cosmetic Vinegar.

BEAUTY IS AS BEAUTY DOES

And while we are speaking of the beauty of your hands, let me add one word about how you use them. Like your face, your eyes, your voice, your hands are part of the language by which you express the essential you. They, too, are your ambassadors to the world. If they are restless and fidgety, if they clutch each other tightly when they should lie soft and relaxed, above all if they are nail-bitten or cuticle-plucked, they reveal a tense, anxious, self-conscious you instead of the poised, attractive person you would like to be.

No woman need ever regret that her work makes impossible those excessively long, conspicuously colored fingernails. They may be advertised as high fashion, but they are not necessarily beautiful. They tell the world only that they are useless hands, incapable of such good tasks as cooking, cleaning, gardening, sewing or typing or playing the piano! Human hands are beautiful for their strength and skill. Make your smooth, well-cared-for hands an expression of your real self.

CHAPTER 17

Pedestals of Beauty: Your Feet

It is no use to talk of beauty of the body, or even of the face, without talking of the feet.

The feet are the pedestals of beauty. Your posture, your contours and proportions, your grace of movement all depend, finally, on your feet.

And your face depends upon your feet! You do not need me to describe for you the look of strain, of misery, of a woman whose feet hurt.

I know I am talking to myself when I ask you to give up your pretty shoes, but at least you can make the reasonable compromise of wearing intelligent shoes during the day, and save your pretties for the evening.

30,000 STEPS A DAY

The human foot is one of the most remarkable structures in nature. Remember, it is the support of a two-legged creature. Unlike the paw or pad or hoof of a four-legged animal, each foot must bear and balance the entire weight of its owner in every step he takes, and that means thousands of steps each day. A normal active child takes 30,000 steps a day. How many steps do you take, on those long-suffering feet of yours?

Let me tell you about the beauty of your feet. The foot is a marvel of engineering. It is a structure of 52 bones and 214 ligaments. Each bone individually is small, delicate, fragile. Each ligament is a thin thread of connective tissue. The muscles of the feet are slender bundles of muscle fibers. The skin of the feet is so thin as to be nearly transparent, except for the sole, which is specially adapted for friction with the ground. It is thickened and it is also ridged, a perfect non-skid surface. It is padded with cushions of tissue at heel, toes, and metatarsals to protect the fine bones and joints from impact with the ground.

This perfect structure was adapted to run bare on soft earth, to grip rocky surfaces, to balance on slopes and steep inclines. And what have we done to it? We have encased it in constricting footwear and made it walk on hard floors and pavements.

FREE THESE POOR PRISONERS!

Those pointed toes that cramp and crush the tender bones and distort the fine flexible joints! Those high heels, that throw your weight all forward on the delicate metatarsal arch that was never meant to bear it. Those needle-thin stiletto heels!

An English study tells us that a girl weighing 112 pounds, wearing stiletto heels, hits the floor with a pressure of one ton per square inch each time she takes a step. A man weighing 224 pounds in ordinary shoes exerts only 28 pounds of pressure per square inch when he walks.

If you could see yourself walking in such shoes, you would know what they do to your posture and your body's natural grace of movement. If you have ever caught a glimpse of your face at the end of a shopping trip in such shoes, you would realize what the strain does to your looks.

But you do not need to ask your mirror what these shoes do to your feet. Your feet tell you, by their excruciating agony. They tell you by the corns, the calluses, the distortions that end, in many cases, by virtually crippling their owner for the rest of her life, just like the Chinese women of the past.

"Sittin' shoes" are for sittin'

My Southern women friends call these shoes their "sittin' shoes." They do not expect to walk in them. But in our big cities I see women of all ages, sizes, weights, staggering along the streets in those impossible shoes. If they could see themselves, especially from the back!

For going out, for dancing, be pretty, be foolish, wear your stiletto heels and pointed toes. Save your "sittin' shoes" for frivolity.

But save your feet, your precious irreplaceable feet, for well-being and beauty. For daytime, for working around the house, marketing, going out with the children, wear shoes shaped to your feet, flexible, soft, roomy to give those toes the movement they crave when you walk. And be sure to have heels of the right height for your proper balance.

The new, improved Space Shoes, as they are so rightly called, are like gloves on your feet, with space where it is needed and support where it is needed. They restore those sad, misused, abused feet to normal functioning and comfort. And the benefit to your beauty is incalculable.

I have heard women say these shoes are ugly. I do not agree. They are no stranger looking than those so-called "pretty shoes" on pitiful suffering feet. I know elegant women who wear their Space Shoes with tweedy skirts and sweaters and country style suits, and I see these shoes often on shipboard and in European resorts. These smart women do not feel they are making any sacrifice of their good looks. On the contrary, the fine carriage and graceful walk of a well-shod woman is a tremendous *plus* to her good looks. And what it does for her face, in removing the lines of strain and pain, I hardly need to tell you.

I know these shoes are expensive. For those who can afford them, I consider them a highly worthwhile investment in good looks, good health, and good temper.

And here is great news, in tune with our do-it-yourself days: Alan E. Murray, who invented these shoes, has now made a do-it-yourself kit. You can make your own, with no special shoe-maker's skill, at a fraction of the cost. I urge you to make yourself a pair of Space Shoes and enjoy this comparatively inexpensive adventure in saving and restoring your feet.

FOOT TREATS

The good nutrition for your good looks, in the Cosmetic Diet, will automatically do two important things for your feet. It will feed those fine bones and muscles and springy cartilages, and thus strengthen and beautify the feet. And by relieving you of extra pounds it will lighten their burden. With exercise and your improved circulation and muscle tone, you will give your body the springiness in movement that will make it not a dead weight on your feet, but a partner to them. Every muscle in your body will help your feet to carry you with ease and grace. With your new contours and your new posture you will actually be lighter on your feet, even if you do not lose an ounce.

In proper shoes, every step you take is a strength-building, circulation-stimulating exercise for the feet. But here is a special foot treat:

Walk barefoot on sand or on grass. In Europe there is an old tradition that walking barefoot in the grass with the cool dew still on it brings magic benefit to the feet, and once I actually saw a group of nuns doing this. They were walking barefoot on a dewy lawn, a perfect picture of grace and peace. Whether or not there is any magic in the dew, I can assure you that its cool moisture and the softness of the grass together will give your feet a refreshing treat that is like magic, and it will do the same for your spirit.

Here is a quick foot muscle toner, given to me by a French ballerina; I know of none better, and it takes only a few moments to do. Run cold water, as cold as possible, into the tub to a depth of a few inches, so that when you stand in it it will come just to the curve of your calf. Now, steadying yourself with one hand on a bar or the wall, stand in the tub and rise on your toes, as high as you can, then down again. Do this twenty times, morning and evening. You will find it wonderfully strengthening and stimulating to those hard-working foot muscles that must carry you about all day.

Most important, give your feet a long holiday from spike shoes. In good shoes your feet will shed their corns and calluses and regain their strength and springiness. Save your pretty shoes for fun, and you will have pretty feet to put them on.

CHAPTER 18

Your Beauty Sleep

Here is a surprising discovery about sleep that has come out of the sleep laboratory of Dr. Nathaniel L. Kleitman of the University of Chicago:

The body needs only rest. *It is the brain that needs sleep.*

We now have proof that the body can go without sleep for prolonged periods, and not suffer any damage. Dr. Kleitman, who holds the world's record for intentional sleeplessness, has made himself the guinea pig for many stay-awake experiments. Once he went longer than 200 hours—nearly nine days and nights.

And what happened to Dr. Kleitman physically? Nothing very much. His heart rate, blood pressure, and red blood count remained normal. He did not even lose weight!

The one body system that gives way is the nervous system. The eyes see double, movements become uncoordinated and fumbling, the temper becomes touchy and irritable, and eventually all judgment and self-control and grasp of reality are lost.

Now do you see why loss of sleep, or unrestful sleep, is so devastating to your looks? The weary, uncertain brain and nervous system, struggling to perform the day's tasks, trace those lines of tension and strain on your face. Touchiness, irritability draw those expressive muscles taut around the eyes, nose and mouth. And when sleep-cheating is habitual, the ugly lines become permanent, the muscles become fixed in the expressions of tension, strain, and irritability.

I tell you this first, and I consider it so important, because it may help to free you from one of the biggest causes of sleeplessness, and that is fear. Fear of losing sleep, fear of the harm that losing sleep can do to health, is what keeps so many people from sleeping.

Scientists assure us that muscles, senses and the body in general all recover from fatigue merely by resting. So as you lie awake, remember that your body is resting and recovering from its fatigue, and instead of worrying about how you will feel the next day you can lie and think your pleasantest thoughts. And then, believe it or not, you will probably find yourself drifting gently off to sleep again.

For this is the second exciting bit of news: *it is the body that puts the mind to sleep!*

How to go to sleep

Here is how we actually fall asleep. While we are awake, messages are constantly going back and forth between the brain and the body. The tension of each muscle, the changing sensations on the skin, sounds and sights and smells are telegraphed to the brain, and the brain sends out its messages to the muscles to perform movements. When the messages from the body slow down, the return messages from the brain also slow down.

As one scientist explained it, this process of falling asleep is like the dwindling conversation between two sleepy people. When the body and mind stop talking to each other you are asleep.

The customary way of going to bed in leisurely fashion helps the body to put the mind to sleep. By lying down, you invite your muscles to relax. By darkening the room and closing your eyes, you shut down the communications from the sense of sight. By covering your body you protect the skin from exposure to cold or other disturbing sensations that would alert the brain.

A quiet room helps to cut down the messages from the ears to the brain. Perhaps your room cannot be absolutely quiet—few of us enjoy that luxury. But if the sounds that come to your ears are familiar and monotonous ones, your brain can ignore them. That is why city folk sleep through traffic noises, and country folk are not disturbed by the ordinary night sounds of rustling trees and shrill insects. If you are used to them, these are actually soothing sounds.

But the most important part of this preparation for sleep is the relaxation of your muscles. When the muscles are tense, they continue to send wakeful messages to the brain, and the brain continues to answer them. And so the restless chattering of the nerves keeps on, like a broken record that keeps playing over and over again to no purpose.

Once you learn to relax your muscles, the messages slow down, and at last they stop. The phonograph stops playing. Your brain can drift blissfully into gentle, restful sleep.

LEAVE TENSIONS BEHIND

Well-nourished muscles that are healthily fatigued will relax of their own accord the minute you let go and relax. But the stresses and strains of some women's jobs accumulate to such a degree that they do not relax but instead take their tensions to bed with them.

If you are one of those, then for heaven's sake learn to relax your muscles. Never, never forget that relaxing muscles gradually put your mind to sleep. When body and mind stop talking to each other, you *are* asleep.

When you lie down on your bed, your muscles do not relax all at once. They let go in stages, first the large muscles of the torso and limbs, then the smaller muscles of the hands and feet, and finally the very fine muscles of the face, around the mouth and eyes, lastly the eyelids. The face of a woman in healthy deep sleep is one of repose, without tension lines.

You can consciously persuade your muscles to relax. Two of my favorite methods I have already given you for relaxing during the day; these are also excellent for preparing you for a good night's sleep. One of these is to stretch out on the beauty board, as they do on beautyfarms, ten to fifteen minutes with your feet elevated above your head. This can do wonders with the least amount of effort on your part. It relaxes legs, trunk, and indeed the entire body.

The other, also an easy one, is the Swing, Sway and Slump

method: stand loosely with your feet apart and your hands hanging, and swing your body slowly and easily, left, right, left, right (see Chapter 7). Do this fifty to one hundred times, and you will slip into bed ready for a deep sound sleep.

Once in bed, your body does the rest; it has excellent natural ways to relax. One of them is the yawn, the deep, deep breath that expands the rib cage as wide as possible, and then expels the breath. With the end of the yawn, all the muscles of the torso let go, and that is the beginning of the body's normal relaxing sequence.

The impulse to yawn and stretch is very infectious. After a while all you have to do is *think* of the words, and you will find yourself performing the acts.

LET WORRIES WAIT FOR TOMORROW

You can teach your mind good behavior at bedtime. Many great minds have perfected the art of going to sleep at will. Winston Churchill could do this when he was Great Britain's leader during World War II. In the midst of his country's most terrible ordeals, even if he had as little as ten minutes to spare during a day of desperate planning and conferences, he would undress completely and get into bed. There he emptied his mind of his many weighty problems, and went instantly and deeply asleep. When he woke he was thoroughly refreshed and ready to take up his burdens again. To this day he naps every afternoon.

Don't be the slave of your anxieties at bedtime. Put them off until morning. This is when procrastination is not a thief of time, but a friend of sleep. Remember the motto of Scarlett O'Hara, the heroine of *Gone With The Wind*. When a troubling thought came to her mind she would say, "I'll worry about that tomorrow."

LET'S LOOK AT YOUR BED

If the face you see in the mirror each morning is tired and unrefreshed, then I ask you to turn from your mirror and look instead at your bed. What do you see?

It is unbelievable how many people sleep in a bed that is too soft or too hard, too short or too narrow, a bed that sags in the middle or one that is bumpy, or a bed that creaks and groans each time the sleeper moves.

We all move about when we sleep. We change position thirty or forty times a night. And this is not restless sleep—on the contrary, it is the most restful. To sleep literally "like a log," never moving all through the night, would leave muscles cramped and limbs numb from lack of circulation. A good bed must allow room for moving, and it must provide even support throughout, wherever the heaviest parts of the body happen to lie.

Here are the four vital points at which the body needs support for beautiful sleep: the neck, trunk, pelvis and legs. If a bed is uneven, hard in some places, soft in others, sagging at center or sides, some muscles in the body are never able to relax completely, whatever position the body assumes.

And while you are looking at beds, look at your husband's bed, and those of your children. Even a good bed may be too small. Americans have been growing larger with each generation—there were 35 percent more six-footers in the Second World War than in the First! Yet beds are still made in the standard length of 75 inches. For deep sleep, a bed should be six inches longer than its occupant. The average single bed is at least three inches too narrow for an adult sleeper.

ONE-MINUTE TEST FOR A GOOD BED

A firm mattress is better than a soft one. The bed board—a slab placed between mattress and spring, which physicians advise for people suffering from back ailments—has come into use with many people who have nothing wrong with their backs but who find that they sleep better on a bed that gives them firm support. The bed board gives them at a modest cost many of the same benefits as so-called "orthopedic" mattresses which are constructed to prevent sagging in the center and on the sides. If you can't afford a new mattress, at least get a fiber board and slip it between mattress and spring.

A mattress is now available with a fiber board built in between two layers of coils. Another mattress is kept firm by resilient steel supports around all four edges. The designer Henry Dreyfuss predicts that beds will eventually be made with button controls by which the sleeper can adjust the mattress to just the degree of hardness or softness that he prefers.

That bed of the future is still to come; in the meantime, make yours as comfortable as possible. There are already dozens of devices for luxurious sleeping. I suppose the original Eve slept on a bed of leaves in a hollow scooped out of the ground. But you modern Eves can have your choice of a mattress that rises up under your head or your knees at the touch of a button, even one that oscillates and rocks you to sleep. A good bed, one that will give you restful sleep, is no luxury but a necessity. Here is a thirty-second test for a good bed—try it now, on your bed and your husband's and children's beds:

Do you lie *in* the bed, or *on* it? If you lie *in* it, sinking in so that your spine curves, it is a *bad* bed, and make no mistake about it. If you lie *on* it, then it supports all your vital points which should be supported, and it is a good bed if it is also large enough and without bumps.

Try this test in the shop before you buy a new bed, mattress, or spring.

What kind of pillow?

Once you are on your comfortable bed, find the position that is most restful for you. Stretch out your whole body; let the arms lie idly on either side; do not cross your arms or hold them over your head for any length of time; this prevents even circulation. Above all, do not have any thick pillows under your head. They interfere with circulation throughout the head, and more than anything they are responsible for wrinkles around the neck and double chins.

Actually only the smallest pillow is needed for the head. Some fastidious ladies carry their own small "anti-double-chin" pillow in all their travels, and on some beautyfarms, little, fat pillows are used which fit under the neck. This keeps neck and chin in perfect position.

If no such pillow is around, simply make a roll out of a small bath towel and put it under the back of your neck. There is no question but that placing your face in an awkward position and lying on the same side of your face, year after year, can cause a flattening of certain muscles and change your facial contour. See if you have deep wrinkles and folds when you awaken. If so, get a small pillow and stop sleeping in a cramped position.

SLEEPWEAR

I am all for the Bikini bathing suits. The skimpiest and most elegant ones I saw in St. Tropez, on the Riviera. Now I wish some designer would design the briefest and most comfortable sleepwear. The less you wear while sleeping, the more fresh air can caress those millions of pores of your skin, and let them breathe. The less you wear when sleeping during the warm days, the more rested you will look and feel next morning. Some have suggested that we should sleep in the "raw." That, I believe, is all right for those who sleep alone. However, it is not very esthetic unless you look like Princess Grace.

FOODS FOR TRANQUILITY AND SLEEP

I might well have begun this chapter on sleep with nutrition, because a well-nourished, relaxed body goes to sleep without difficulty, but I was anxious to bring you the new things from the sleep laboratories to remove your fear of not sleeping. Now let us see what food can do to promote your beauty sleep.

Sleeping pills will not give this kind of natural, restorative sleep. Doctors prescribe sleeping pills in times of emergency or special situations when this temporary aid is needed. But countless women, I grieve to say, come to depend upon drugs for what should be natural wholesome rest, and they demand renewed prescriptions from their doctors.

This is a crime, indeed a sin, against their good looks, when good sleep is so easily within their reach!

Taking something light to eat or drink at bedtime is the time-honored aid to good sleep. There are sound physiological reasons for this. One of them is that food in the stomach sets the digestive processes in action, and the circulatory system automatically sends more blood to the digestive organs and less to the muscles. Almost everyone has had the experience of feeling sleepy after a meal.

A great many foods that are part of a wholesome diet contribute to the healthy relaxation of muscle and nerve, but three are especially valuable. These are vitamin B-6, calcium and vitamin D. Foods especially rich in these are my favorite tranquility foods.

Vitamin B-6 appears to be a specific sedative for twitchy nerves. There is, in fact, a close connection between the entire vitamin B group and the health of the nerves, and since the B vitamins are best taken as a group, called the vitamin B complex, all foods high in B vitamins are good tranquility and sleep-producing foods. These include our old friends, food yeast, wheat germ, unsulphured molasses.

A lack of calcium may be one of the hidden causes of insomnia, and this is completely unnecessary in the face of our abundance of calcium-rich foods like milk, cheese, yogurt, very fine bone flour, and so many more. Plain hot milk is a potent tranquilizer at bedtime.

Vitamin D, the sunshine vitamin, is essential to the body's ability to absorb and use calcium. This vitamin is formed in the skin when exposed to sunshine; as a food it exists naturally only in certain fish and in caviar. When did you last eat caviar? Better and more reliable sources of this vitamin are irradiated or vitamin D milk, and cod liver oil capsules or concentrates.

Sleep is Nature's sweet restorer. Never forget that it is during sleep, the blessed state of physiological unconsciousness, that your mind and nerves, masters of your whole bodyhouse, re-charge and rebuild themselves.

Remember how the wise Dr. Carrel expressed it, "And the body does it all in silence." It will not do much good, I know, but I repeat, real beauty sleep is the "early to bed" kind; it is during the magic hours of the night that all nature rests and takes a breather. During this period throughout nature, the miracle of being reborn takes place. How often we lucky people with gardens observe that stalks shoot up, buds burst wide open overnight! All nature and all animal life takes its beauty sleep early and at the first peep of dawn, they awaken lustily and gratefully to welcome the rising sun.

MENTAL COCKTAILS

Some approach life as lovers and others as accountants. You have heard me say this before, but I believe it bears repeating. So much of the beauty of really beautiful people comes from their vitality of spirit, their love of life! Yet there are times when all of us feel the need of a lift when things do not go as we wanted them to; when we are disappointed in people, or when we are tired and our work and responsibilities seem heavier than usual. At such times we all need a new source of courage and spiritual energy.

Many good women of the past, in times of difficulties and when life was at low tide, would go to their Bible for new hope and inspiration and when we were young and immature we used to smile at such simple faith, but today Dr. Carl Gustav Jung, the wise patriarch of Zurich, reassures us that those blessed with a great faith are indeed the fortunate ones. Dr. Jung in his big practice discovered that those blessed with faith even recover more readily from their ills than those who have none.

Dr. E. Jacobson of Chicago has written many fine books about the power of mental images. If we can replace the mental image of the thing that worries us with the image of something happy, beautiful, serene, then we have gained release from anxiety and with such release and refreshment, we are able to tackle our problems. *I believe you can banish the blues by consciously, deliberately turning a switch in your mind from unpleasant to pleasant thoughts. I know this can be done for I have done it a thousand times and so have many of my students.*

Reader's Digest, a few years ago, reprinted my "Mental Cocktails," as I call them—a collection of inspiring thoughts by people who faced the same problems we face today. I have my own personal mental cocktail book. It is a small, worn leather-covered album in which I have written and pasted helpful thoughts from the Good Book, philosophers and poets, also extracts from letters of friends and dear ones.

You can have your own book of mental cocktails. It is a special recipe book that you can begin to write any time, and consult any time. You can learn to choose your spiritual food as you now choose the food for your body. It is probably more difficult, but it can be done.

To get you started, let me share with you some of my own mental cocktails from my little book, which is always on my bed table:

When sleep doesn't come readily:

> If slumber should forsake
> Thy pillow in the dark,
> Fret not thyself to make
> How long thou liest awake.
> There is a better way:
> Let go the strife and strain,
> Thine eyes will close again
> If thou will only pray.
> Lord, Thy peaceful gift restore
> Give my body sleep once more:
> While I wait my soul will rest
> Like a child upon Thy breast.
>   *Henry van Dyke.*

If you are worried:

> If, when you look into your own heart,
> You find nothing wrong there,
> What is there to worry about,
> What is there to fear?
>   *Confucius.*

If you have regrets:

> Finish each day and be done with it—
> You have done what you could.
> Some blunders and absurdities no doubt crept in;
> Forget them as soon as you can.
> Tomorrow is a new day;
> You shall begin it well and serenely.
>   *Ralph Waldo Emerson.*

We are the builders:

> Every man is the builder of the temple called his body—
> We are all sculptors and painters,
> And our material is our own flesh and blood and bones.
> Any nobleness begins at once to refine one's features.
>   *Henry David Thoreau.*

My favorite:

Lift mine eyes from the earth and let me
Not forget the uses of the stars.

Forbid that I should judge others,
Lest I condemn myself.
Let me not follow the clamour of the world,
But walk quietly in my path.
Give me a few friends who will love me for what I am,
And keep ever burning before my vagrant steps
The kindly light of hope.
And, though I come not within sight of the castle of my dreams,
Teach me still to be thankful for life,
For time's olden memories that are good and sweet;
And may the evening's twilight find me gentle still.

Max Ehrmann.

For the pain that is hard to bear; the loss of a loved one: Remember,

What you love *eternally*,
Is *eternally* yours.

And here are the wise words from Dr. Albert Schweitzer, one of the great men of our time:

Sometimes our light goes out,
But is blown again into flame
By an encounter with another human being.
Each of us owes the deepest thanks
To those who have rekindled this inner light.

Perhaps you can rekindle the light for someone by passing along the recipes from *your* book of mental cocktails that have lifted your spirit.

There is a very old, but very true Chinese saying:

Better to light one candle,
Than to complain of the darkness!

CHAPTER 19

Exquisite Cleanliness

Hygeia, the daughter of Aesculapius, was also the Goddess of Health, and for centuries Hygeia has been the symbol of physical perfection and beauty through personal hygiene, which above all means exquisite cleanliness of body, inside and outside. To my mind, there is no greater enemy to a woman's happiness and good looks than internal uncleanliness, or constipation, as that ugly word describes it.

Dr. Charlotte West, in her famous book, *Ageless Youth* says: "Constipation is probably so little heeded because it rarely gives rise to actual pain; it does give rise to a vast amount of physical discomfort, however, and what should interest us most is the health and beauty defects resulting from constipation. These often cause genuine unhappiness. Who can be attractive with an offensive breath, a malodorous body, a muddy skin, dull eyes, a listless manner and dullness of mind?" Then Dr. West goes on to blame the overrefined, "empty" foods, too little exercise—especially walking—and modern labor-saving devices which relieve women of physical work, but also prevent the development of firm abdominal muscle tone.

I could not possibly write a book on beauty without saying that a healthy intestinal tract, which empties itself at regular intervals, is of greatest importance not only for a radiant complexion, but for your whole beauty ensemble. The best way to banish this evil forever is to apply all the methods which science has given us.

If you are one of the unfortunate ones who have suffered from constipation for a long time, you should first of all have your doctor give you a thorough examination to make sure that there is nothing organically wrong with your digestive apparatus. No doubt, your doctor will recommend more bulky diet which you must be sure to follow. You will also have to learn to use more vitamin-rich and protein-rich foods to create the right medium for a strong and healthy intestinal life. Remember there are millions of beauty-promoting bacteria living at all times in your intestines, but there are also many harmful bacteria which multiply fast, cause putrefaction, rumbling, and unlimited amounts of gas, chiefly because of a vitamin, protein and bulk-poor diet.

Simple people in the Balkans knew this instinctively and always included sour milks and black bread in all their meals, and I was amazed that nutritionists like Dr. Menshikov in Moscow insist that Russians go back to their old habits and make sour milk, kumiss, yogurt, curds (lean cottage cheese) and their black bread a part of every meal. These humble foods are the most natural and wonderful foods for feeding the friendly bacteria in the twenty-eight foot intestinal tract, and also the best foods for overcoming beauty's Enemy No. 1, the incomplete elimination of waste products. This is the laziest and easiest way. There are others:

A CLASSIC EXAMPLE

At the famous Mayo Clinic they fed a group of volunteers the foods which usually are served at American homes. Meals consisted of white bread, beef, cornflakes, potatoes, rice, sugar, skim milk, cheese, butter, gelatin, canned fruits and vegetables, cocoa and coffee. All these foods are miserably low in vitamin B-1, and promptly all of these volunteers became irritable, quarrelsome, depressed and sluggish. Some developed extreme tiredness, sleeplessness and, what is of greatest interest in this lesson, on this diet which millions of Americans eat every day, all those volunteers became constipated. By the twenty-first week, bad headaches and vomiting began and the experiment had to be stopped. Within a few hours after these volunteers were given vitamin B-1, they became cheerful and lost their tiredness, and all the other symptoms disappeared one by one. This should prove to you how important vitamin B-1 is to normal elimination.

NATURAL LAXATIVE FOODS

Food Yeast is a natural beauty laxative because it is so rich in B vitamins. By all means add a teaspoon of good-tasting food yeast to fruit juice, tomato juice, milk and other beverages. Use it daily and be generous with it.

Dark Molasses is one of the finest natural laxatives of all times, as our grandmothers knew. Their favorite complexion cocktail was old-fashioned molasses and sulphur. We no longer need to take this evil-tasting combination; the sulphur we get in young radishes, celery and green peppers, and the molasses, the darkest you can buy, can be mixed with all sorts of foods and used in place of empty white sugar.

Honey is another beauty laxative. It is so mild that pediatricians recommend it for babies. An interesting combination of honey and molasses, half and half, provides the vitamins and iron richness of molasses with the gentle mildness of honey. Thousands of my students enthusiastically use this honey-lass combination for all sweetening purposes.

Yogurt, besides being a delicious food, is also very helpful in cases of faulty elimination. The bacteria in this cultured milk utilize the sugar in milk and convert it into beneficial lactic acid. Milk sugar also helps to make soft bulky stools which are passed with great facility. The friendly bacteria of yogurt also synthesize the B vitamins so important to good elimination.

Wheat Germ is by far the most valuable of all cereals for its vitamin B and protein content and is also a beauty laxative par excellence. When you use the fresh and vital kind, available in paper bags from your health food store, such "live" wheat germ, sprinkled freely on your morning cereal or into fruit juice, makes a fine self-starter for lazy bowels.

Quick Salt Water Flush. This efficient flush is recommended by Dr. E. V. McCollum of Johns Hopkins, and also by Dr. Victor Heiser, author of *An American Doctor's Odyssey*. Simply add two rounded teaspoons of salt to a quart of very warm water and drink the whole quart on an empty stomach the first thing in the morning. In about thirty minutes a copious flushing will result. Be sure not to eat breakfast until after you have flushed. For a more pleasant-tasting quick flush, many of my students put three level teaspoons of vegetable salt into a quart of very warm water and drink the entire quart. Such a flushing taken occasionally, is harmless and thousands swear by it. It should not be taken habitually because the water-soluble vitamins are also flushed away.

Natural Herbs. Following a highly nutritious diet, such as the Cosmetic Diet, should automatically banish constipation. The ideal way is to get along without any special help, but for those who for some reason are not eating intelligently and, therefore, suffer from occasional constipation, instead of synthetic laxative pills, I recommend a combination of dried, natural herbs which I discovered in Switzerland. It is as natural a formula as I could find and is made up of 17 crushed herbs. Thousands of pounds of these herbs were formerly imported into this country, but since this formula became such a phenomenal success, it is now made here. So, if you must use a laxative occasionally, try this Swiss formula. It is obtainable at all health and diet shops and some drug stores. On one of the chic beautyfarms they make a laxative tea and serve it before retiring. They coyly call it "ladies' tea," but it is nothing else but a brew made with Swiss Kriss herbs. For my favorite beautyfarm laxative, follow the recipe for California fruit balls on page 341.

Permanently overcoming faulty elimination is entirely possible. Be patient, re-read these recommendations and follow the Cosmetic Diet. Be sure to be generous with the B family vitamins, especially in food yeast and fresh wheat germ. Also, make use of dark molasses and that custard-like food, yogurt. If you cannot obtain wholesome whole grain bread, learn to make your own. It is news to most Americans, but the black bread which the terrifyingly vital Russians eat daily, contains, believe it or not, black molasses!

Part Four

AT HOME WITH BEAUTY

CHAPTER 20

The Family Dinner Table

You probably wonder why I want to talk to you about your family in a book on beauty. I feel that I must because some of the greatest handicaps to beauty are the many tensions, anxieties, and needless arguments within families.

Only in a tranquil, happy home and in a climate of family love can a woman's beauty blossom and thrive.

Just for curiosity's sake, let us assess the climate in an American home today. Let me demonstrate what television shows us as happening at a family dinner.

Father arrives.

MOTHER: Oh, there you are. Sorry, dear, but Junior has to go to a club meeting, so we started.

Father sits down.

FATHER: Where is Mary?

MOTHER: She and some of the kids went to a movie; they said they'd have supper at a drive-in.

Junior rises.

FATHER: Where are you going, son? I haven't had a chance to exchange a word with you. Besides, you haven't finished your food. I don't like you rushing off like that.

Junior looks at Mother; Mother winks reassuringly.

MOTHER to Father: Never mind, dear, he's in a rush. (*Turning
   to Junior*) Run along, dear.
   Mother rises.
FATHER: Where are *you* going?
MOTHER: Sorry, dear, I better take Janie up to bed—she's had a
   slight cold coming on.
   Mother and Baby disappear.
   Father left alone at the table—closeup of his perplexed face.
   Everyone laughs.

Perhaps you think this is an exaggeration. Maybe this does not
happen in your home. I sincerely hope not. But I did not invent
this. It is a scene from a popular weekly television show I saw
recently at the house of friends. It was not intended as an attack
on the American home. It was advertised as a heart-warming family
comedy and it was meant to make the audience laugh. It is ironic,
but it should give us pause.

No wonder we have such a divorce rate; no wonder we have so
many delinquents; no wonder we have the high incidence of mental
illness.

A great deal of the blame can be traced back to these restless
family dinners.

In the scene just narrated, father seems to be the principal
loser. But actually it is the mother who is the real loser, and when
mother has lost something, the whole family suffers.

I cannot help but look back into the carefree days of my own
childhood. I remember my father at the head of a big oval oak
table, and my mother ladling soup from the huge tureen, while
we five boys and five girls sat quietly in our places. My mother was
a wise woman; before eating she always created an atmosphere of
peace and quiet by folding her hands and saying Grace.

I remember that atmosphere of warm security that nourished us,
a nourishment no less important to us growing childern than the
fragrant, wholesome soup.

We can never turn the clock back, but something good has been
lost when the whole family can no longer sit down and enjoy
"breaking bread" together. I believe this must be regained; I
believe that when American women see how much they have lost,
they will address their minds to regaining it.

ARE YOU A DP?

I am sorry to say that many American women are displaced persons. The exploding American home has stripped them of so many of their functions that they are no longer sure of their status and dignity. They hardly know where they belong or what is expected of them. They show it in their anxious, harried faces. That is not the way to beauty.

As a recent writer observed, "American women have gained control over half the national income, but in the process they have lost control over their homes and children."

I will not join the throng who are so quick to blame the American woman for everything that is wrong with life. This busy rich land is so full of ready-made entertainments and activities, so occupied with comings and goings, that it is hard for the home to hold its own against all the distractions. It takes a woman of clear vision, who knows what is at stake for her and for her family, to put up the barricades and keep her family life from disintegrating before her eyes.

There are such women; perhaps you, reading this book, can count yourself one of them. Perhaps your children actually prefer to come home to dinner, despite the many other deceptive temptations, because dinner at home is a happy occasion and you have taught them good manners, the kind of manners that grow out of love and consideration for each other.

And this I urge strongly: put Father back at the head of the table. The most advanced psychoanalyst would tell you that children need to rely on the strength and authority of a father—strength to protect them, and authority to set limits to their liberty and keep them from getting into trouble.

Child psychologists today advise parents that harshness is not necessary, but firmness is as necessary as it ever was. Here is the way Dr. Richard E. Wolf, a pediatrician and a father, described the father's role in his article, "Being a Father Today," in the *Encyclopedia of Child Care and Guidance:*

"A child needs both Father and Mother, and he needs them to be different. To a boy and girl a father represents a man's strength and wisdom, his knowledge of the world and its workings, his judgment based on experience outside the home. They need to hear his voice in family decisions as well as their mother's. They need to see in him the protector and provider for Mother and children. From him they take their model of manhood, and from him they learn an attitude toward women. If mothers do all the managing while fathers sit by, both girls and boys may suffer a confusion about their own status which will handicap them in their relationships as they grow up."

Our overfed and undernourished children

There must surely be something wrong with the dinner on the table when we read reports of the poor health and especially the poor nutrition of our young people today. How is it possible, in this land of plenty?

A few years ago, after a ten-year study of 2,536 boys and girls between the ages of thirteen and twenty, Dr. Pauline Berry Mack concluded that our children are "gravely undernourished."

Nearly half the girls were getting less than the minimum requirement of protein; the boys had only a slightly better record. Every one of these young people was living on deficient amounts of calcium and phosphorus, and it was no surprise that only seven girls and twelve boys had perfect teeth. Dr. Mack found 49 percent of the boys and 48 percent of the girls suffering from "nutritional nerves"—fidgeting, twitching, blinking, nail biting. As we would expect, their diet was seriously lacking in the B vitamins. Three-fourths of these adolescents were suffering from eye troubles traceable to poor diet; rough skin and acne were prevalent, especially among the girls. There were grave shortages of vitamins A and C.

In another study of 4,458 children, 56 percent failed to meet minimum health standards.

These, and the adolescents in Dr. Mack's study, were not underprivileged children. They were an average lot of American youngsters drawn from high and low income families.

What is wrong here? How can a mother hope to compete with the seductions of television commercials promoting foodless foods, the candy bar and soda pop vending machines, even in the schools, the hot dogs and greasy hamburgers and the mountains of French fries, potato chips, ice cream sodas and pizza pies?

I do not say it is easy. But is the food on your family table compensating for this? And what about a mother's own example? Earlier in these pages I quoted studies indicating that the mothers of these teen-agers were eating no better than their daughters.

THE POWER OF THE HOME

Children are bound to be tempted by influences outside the home. Parents have always had to cope with this problem. But never, never forget that the home influence is the strongest influence. The home wins out in the end.

Studies of college-age boys and girls indicate that they follow in their parents' footsteps. For better or for worse, they adopt their parents' preferences in reading matter and entertainment, living standards, political and religious beliefs, and patterns of eating and drinking. The foods mother used to serve become their favorites for life. The manner in which she prepared and served them come to be potent symbols of home, security and mother herself.

The distinguished anthropologist, Dr. Margaret Mead, puts it this way in her article, "Family Life Is Changing," also in the encyclopedia for parents that I mentioned above:

"A man who has grown up watching his mother simmer a meat stew on a wood stove in a farm kitchen may be poorly prepared to feel that his wife, in a smart housecoat serving precooked food in a dinette, *is* a mother at all."

I am inclined to agree with that man. The pretty housecoat is all to the good, but the *precooked* dinner and the dinette, more like a booth in a juke joint than a dining table in the home, are part of what is wrong with our American homes. What is there to choose for our teen-agers between a frozen dinner in a dinette and a hamburger in a luncheonette booth?

NUTRITION AND PROBLEM CHILDREN

The evidence is piling up that the basic difficulty with problem children may be nothing else but nutrition.

In the schools of New York and many other cities the teachers found out years ago that many of their most difficult children were those who came to school without breakfast. When the school lunch programs were instituted, however, the miracle that was expected did not quite take place. Many of the children would not eat the tasty nutritious food that was placed before them—because it was not like the food they were accustomed to at home. In some states the state universities have undertaken a food re-education program in the homes in order to solve the nutrition problem of the children at school.

Recently I read an amazing report of how a change in food transformed a child's personality. The story was told by a Los Angeles dentist, Dr. Donald Shriber, of an eight-year-old boy who came to his office every three months with between three and five new cavities to be filled. Worse than the condition of his teeth, however, was the child's behavior. He kicked, screamed, bit the dentist's hands.

Then the dentist prescribed a diet free from sugar and white flour. Six months later there were no new cavities, a year later only one. Astoundingly, the boy's behavior had also changed from wild hysteria to cheerful cooperation. In school he was able for the first time to keep up with his class. At home he had all but stopped quarreling with his sister. His continuous colds and sore throats virtually disappeared, as did his dependence on laxatives.

This is an unusually dramatic case, and not all youngsters may respond so promptly. But I deeply believe that many emotional problems, with adults and even more with children, begin with food. And they can be ended the same way.

THE EMOTIONAL POWER OF FOOD

Do not expect overnight miracles when you set about changing your family's eating habits. Above all, do not court disaster by announcing that you are making changes.

If food were merely food, your task would be simpler. But the psychiatrists and psychologists tell us constantly that food is much more than nourishment. It is pleasure, gratification of the senses. It is security. It often masquerades as love.

Dr. William Kaufman, an internist practicing in Bridgeport,

Connecticut, made a fascinating study of ways in which human beings unconsciously make foods serve these other purposes. His report, which he delivered a few years ago to the American Association for the Advancement of Science, was based on records kept by 1,200 of his patients over a period of twelve years. Under the title, *Some Emotional Uses of Food*, he classified foods according to the emotional purposes for which people tend to use them.

When people are under emotional stress, says Dr. Kaufman, their consumption of the "security foods," milk and milk products, tends to rise. This, I am happy to observe, is all to the good!

But hear this: "Similarly, if we are thwarted, or if we have failed to gain the approval of others, or if we feel sorry for ourselves, we unconsciously seek gratification by eating more of the reward foods—such as chocolate, hot dogs, candy."

Does this explain some of the teen-agers' bad eating habits?

"Grown-up foods, such as coffee, tea, or beer—foods which once were forbidden to most of us" also exert a strange fascination for some adults. How much more for teen-agers!

And exhibitionistic food habits, such as splashing ketchup, mustard or black pepper on all dishes whether they need the seasoning or not.

Then come the fetish foods: "Many of the highly advertised foods become fetish foods. Some children don't feel strong unless they have Wheaties, Breakfast of Champions."

Even the younger set has its emotional foods!

DEALING WITH YOUR TEEN-AGERS

You have one other powerful string to your bow, especially with that most rebellious age, the teens. Your adolescent boy wants to be physically strong, muscular, a good athlete; he longs for a sturdy manly physique. Your adolescent girl yearns for a lovely skin and a pretty figure.

You, and you alone, have the kitchen magic to give them these treasured gifts.

They will not like to be told. They will not like to be ordered to eat what you know is *good* for them. The adolescent years are years of feeling and testing one's independence. Respect this in your boy and girl. You would not want your boy to be a mother's baby, nor your girl to have no judgment of her own.

Make up your mind that you cannot achieve your objective by force. You want not obedience but cheerful intelligent cooperation.

Your man can charm his boy into eating the foods that are good for him. Once father is convinced, son will soon follow the manly example. And you yourself can conspire with your girl for her good figure and fresh, blemish-free complexion.

I know many mothers who did wonders for themselves and their young daughters by dieting together (I dislike the word, but actually it means eating sensibly together), and mothers who made good cooking and nutrition wisdom so attractive that they had their daughters in the kitchen with them as willing apprentices.

With your womanly wisdom, and your tact, you can accomplish this transformation of your family's ways any time you put your mind to it.

CHAPTER 21

A Beauty Spa in Your Bathtub

There is no other single item in the world that can compare with the beauty-giving value of water. Each time you step into your bath you are joining the sisterhood of beautiful women from Cleopatra to Mary, Queen of Scots. The use of water for beauty is as old as the first Eve who saw her face in a clear pool of water, and as modern as your clean white bathtub. The Greeks, who worshiped beauty in all its phases, made fabulous statues of their great beauties, their favorite was Aphrodite surprised in her bath. The great Greek temples to Aesculapius, who was the god of medicine, were always built around watering places, either by the sea or where mineral springs bubbled from the earth. The Greeks firmly believed that all medicinal virtues contained in herbs and stones were to be found in natural spring waters.

NATURE'S GIFTS TO BEAUTY AND HEALTH

The ancients also knew that water, sun and air were nature's free gifts to health and beauty. They could not explain scientifically, as we can today, why these elements are so beneficent to man. They could only guess at the physiological reactions of the body to changes of water temperature, to the friction of rubbing and scrubbing, to earthy minerals in the waters. They knew nothing of the gentle radioactivity of some of the springs, and the health-giving effects of these small amounts of radioactivity where circulation is poor.

They accepted these benefits as the free gift to man from their gods on Mount Olympus.

Not only the Greeks, but peoples all over the world recognized these blessings of water. The Japanese especially are famous for their love of bathing, which goes back to their ancient days. Their natural hot springs were discovered long ago—the village folk used to soak in them in midwinter, melting away the aches of hard-working muscles and arthritic joints, bringing the circulation back to chilled skin.

The American Indians knew and used our famous hot springs in Arizona and California for hundreds of years. The Indian medicine men knew a good deal of empiric medicine, along with their incantations and ritual dances to cure the sick. They had a bathing ritual very like the famous Finnish, Turkish, and Russian baths. They, too, used heat to bring on a sweat, followed by a plunge into a cold stream—or a roll in the snow—for that sharp shock that sends the blood racing through the body.

I said earlier that I envy Russians their walks. I envy them their spas and health resorts, too. They inherited a few elegant watering places from the Czarist regime. Today the Russians have more than 2,500 spas—their doctors have a different resort to recommend for every kind of ailment! They have even created a new medical specialty, a science called koorortology, from the German word *kurort*, which means health resort.

The spas of Europe have been gathering places for smart people for many centuries, and they still are. People with money still go each year to "take the cure" at such famous bath resorts as Carlsbad, Baden-Baden or Aix les Bains. Our American spas, which contain some of the finest waters, used to be popular. Unfortunately, with our "time is money" obsession, the popularity of our watering places has declined.

Now, I am happy to say, there is a revival. There is no reason why every American woman and her husband should not spend their holidays at resorts where medical, nutritional, and beauty specialists will prescribe for her figure, her complexion, her hair, and her man's good health and vitality.

Recently a news magazine published a picture of Aldous Huxley, the distinguished English writer now living in California, at one of these spas in the desert. He was there to gain weight, along with other celebrities who were there to lose it. They all dieted and exercised together, and the photograph shows them enjoying the warm rays of the sun.

That is all to the good, but there are as yet not nearly enough resorts for the millions who need this relaxation.

Start your own beauty spa

But you need not wait for more mineral springs and bath resorts to open. You can begin right now to enjoy the benefits and pleasures of the spa in your own home. If you live in the suburbs —as more and more families are now doing—you can go even farther, and make a spa for yourself and your man, for your whole family, in your own home.

Perhaps you have read about the new vogue for fabulous bathrooms nowadays, modern versions of the magnificent Roman baths. We are very admiring of those Roman baths, but we tend to forget that most Romans never saw the inside of one of them.

The familiar bathtub in your efficient American bathroom can be filled with beauty. Let me tell you some of its marvelous possibilities.

Beauty in your tub

The best things in life are free, and one of the greatest gifts is clear clean wholesome water. We are told that all life started in water, that we came originally from the sea. Each of us, we might say, is a miniature ocean enclosed in skin. Even our skins have their salty water content, within each cell and in the fluid-filled intercellular spaces. Water is essential to the life of every cell. It is essential both inside and outside.

If you have thought of your bath mainly as a Saturday night affair, let me tell you that cleanliness is only the first function of your beauty bath. For by changing the temperature and length of your bath, and by adding mineral salts, oils, unguents or cosmetic vinegar, you can make your bath serve a whole spectrum of relaxing and beautifying experiences.

Your bath can give you stimulation or rest; it can be invigorating or relaxing. Your bath can become a wholesome tranquilizer and sleep-inducer, much better than those questionable drugstore tablets.

The most important value of your bath is its action on your circulation, especially the circulation to your skin, in the tiny arteries and veins and capillaries that carry beauty and new life to every cell.

This peripheral circulation, as it is called, is of great importance to the whole body. It is so important, in fact, that physicians of other times and other lands prescribed for serious diseases by stimulation of the peripheral circulation. Your vigorous rubbing and scrubbing rubs away all the dry and dead cells on the surface, that invisible scale that our skins are constantly shedding. Such a simple device as a bath brush brings out all the freshness of your new skin.

And that is not all. By its relaxing effect your bath can smooth away lines of tension from your face, and the tensions between shoulder blades which are deadly to proud posture and free movement.

ACCESSORIES FOR A TUBFUL OF BEAUTY

Cleopatra's secret of keeping her skin exquisitely soft and perfumed is no secret to modern women. More and more women use scented bath oils today because they soften the skin and the delightful odors are relaxing to weary spirits.

Any woman's skin can become softer and smoother by adding a tablespoon of scented oil to her tub. If you cannot afford those on the market, do as the Indian women do and make your own specially scented bath oil with a base of sweet sesame oil, the same oil which helps your skin so much from the inside. There are bubble baths, foam baths and body lotions. Try them all—these luxurious touches make you feel pampered and beautiful. Yes, your psyche also needs nourishment; this can make a larger contribution to your feeling your best and looking your best than you may have realized.

And now a serious note. More and more women complain that bathing gives them a dry flaky skin. Long ago the beautiful Queen Elizabeth of Hungary suffered so much from very dry skin that she put her chemists to work; the formula they came up with, which would forever prevent her skin from drying, was called Budapest Water. Hungarian beauties use it to this day. Let me give you the formula; it is easy to make. (See page 358.)

And here are a few more inexpensive accessories that will turn your bathtub into a beauty spa deluxe:

A large wash cloth or, best of all, a *Loofah*, which is a sponge or mitt made of vegetable fibers, to provide stimulating friction on your skin.

A rolled towel on which to rest your neck, or a foam rubber cushion, small, covered with toweling or plastic (you can make this yourself).

A tub tray that fits across the sides. This is optional, but it helps you use and enjoy the longer bath routines. With the tray to hold your tools, you can manicure, pedicure, set your hair, attend to other grooming chores.

A bathtub seat, also optional, to make footbaths comfortable.

And that's all, plus your soap, water hot and cold, and *time*.

I urge you to take more luxurious and relaxing baths; it is one of the best investments you can make. Ignore the phone, ignore the family, ignore "togetherness"; this is your time to relax, recharge. On an old jade bathtub of a Chinese Emperor they found this inscription: "Renew, rejuvenate thyself daily." That is what I would like to put on your bathtub.

BEAUTY RITUAL

This can be taken Saturday night or any night during the week. You can turn this ordinary bath into one of pleasure and luxury. Make the water comfortably warm, not hot. If the water is hard, use a water softener, bath salts, a handful of oatmeal in a bag or whatever pleases you. Have a coarse wash cloth, a friction sponge or a Loofah, a nail brush, pumise stone for the feet, and a good super-fatted soap all arranged in one tray.

Let the warm water envelop and relax you for at least five or still better, ten minutes. Then rub and scrub every inch of your body so your skin becomes shining and clean, but this is almost incidental; to make an ordinary bath a bath of beauty you must stimulate the skin and peripheral circulation to bring your beautystream to every inch of your skin. This rubs away the dull dry veil of old skin cells and exposes the new, young, and soft skin.

End this bath by letting the warm water slowly run out and turn on the cold water full force, splashing cool water all over. If you are a shower fan, after this warm bath stand up and take a cool-to-cold shower, then rub yourself dry until you are pink and glowing.

QUICK STIMULANT BATH

Take a three minute shower as hot as it can be borne comfortably, then turn on cool water and gradually let it get colder and colder, for just one minute, and emerge rosy and red. Dry vigorously and follow with cooling lotion.

LUXURIOUS MILK BATH

A most soothing, smoothing and luxurious bath, equaling if not surpassing the famous Anna Held Milk Bath, is now yours for a few cents, right at home in your own bath tub. All the ingredients for this milk bath are on your pantry shelf.

Take a piece of muslin or double cheesecloth the size of a man's handkerchief. Put into it one heaping cup of powdered skim milk, one cup of ordinary oatmeal and one cup of ordinary laundry starch. Tie the muslin into a bag and you are ready for an experience. Fill your bathtub about two-thirds full of warm, not hot, water and swish the muslin bag back and forth in the water. When the water is milky white, lie down in the gentle liquid and relax. Then rub and scrub yourself with the muslin bag; the water will become increasingly white and soft. After twenty or more delicious minutes of floating in your milk bath, dry yourself gently. Your skin will be smoother, softer and whiter than ever before.

Relaxing bath

American Indians, long before the white man came, made use of the relaxing and healing power of their hot springs. For their muscular pains and exhaustion, the Indians would sit in hot spring water, not just for minutes, but for a half hour to an hour. In our busy lives we lose sight of the fact that hot water when applied long enough, draws tension and congestion away from our inner organs; blood vessels relax, circulation is speeded up; arms, legs and the entire body become flushed with red blood. In such a bath we are actually *forced* to relax. Not all of us can go to healing hot springs, but we can get the benefits of hot water plus a handful of mineral salts in our own bathtubs. The most important factor for a soothing and relaxing bath is the temperature. Mother Earth controls the temperature of her natural hot springs, but you can control it with an inexpensive bath thermometer, the same one that you use for baby's bath. Simply fill the tub two thirds full of good warm water and add half a cup of mineral bath crystals. Lie in it and relax. It is important to keep the water at one hundred degrees. Your floating thermometer will tell you if you have to add more hot water and so you will be able to relax completely for thirty minutes or more. Do as the Indians do. Soak a towel in cold water, make a roll and place it at the back of your neck and relax, let go and enjoy this one-hundred-degree bath at least once a week or whenever you have need for deep relaxation.

Tranquilizing bath for deep sleep

It is not generally known that one of the great advocates of baths for many good values to health was Dr. Simon Baruch, the father of the Bernard Baruch. This bath is the one Dr. Baruch recommended for quieting jangled nerves, and especially to encourage restful sleep. As he pointed out, it is extremely simple, but it is rarely done correctly.

Fill the tub with water between 100 and 102 degrees, only a few degrees above body temperature, but it is important to have the temperature right, neither warmer nor cooler. The tub should be full enough so that you can lie in it fully submerged up to the chin. Put your rolled towel or plastic-covered pillow behind your head, and rest in the water for at least ten minutes, up to thirty minutes if you have the time.

This bath will relax and soothe all the nerve endings in your skin, as well as your muscles. It lowers the blood pressure, and after the first few minutes your breathing will become slow and deep. When you step out and pat yourself dry, you will be ready for a night of deep and tranquil sleep.

A SITZ BATH FOR ADAM

Hot baths are wonderfully comforting and relaxing. Take them whenever you are tense, tired and out of sorts, but remember that it is cool to cold water which peps you up. At the famous water *kurort* in Woerishofen in Bavaria, they call this bath the youth bath because the increased circulation to the vital centers helps to keep a man young. They even have special sitz bathtubs for this ablution.

Here is how the tired husband can get the beneficial effects of plain cold water without a special bathtub: Let the cool water run into the tub until it is about half full. The idea is to concentrate the water as much as possible around the "sitz." Sit in this cool water for three and not more than five minutes with knees drawn up so that only the feet and "sitz" are in the water. The cooler the water, the greater the benefits. Jump out of the tub and rub dry with a coarse bath towel. It is amazing how this sitz bath can refresh you. I gave directions for this sitz bath in my book, *Look Younger, Live Longer,* and since then, thousands have thanked me for the benefit they received from this simple five-minute bath. For many men this has taken the place of pink pills, benzedrine and other stimulants. Take this two or three times a week or whenever you feel the need for a lift.

Another ancient refresher for weary Adams was told to me by a Scandinavian friend; it was handed down from the days of the Vikings. If you haven't the time nor a bathtub for a sitz bath, simply immerse the scrotum in very cold, even ice water, for one or one and a half minutes. It is a quick and simple way of increasing local circulation.

CHAPTER 22

Your Man

Is your husband in love with you?

I know this is a most personal question. Yet I cannot talk to you about beauty without talking of the greatest beauty-giver in life—Love.

If you have a man to love who also loves you, I hope you take good care of him. (And if you are without a man of your own, perhaps you will find here some clues to the womanly ways that win and keep a man.)

When I urge you to take care of your man, I do it as a reminder, because frequently people who have lived together for a while begin to take each other for granted. Still later, when the children have grown up and married, they confront each other almost like strangers. And I wonder if you know that there is a peak in divorces among people who have been married twenty years? I sincerely hope this does not happen to you. Take a good look at your man and listen to him, let him do the talking for a change. What do you see and hear?

You may see thinning hair and a thickening waist. Can he still get into the suit in which he was married? You may hear minor complaints, aches and pains, the creaking of a body that is no longer joyfully active—a sure way to grow old young! You may hear and see signs of poor digestion, possibly of ulcers. Take note of them. Nothing is clearer in medicine than the connection between food and the emotions.

You may worry about his taking an extra drink somewhat too often. Take note of this sign, too. Dr. Roger J. Williams, who has done brilliant work in biochemical research, tells us that alcoholics are hungry, malnourished people. He says that in our American diet of high fats and overrefined starches and sugars, the hypothalamus—that center in the brain that guides the appetite—is starved for the relatively large quantities of minerals, vitamins, and amino acids that it requires. He believes that much alcoholism could be prevented, as well as cured, by sound nutrition which interestingly enough includes a tablespoon of golden vegetable oil, plus a vitamin concentrate, especially high in vitamin C. Should you be so unfortunate as to have an alcoholic problem in the family, I strongly suggest you read Dr. Williams' book, *Nutrition and Alcoholism*.

You may see your man constantly tired, sleepless, anxious, irritable. All the signs of psychiatry today point to the connection between healthy body chemistry and health of the mind, emotions, and behavior.

You may be troubled (perhaps he is, too) about a seeming loss of his masculine powers; this, to a man, is a profound anxiety. Yet this too is most often a result of tension, lack of energy, deficient nutrition—and deficient love.

Finally, you may be worried about his heart. What wife today is free of this worry?

It is not surprising that bachelors have a shorter life expectancy than married men. Certainly a man without a woman to love and care for him is not the best candidate for a happy, long life. Yet, from the thousands of questions married men ask me, it is evident that they face many problems. No doubt, the strains and tensions of our competitive way of life are to blame, and to change all that is a large order for one lone woman!

USE YOUR WOMAN-POWER

I believe that any intelligent woman has the power to change this hectic pace for her man. It is not as difficult as you may think. Its secrets are right in your own home, in your kitchen, your living room, and the bedroom you share with him.

In my many travels I have found that women—despite all the jokes about their unrealistic thinking—are the realistic, practical members of the human race. Men are the adventurers, the gamblers, often the self-deluders. Women are the ones who recognize a fact when they see it—they seem to have an extra sense!

What then, are the facts behind that big phrase, our hectic "way of life"?

Our country enjoys the highest living standard in the world. Yet in seventeen other countries, men live longer past the age of forty-five than they do in the United States.

Of Americans who live past the age of forty, 50 percent die of cardio-vascular disease—disease of the heart or arteries. And of these, 77 percent die of arterial disease.

In our American high-standard diet, 44 percent of the daily food intake consists of fats.

Compare this with another set of facts:

In Japan, only 10 percent of men past the age of forty die of heart and artery disease.

Only 10 percent of the Japanese food intake is fat.

What do these amazing figures tell you? Apparently a man's chances of dying of cardio-vascular disease are almost exactly as great as the percentage of fats in his diet.

Compare this with another finding, revealed during a recent conference at the New York Academy of Sciences on "Culture, Society, and Health." The increase in heart disease deaths among young American men—the "epidemic," as the medical world is beginning to call it—can be traced directly to changes in living habits in the past thirty years.

"Lack of exercise, coupled with rich snacks in front of television screens, may be a major factor," reported Dr. David M. Spain, pathologist of Beth-El Hospital and Columbia University College of Physicians and Surgeons.

There you have the man-killing American "way of life," pinned down to a few facts as simple as your own grocery list!

A NEW DEAL FOR HUSBANDS

A leading women's magazine has been telling us for years, "Never underestimate the power of a woman." I never have, and neither do most men. In my observation, it is the women them-selves who fail to understand and use their power.

Once it was said that there was a woman behind every man—presumably, it was she who gently, subtly directed him. That was in the days when women were slaves to housekeeping and child-rearing.

Today women are emancipated. They go out into the world, the equals of men. And now it seems there is a woman in front of every man, shaking a finger before his face and telling him what to do.

That is the picture that I see, rising from the mountain of letters I have received through the years. "Dear Gayelord Hauser, How can I get my husband to take care of himself . . . to diet . . . to relax . . . to exercise . . . I keep telling him . . . etc. etc."

What has happened to the ancient feminine art of "getting around" a man?

I have a secret to share with you. Do you know the one complaint that men most often make about their wives? They say, "If she would only stop nagging!"

When a man says that to me, I see again that mountain of letters that show the other side of the picture, the letters from wives that say, "I *keep telling* my husband . . ."

Every woman knows that when she "keeps telling," she is nagging. Every woman knows in her heart, too, that nagging—or if you prefer, telling over and over again—does no good. Why does a woman continue to do this when she knows it accomplishes nothing? Does she do it, perhaps, to relieve her own tensions and irritations?

I am afraid she does. And I ask you, all you wives who love your husbands and want to take care of them, wouldn't you do better to find some other way of dealing with your tensions, instead of working them off on your long-suffering men?

Remember, constant dripping wears away a stone! Constant nagging wears away the most patient man. Sooner or later he will flare up in answering irritation, and there will be a needless quarrel. Many husbands simply protect themselves by retiring behind the newspaper and turning a deaf ear. A wife may "keep telling" her husband, but he is no longer listening.

No, telling him does no good. You should know that a man

does not like to be *told*. He does not *need* to be told. He knows all too well about his waistline, his flabby muscles, and the menace of a heart attack.

A man needs to take for granted in himself his manly strength and vigor. When you tell him that he has to watch his diet, watch his weight, watch his health, you undermine that belief in his manliness. You make him feel soft, unmanly—womanish! That is why he bristles with irritation, or turns a deaf ear. He has to protect his ego.

If you are a womanly woman you cherish the manliness of your man. You want to build up that ego, not break it down. You will quickly realize that what he needs from you is not talking about his health, but doing something about it.

If you have been trying to change his ways with words, give it up. Slip into a new gear. Change to the gentle, artful persuasion that only a woman knows how to do. Change his ways without even letting him know it.

You have the power to do this. You are still the mistress of the home. Above all, you are the queen of the kitchen, where so many of the sins of our modern way of life are committed.

You alone have the power to cook lean meals for him, without making announcements that will challenge him to resist. You alone can bring him serenity in his leisure hours. You can even get him to exercise, if you are wise in the way you go about it.

Remember, you are his new wife, who never nags. Give up "telling him" to take care of his health. Let him forget about his health while you take care of it for him.

THREE GIFTS FOR YOUR MAN

In the fairy tales that we loved as children, there were always three magic gifts by which the prince made his way through perilous adventures and returned to his princess, to live happily ever after. Here are the three magic gifts you can give to your man:

Give him a new heart, one that will enable him to work and reach his life's goal.

Give him a new waistline, his youthful looks and vigor restored.

Last, but most important, *give him a new wife*, yourself transformed within and without.

By giving him these three great gifts, you will give yourself the greatest gift of all, a new husband, a better companion and a better lover, one whose pride and pleasure in you will keep you young and beautiful.

The new wife that you are going to be, the one that consciously and intelligently cultivates beauty within and without, has been the subject of this book. If you have come with me this far in its pages, you are already creating the third magic gift.

And this new wife, who now knows the power of good nutrition, also knows the power of her womanly wisdom to create for her man the other two gifts.

A NEW HEART

Here is good news: You can do, not merely something, but very nearly everything, about this way of life that threatens your man.

What I am about to tell you is vouched for by serious, conservative scientists. It is a hypothesis so far, but a strong and positive one.

Arteriosclerosis, the arterial disease that is the unrivaled, number-one killer today, can be foreseen, can be prevented, and sometimes it can be cured. Dr. Harold Thomas Hyman, whom I have quoted earlier in this book, greets this hope as "lighting a hitherto cheerless chamber with the first rays of hopeful prognosis."

Arteriosclerosis is a sort of porridge that forms in the arteries. It leads to a thickening and stiffening of the arterial walls that cuts off circulation to the heart. It does not have a single cause, but a combination of them. Inherited factors, and certain metabolic diseases, such as diabetes, make some men more susceptible than others, as is true with most diseases. But the crucial combination of factors are these: sedentary occupation, overweight, possibly with low thyroid function, and the stress and strain of modern living.

Dr. Hyman points to the "lush American diet" compared to the frugal diet of Chinese, Japanese, Italians, among whom heart attacks are relatively rare. As the immediate causes of arteriosclerosis he lists: "Sustained and prolonged hyperalimentation (overeating); excessive salting of foods; and undue dietary dependence on concentrated carbohydrate foods and on saturated fats which, in the process of refinement, have lost certain essential amino acids, minerals, fatty acids and vitamins."

Most doctors now make the test for the cholesterol level in the blood, and if the level is above normal, they prescribe a diet low in cholesterol-producing foods, mainly the fats. An exciting and more exact test, called the lipoprotein test, has been developed by scientists of the Donner Laboratory of the University of California, led by Dr. John W. Gofman, author of the valuable book, *What We Do Know About Heart Attacks.* This test is recommended by more and more doctors (Dr. Hyman included), and it is done by a nonprofit organization, the Institute of Medical Physics, Inc., in Belmont, California. If you are at all worried about your husband's heart, I strongly urge you to discuss this test with his doctor. As Dr. Hyman says in his textbook for physicians, it is especially valuable to the doctor in general practice because it gives him a way of detecting, in *advance*, those "overtly healthy individuals" who are *prone* to arteriosclerosis.

A NEW WAISTLINE

You have known for a long time that overweight is a menace to your looks. Now you know also that it is a menace to your man's health and peace of mind. Not only motion picture Don Juans are reducing their waistlines today; all serious men are learning to eat intelligently.

The Senate restaurant offers a special reducing menu; all dishes contain the minimum amount of fat. The official physician to Congress, Dr. George W. Calver, has been urging leaner diets upon representatives and senators since 1928. He worries especially about the freshmen legislators, men between thirty-five and fifty years old. So much of their work is sedentary—and so much of it involves not only sitting, but eating too, at the political banquet tables—that they have a constant struggle against excess pounds. Dr. Calver enlists their wives and even their secretaries in keeping track of what his charges are eating.

Lyndon Johnson believes that his heart attack saved his life. After he recovered, he wondered whether it could have been prevented. His doctors told him that the same regime he had to follow to prevent a recurrence might well forestall a heart attack in the first place. He had been working at a breathless pace, without pause for relaxation or exercise. His breakfast was coffee and cigarettes, his lunch a hurried hamburger, his dinner a heavy meal of fried meats and potatoes. One of his new rules is to keep down weight: The tall Texan (he is six feet three) reduced from 202 to a lean 174 pounds. A second rule is that he must have no more than 50 grams of fat each day. Mrs. Johnson promptly equipped her kitchen for leaner cooking.

The one and only way to reduce, as we all should know by now, is to eat less. The same philosophy that you read in Chapter 9 for your looks, applies to your husband's new waistline.

IF YOUR MAN IS SEDENTARY

The second step, both to trim looks and good health, is exercise.

Men were hunters before they were farmers, and farmers before they were businessmen and desk-sitters. The human body, Dr. Laurence E. Morehouse tells us, was built for the rigors of the hunt. This professor of physical education at the University of California reminds us of what I have already mentioned in urging you to exercise for your own sake:

"Movement of the skeletal muscles in man not only performed his external work in primitive days, but also acted as supplemental heart muscles in moving fluids through the body. The modern sitting man relies on his heart muscle alone to pump fluids which support the internal environment of the body. The heart cannot do the job of circulation without the aid of other muscle pumps and sitting man soon begins to suffer."

Sitting, man soon begins to suffer. Mighty important words these, and the shouting will become louder and louder, because movement or exercise is important not only for your man's heart, but for every part of his body—even his hair!

From many years of experience, however, I have learned that you cannot force a tired, flabby body to exercise. How many mechanical exercisers, stretchers, bicycles and rowing machines are gathering dust in American attics and basements! Many homes have one or two in the storeroom. All these appliances cost money, and they were bought with the most earnest resolutions.

But resolutions are not enough. Your husband, first of all, needs new energy. You must build up your man's body to the point where it will demand exercise, so much so that exercise will become a pleasure.

Remember the pleasure-pain principle, our deepest motivation.

Begin your magic, right in your shining, push-button American kitchen. Right there is where you can create your man's new waistline and his new heart.

MAGIC IN THE KITCHEN

You are going to give your man, not a diet, but a new way of eating. You are going to put before him tasty, delicious meals, rich in proteins, vitamins, minerals, fatty acids, low in sugars and starches and especially lean in fats. You are going to replace the refined sugars with natural sugars, full of their own good minerals and vitamins, and the refined starches you will replace with the whole, natural variety. You are going to replace the killing, hard fats with liquid vegetable oils that contain the life-saving, essential fatty acids. You are going to stop oversalting, oversugaring, over-cooking and flavor his food instead with delightful spices, herbs and flavors.

With even a single change in his menu, the change from hard fats to vegetable oils, you can protect the health of your man's arteries at the same time as you relieve him of those extra inches around his waistline. And with the change of the whole spectrum from empty foods to sound nutrition, you will give him new vigor and zest for living. You will boost his morale along with his metabolism.

So throw away the hardened hydrogenated fats that you have been using as shortening, even if they are vegetable fats. Look at the label on your margarine; make sure it is not the hyydrogenated kind. Throw away your frying pan. Have your butcher trim the fat off the meat you buy, or sharpen your best knife and trim it off yourself.

Soya oil, which the Japanese housewife uses, sunflower oil which the Soviet Ministry of Nutrition is devoting thousands of extra acres to produce, peanut, sesame, avocado and wheat germ oils are all insurance for your man's heart and general health. Do they have a familiar ring by now? I hope they do, because these are the fatty acids that are part of your Cosmetic Diet for more beautiful skin and hair.

Here let me tell you something exciting that has been recently discovered about wheat germ oil and wheat germ, the two wonder foods I introduced in my book, *Look Younger, Live Longer*. Experiments with athletes show a direct connection between this little heart of the wheat and the stamina of the human heart. At the Physical Fitness Laboratory of the University of Illinois, fitness scores were higher with wheat germ or its oil added to the diet than with exercise alone.

Just one teaspoon of wheat germ oil taken daily increased athletes' physical capacity and endurance by as much as 51.5 percent.

Now wheat germ is rich in vitamin E, and there is one school of thought that considers vitamin E a specific vitamin for the health of the heart. Whether it is this vitamin in the wheat germ or some other factor, it is clear that this food element provides something that gives men added endurance under physical stress. Yet this very precious substance is refined out of American bread and cereals. But you, performing your magic in the kitchen, can easily learn how to restore it to your man's food. You simply add some golden wheat germ oil to your salad dressing. Sprinkle wheat germ kernels over salads and cereals. You can even make a delicious wheat germ pie crust. (See page 331.)

Lecithin is another one of the beauty-full foods I introduced to you in Chapter 7. Dr. Lester M. Morrison, in his fine book, *The Low Fat Way to Health and Longer Life*, describes it as one of the most important nutritional supplements developed in the last fifty years.

I have known about lecithin since I was a schoolboy in Germany. Our family doctor insisted that we children, and especially my sisters, must have it in its natural form of beaten egg yolk, in fruit juice or sherry wine; it was the only form in which we knew it then. In Germany at that time it was considered a very good food for the nerves.

Lecithin is better known now. We know today that it can be a lifesaver because it is a natural emulsifier of fat, and fat is the enemy of the heart, whether it is part of the added burden of over-weight or a direct cause of high cholesterol in the arteries.

I have mentioned that the Chinese and Japanese suffer very little heart disease. It is also a curious fact that in their diet—so poor by our standards—the soya bean has been the keystone. They call it their holy bean, their meat without a bone. It has been their flesh, fowl, milk, cheese, and oil for thousands of years. And here is the most surprising fact of all: The soya bean is one of the richest natural sources of lecithin. I beg you to use soya bean oil; also try some of the soya bean dishes.

Have you noticed that your kitchen magic for your man's health and fitness is not unlike the kitchen magic I have been recommending for your verve and good looks? It should not surprise you.

THE OUTER MAN

Next to loss of sexual potency, a man worries most about losing his hair. Most men do not admit it, but it is one of the questions I am most often asked at my lectures before men's clubs, and today there is a booming business in toupees. Medical science, as a whole, pays little attention to this problem. Yet I think it is important, otherwise men would not spend millions of dollars on useless hair tonics.

The whole question of baldness is confusing. There are many theories. Some researchers claim that men lose their hair more often than women because an excess of male sex hormones affects the quantity or quality of the oil produced in the sebaceous glands of the skin and scalp. The laboratory evidence for this claim is that when the oil was rubbed on the bodies of mice and rabbits, all the rabbits and many of the mice lost their hair in ten days.

When female hormones were injected into bald-headed men, the men stopped losing their hair, but began developing breasts, so obviously that was not the solution. A good endocrinologist can determine whether an excess of male hormones is in fact the cause of your man's falling hair, and can give him a prescription for an oil lotion containing the recommended female hormones in the proper dosage. An estrogenic hair lotion, offered by a New York endocrinologist to be applied directly to the scalp, is reported to be helping some men keep their hair.

Some American doctors believe that a lack of proteins can cause extensive loss of hair, and some Scandinavian doctors believe that too much salt in the diet can cause baldness. According to them, cutting down on salt significantly reduced hair loss. This is right in line with Dr. Eugene Foldes of New York, who has been able to arrest hair loss by reducing the salt content of the body. Dr. Franz Halla in Vienna claims that pork fat has extremely bad effects on hair growth and blood circulation.

Dr. Irwin I. Lubowe, the distinguished New York dermatologist, pays a great deal of attention to nutrition in his excellent book, *New Hope for Your Hair*, and in his discussions on the importance of vitamins he points out that nicotinic acid or niacin causes marked vasodilation of the scalp. This means dilation of the capillaries bringing increased circulation and thus increased nutrition to the hair follicles.

A method closer to home holds out promise that your man's chance for hanging onto his hair is good as long as he keeps the muscles under his scalp in good tone. Dr. M. Wharton Young of Howard University in Washington, D.C., in order to test his theory that good scalp muscles prevent baldness, applied electrodes to hairy and hairless parts on the scalp of balding people. Then the subjects were asked to move the scalp and wiggle the ears. The muscle contractions registered on the machine as electrical impulses, but only in areas with hair; the bald spots showed no movement or muscular activity whatsoever. This proved to the experimenters that it is the muscles under the scalp, with their rich supply of blood vessels, which bring nourishment to the hair follicles in a healthy loose scalp.

According to Dr. Young's theory, massage fails to stop baldness because it does not strengthen the muscles under the scalp. Only exercise can strengthen muscles, in the scalp as everywhere else. According to Dr. Young, this can be accomplished by wrinkling the forehead as hard as possible. At first it seems difficult, but with a little practice it becomes easier.

If your man is losing his hair, tell him about this most important exercise. Here is what he should do:

Pull the forehead up as much as possible without the use of the hands. Then pull it down as hard as possible. He will find as he does this scalp lifting exercise that the ears also move, and that is as it should be. Encourage him to do this exercise regularly, moving his forehead and ears up and down ten times or more, at night, in the morning, and whenever he thinks of it. After awhile he will notice that he can move his scalp and wiggle his ears quite easily. This takes only a few moments of his time and is well worth doing if he wants to stop his receding hair line.

A NEW WIFE

I began this chapter by saying that love is the greatest beauty-giver a woman may be fortunate enough to enjoy. Let me say now that it is also the greatest source of contentment and well-being, yes, and morale, that a woman can give to her husband.

I am not a marriage counsellor. But a vast number of women have written to me, asking for advice in their anxiety, and it is sadly apparent that many American women who truly love their husbands do not know how to show their love. They simply do not understand the psycho-sexual nature of the male.

European women on the whole have had a better education in this respect. There is a gem of Continental wisdom that mothers have passed on to their daughters for generations: A wife should be a chef in the kitchen, a lady in the drawing room, and a mistress in the bedroom.

A man needs to know that he is wanted. The most masculine of men—to quote Dr. Gregorio Marañon—does not aggressively woo women once he is past the hot years of youth. The most masculine man is a faithful, loving, dependable husband and father, who devotes himself to keeping his family safe and cared for. He is not likely to force his attentions, not even on his wife. He needs to be invited and encouraged.

Do you remember to make yourself attractive for him? I am sure you are never deliberately negligent in your appearance. But in the press of housekeeping and child care, perhaps also work outside the home, many women tend to let down their standards at home when they would never dream of appearing before an outsider in pin curls and cold cream.

The fact is that many women who do let down in this way are the first to complain that their husbands are no longer ardent lovers!

Habit and routine are deadly to love. Why do so many men approaching middle years fall prey to temptation outside the home?

Many a man's eyes stray because his love is not courted, but merely taken for granted at home. But another reason for infidelity is that a man is worried about his dwindling potency and is seeking reassurance wherever he can find it.

This is such a sensitive subject with a man that he may never mention it to his wife. He may not even admit it consciously to himself.

There is still a widespread belief that a man's sexual prowess ends with a change of life like the end of child-bearing in a woman. Somehow you should convey to your man that this is simply not so.

Here is what the recently published, medically endorsed book, *Sexual Pleasure in Marriage*, by Jerome and Julia Rainer, says on this troubling subject:

"The theory that there is a male climacteric with symptoms similar to those of the female has long been obsolete. If he suffers somatic ailments or states of depression . . . the causes are not to be sought in a nonexistent climacteric. Neither is a sudden slackening of sexual desire and potency, in a man otherwise physically well, a result of physiological decline. These phenomena have a psychic origin."

In other words, it is all in the mind! A man may lose confidence in his manhood when his wife does not seem to invite his attentions, when she does not bother to make herself attractive, even seductive, just for him. And it is a sad fact, which no wife should forget for an instant, that there are some 25,000,000 women without men in the United States, widowed, divorced, or unmarried, many of whom would give anything to have a man of their own.

No wife can afford to be careless about her man's health, or his happiness, or his love.

FOOD AND LOVE

Can you strengthen your man's sexual powers with food?

Some years back I wrote an article for *Esquire* on the care and feeding of executives. It won a tremendous response and brought me many invitations to lecture to men's clubs. I remember especially a luncheon at the Athletic Club in Philadelphia. As usual I answered all kinds of questions on diet and health, on how to relax, how to get rid of tiredness.

Then there was a lull, in which I could painly hear some snickering from a table at the end of the room. Finally a small, slight man stood up and blurted, "Is there any connection between food and sex, and what should a man eat when his love life is on the blink?"

The whole room shook with laughter, but I admired that courageous little man. He looked tired and worried, but he was the only one who had dared to ask the question that haunts most men past the age of forty, and even some who have not reached that fortieth birthday. I answered him in all seriousness. I told him that, of course, there is a relationship between a man's diet and his sex drive. I said, "I only wish I could give you one potent recipe, food, or formula to make you a romantic, carefree lover, but unfortunately, it is not that simple."

I went on to tell him what I now want to tell you. The search for a more satisfying sex life has been going on ever since Adam found the first gray hair in his beard. The ancient Greeks and Romans had books full of strange formulas for waning sex powers. Some of them contained dangerous poisons—the Roman poet, Lucretius, died of one of these love philters.

And some were frankly based on magic. For instance the early Greeks swore by onions and garlic because both of these root vegetables had the shape of male testes. Another favorite was wine made from the mandrake root, simply because this two-legged root looked rather like a miniature man.

But strangely enough, many of those ancient love potions contained such highly nutritious foods as eggs, snails, fish, all of which are full of vitamins and minerals; liver, the richest source of iron and the B vitamins; wild game, which we know today ranks higher than domestic meats in many vitamins and is also much leaner. Among the vegetables they recommended were cabbage, a fine source of B vitamins and C, and peas which are high in vegetable protein. High on the ancient lists of love foods was honey, one of nature's finest sugars.

Listen, now, to a 2000-year-old tip on foods for sexual prowess: wild honey, ginger, vinegar, wild garlic, shallots, cinnamon, nutmeg, wild seeds, pepper and all heat-producing spices.

Today we laugh at such concoctions. But do you recognize in this list some health-giving, beauty-giving foods? Of course you do. As for the spices, we know today that they stimulate the stomach to produce gastric juice and thus promote good appetite.

Actually we do not need to go back to antiquity to find love potions. In my boyhood days in the Black Forest, the country folk staunchly believed in their "potent potage for lovers," and to this day in some parts of Europe, women prepare this soup when they feel neglected by their husbands. Its chief contents are glandular meats such as liver, heart, tripe, cock's comb and testes, cut up fine and simmered in a powerful broth of onions, leek, garlic, celery root, parsley and every other available garden green. It is a very thick soup and must on no account be strained for, say the peasants, to derive the "strength" from this potent potage a man has to eat every bit, its meats and vegetables as well as its broth.

In France even today, their beloved bouillabaisse is considered a dish for lovers, and as you know, it contains every conceivable fish and shellfish, every nutrition-rich gift of their Mediterranean Sea.

Today we know that there are no mysterious love potions for tired lovers. But we also know that many of those fantastic formulas did really perform miracles, not through magic, but through good nutrition! The good proteins and the high vitamin and mineral content of those love dishes invigorated men in those days as they do today.

And this is the truth about the ancient love potions, which science confirms today. Good nutrition is not only the basis for health and beauty, but also for a healthy and happy sex life.

As a loving and understanding wife you can perform this same miracle for your man. You can sustain his manhood, strengthen his morale, and satisfy his deepest hunger. You need no magic recipes, formulas, or tricks—nothing else but good nourishing food, potent with nature's own potency. That is what science knows about food and sex today.

CARE AND FEEDING OF HUSBANDS

All hard working husbands should be treated and fed as VIPs. Good meals are doubly enjoyed and give double value when eaten in a relaxed atmosphere. Feeding a husband in the modern manner means *cutting down* on hard fats, starches and sugars, and *increasing* the protein foods. (Remember, he needs half a gram of protein for each pound of *his* ideal body weight—not his overweight. If your man weighs 160 pounds, he needs 80 grams of protein every day.) Also, include as many fresh fruits and vegetables as possible. You may have difficulty at first changing your man's eating habits, so use your womanpower—do it gently and gradually. By all means begin by serving good protein breakfasts because this greatly determines whether the day ahead will be hectic or whether things are taken calmly and in stride.

BREAKFAST

Unlimited choice of fresh or frozen fruit juices, tomato juice or fresh fruits in season. (You can make an irritable husband amiable by handing him his fruit juice while dressing; this ups the blood sugar level by the time he comes to breakfast.)

Choice of proteins: 2 eggs: poached, boiled, scrambled or fried in golden oil. Or: omelet, ½ cup cottage cheese, lean broiled meat patty, liver, fish or ham. When bacon is served, make sure it is lean and crisp

Cereals: Serve only whole grain varieties. If he insists on cold cereal, serve it à la mode, fortified with 2 tablespoons of fresh wheat germ and half a cup Hi-Vi lean milk

Breads: Muffins, biscuits—only the whole grain variety. Also introduce high protein wheat germ and soya muffins. Breads are better eaten untoasted. If he insists on toast, make it light brown; only one piece should be eaten and this can be buttered lightly. If a more generous spread is desired, serve homemade lean cream cheese or cottage cheese

Coffee: Freshly made, preferably Swiss coffee made with fresh milk, or tea with milk

> *HI-VI RITUAL:*
>
> So that there is no possible chance of missing any important nutrients, see to it that he takes the prescribed vitamin-mineral concentrates before leaving the breakfast table. It is a wise plan to keep the concentrates on a special tray

LUNCHEON

Choice: Vegetable espresso, tomato juice or hot bouillon, if desired

Choice of proteins: Lean meat, cheese, fish, eggs, cottage cheese. Serve with a portion of green salad or better still, mix the proteins into a bowl of crisp salad greens and marinate with golden oil dressing

Add: One slice of good bread or a muffin, lightly buttered

Beverage: Choice of coffee, milk, tea or yogurt

MIDAFTERNOON

To prevent any let-down, choice of a glass of vegetable espresso, carrot, celery or apple, or a glass of milk, yogurt or tomato juice, fortified with a teaspoon of food yeast

DINNER

Give your husband a chance to unwind. Serve a cool, non-alcoholic vegetable or fruit juice cocktail.

Choice of: Lean meat, fish or fowl—broiled, baked or stewed
Mixed green salad with golden oil dressing
One or two short-cooked green vegetables. (Twice a week, a Light-hearted Baked Potato.)

Dessert: Fresh fruit, compote, honey custard; occasionally, open-face fruit pie or lean cheese with an apple or pear

Beverage: Small demitasse, milk or yogurt

BEFORE RETIRING
A glass of lean milk, cottage cheese with cracker, yogurt or hot Swiss broth

CHAPTER 23

Your Beautyfarm

This is what happens if you are so lucky and so rich as to be on a beautyfarm. When you arrive you are shown to your bright and airy room. Perhaps there is an Aubusson rug on the floor and a Chagall painting on the wall. After you have unpacked, the staff doctor comes and examines you, unless you have brought a letter from your own doctor saying that you are in good health.

The next morning your breakfast is served to you in bed by an attractive maid and on your tray, set with very fine silver, very fine linen and a beautiful flower, will be a bowl of fresh fruit, some scrambled eggs and one slice of protein toast, plus coffee with hot milk (this is a modern beautyfarm breakfast—the day of coffee and fruit juice is passé). On your tray you will also find your program of activities, your beauty menu for the day.

Right after breakfast you will be asked to put on your exercise suit, a leotard, which the beauty institutes have taken over from the ballet and dance schools. Over this you put your robe and now you are on your way.

Before your exercise session a nurse or a rather determined woman—the exercise director—will make a record of your measurements. There will be no secrets: the exact weight and measurements will be put down in black and white and the woman in charge will inform you just what your ideal measurements and weight should be. Then your posture is carefully noted. On California beautyfarms you are asked to walk and they take a film to see you in action. After that a beautician looks over your skin, hair and nails. Your plus and your minus points are recorded and finally the "work" begins.

One farm has a "beauty barn" where you are pommelled, steamed, oiled and brushed. After your first workout—about eleven o'clock—you are served a cup of hot broth with an egg yolk or a fresh vegetable espresso so that you will not be too hungry by one o'clock. The time before lunch, about an hour, is your own. You can swim in the pool where you may be given some special underwater gymnastics; some have pools with hot and cold water springs. If you are more than ten pounds overweight, the physical education director will map out a walk for you of two or three miles, according to how much you have to lose. So that you will not feel sorry for yourself, one of the instructors or one of the other guests will accompany you on a lovely country road.

LUNCH ON A BEAUTYFARM

Lunch time is picnic time on a beautyfarm. A beautyfarm in Palm Springs, California, arranges interesting picnics for their clients. They serve the finest, freshest salads, fortified with the most delicious forms of protein: chicken, lobster, eggs, fish and gelatin-tongue salads, and always big bowls of lean cottage cheese. There is unlimited choice of salads made with golden oil dressing, but only one piece of high protein toast, wholewheat bread, rye bread or soya muffin is allowed. There is always steaming hot vegetable broth, hot fortified tomato juice or Swiss broth, which is a great favorite. For dessert there are bowls full of fresh fruit or Lady Mendl compote. Beautyfarm beverages are: clear coffee, Swiss coffee, fortified milk, yogurt, English tea, rose hip tea, peppermint tea, papaya tea, fresh fruit juices or vegetable espresso.

After lunch you are glad to retire to your room. You will be tired and you will probably take a nap. Ann Delafield, the dean of physical education, suggests that every woman, before retiring or resting, should take a fifteen minute refresher on the beauty slant

and let the law of gravity put her posture into beautiful alignment. This is done on many beautyfarms.

After the noon siesta, you look at your program for the day. The
afternoon will be dedicated to more beautifying. There will be
fragrant oil of rose geranium baths or herbal facials, hair brushing
under the trees, manicures, pedicures. There may be tennis or
more swimming. You will be on the move every minute—there is
never any time for boredom and among the ladies there is a
splendid spirit of camaraderie; they are all there for the same reason
and the favorite conversation is: how are *your* measurements; how
much did you lose? There is also a friendly spirit of competition
which makes even reducing easy and more like a game, and of
course, the luxurious surroundings, the beautiful service, the lean
food and the absence of family duties are other reasons for the good
results.

Besides the tennis courts, swimming pools, nearby golf courses,
there are wonderful walks and it is amazing how gladly women will
walk when they have good shoes and good company.

At five o'clock you return to your own room, this time to freshen
up. You are expected to change for dinner; the early beautyfarms
expected guests to dress, but this is no longer obligatory, they discovered the ladies often were too tired. However, the guests always
change from their daytime costumes. Slacks are not permitted in
the dining room.

Ever since I introduced vegetable juices at the Main Chance
Beauty Farm, all the other beautyfarms here and abroad have taken
advantage of this idea. Cocktails, about half an hour before dinner,
consist of foaming glasses of fresh vegetable juices. The most popular combination is carrot, celery and apple juice. Some of the
women are so hungry they drink two glasses right from the spout,
and that is all to the good because the natural sugars of the juices
raise the blood sugar level, a sure and natural way to prevent
overeating at the dinner table.

LE DINNER EST PRÈS

Beautyfarms outdo themselves to give the guests beauty-full and
satisfying dinners: broiled livers of all kinds; chicken livers en

brochette or parsleyed calves' liver are served several times a week; broiled chicken, broiled lobster tails, lean sirloin steak are also favorites. There are always two freshly green sautéed vegetables. The desserts are all delicious, with a choice of fresh fruit sherbet, apricot mousse, exotic fruits or fruit pies made with thin shells of coconut or wheat germ crust.

The ladies all enjoy one generous portion of everything. For the newcomers with overstretched stomachs there are always trays full of crisp, chilled finger salads made up from fresh bits of cauliflower, sliced green and red peppers, radishes, celery hearts, young onions and green olives. These can be eaten freely without conscience trouble. There is never any difficulty about overeating at beautyfarms. The ladies watch one another and the hostess is usually a good-looking dignified woman who keeps a watchful eye on her charges.

After dinner the women gather in the beautiful salon for cards, conversation and perhaps some fine music. Time never hangs heavy on a well run beautyfarm. Even the evenings seem to pass too quickly. The women are naturally tired and glad to retire about ten o'clock. There is always a nightcap choice of half a dozen fragrant teas: linden, verbena, licorice, papaya or hot Swiss broth. And then to dream in your own comfortable room on your own comfortable bed until the next day.

This gives you an idea of what it is like to be a guest at one of the luxurious beautyfarms: the service is fabulous, the food superb, the setting is beautiful.

But there should be beautyfarms for all the lovely ladies in the land, not only for millionairesses. And I predict there will be many more in the future. I hope that I can help to speed up the day.

In the meantime, let me assure you that any woman can establish her own miniature beautyfarm right in her own home. You won't be pampered, you won't have your breakfast served in bed, but you also won't have to pay five hundred dollars a week!

A BEAUTYFARM IN EVERY BACK YARD

It is the easiest thing in the world for you to have a miniature beautyfarm in your own back yard. Even if you have only a small piece of land, you possess the important beautyfarm needs already: sun, soil, air and water.

To let the sun caress your body you turn a sheltered corner into a suntrap with a sheltering trellis against the wind or prying eyes, or if you prefer you can make or buy an aluminum-coated sun reflector which keeps drafts away, and gives a golden tan without harmful chemicals in a few days' time.

Be careful with the sun. Always oil yourself with your cosmetic mayonnaise. Follow the sun-exposure schedule faithfully. Begin with no more than twenty minutes and turn from side to side so you will tan evenly.

You will need a Beauty Slant board for your beautyfarm; cover it with plastic to protect it against the elements. You can get double benefits if you do your sunning in the beauty slant position and let the law of gravity work for you at the same time. Be careful not to go to sleep in the sun.

For exercise: a hanging bar for you; for your Adam it will be a chinning bar. Get him to put up a punching bag for himself; it is excellent rhythmic exercise for his arms and torso muscles and a first-rate tension releaser.

Iron dumbbells in different weights belong on every beautyfarm. Muscles become firm twice as quickly with these; ten minutes a day strengthens your man's arms and they are very valuable to you to keep the bustline high. Five-pound dumbbells are best for him and two-pound dumbbells are best for you.

Add the beauty gift of water to your private beautyfarm. A wonderful investment would be a small swimming pool. I believe there is nothing that can give more pleasure to the whole family. It does not have to be a big expensive one. Investigate the round, oval and free-form pools. There are companies that install these in one day: they bring the cement ready-mixed and blow it over a steel frame fitted into the excavation. If you say that a pool is too expensive, I say so is a second car. A pool is a much better investment for health and good looks than a second car. If a pool is out of your reach this year, then install an outdoor shower, a great comfort and wonderfully refreshing. Remember, cool water peps you up, warm and hot water relaxes.

With a few dollars and a dash of imagination you can make an ordinary back yard into a pleasure and beauty-giving beautyfarm.

Your beautyfarm kitchen

Any good cook can become a beautyfarm cook.

I will go further: anyone can become a beautyfarm cook if she wants to be one.

You need no elaborate Cordon Bleu cooking courses. You need no education in the blending of great sauces. All you need is a love of good beauty-giving foods, a few good cooking utensils, and a short list of essential supplies.

Your cooking pots are an important key. Most women use too much water in cooking because the food burns in their ordinary pots. Avoid both the burning and the loss of essential vitamins and minerals by having heavy cooking pots with close-fitting lids that are also heavy enough to stay down. You need at least two of these heavy saucepans for your vegetables; in California we use enameled cast-iron pots and lids, in New York we use heavy stainless steel. These pots are a bit more expensive than thin light weight enamel, but they last forever, and are a good investment. You will need several appliances to help you save time and valuable nutrients.

A *liquidizer-blender* is what most beautyfarms use. This is a sturdy and versatile hi-vi food and beverage machine with a sturdy motor of many speeds. The machine grinds, chops, whips and even turns nuts and seeds into delicious butters and spreads. The liquidizer is a wonderful avante garde device.

You need the most *modern juicing machine* to make the important vegetable espressos. (Buy a simple sturdy machine which can't vibrate and is easy to clean.) Every woman in search of a good skin should have a pint of carrot, celery or apple espresso each day.

A *stainless steel vegetable shredder* is also a good investment. When vegetables are shredded they can be sautéed in five to seven minutes, as the Chinese now do. Use a bit of golden oil or a bit of broth.

And every kitchen should have *a set of sharp stainless steel knives* for cutting off all visible fat from all meats. Beautyfarm cookery is lean cookery.

You will also need *a fine stainless steel strainer* to remove fat from gravies (pour over ice cubes). For making quantities of

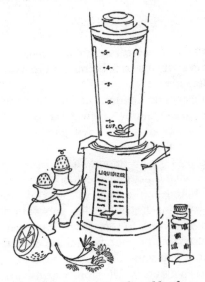

Beautyfarms use liquidizer-blenders

delicious yogurt you should invest in *a large, open-mouthed thermos bottle* or still better, *a yogurt maker,* for making fortified, plain or fruit-flavored yogurt.

Now look at your pantry shelf

Throw out all the hard, hydrogenated fats, empty white sugar and bleached flour. Put in their place the golden oils, whole grain flours and natural sugars: honey, brown sugar and unsulphured molasses. Also try the new sweet licorice and the delicious carob flour. You will find a long list of interesting and romantic foods for your pantry in Chapter 7, "Romantic Foods."

Always keep a supply of flavorsome herbs and spices of all kinds in your kitchen. By all means use fresh herbs if you have a garden; if not use the dried ones, but be subtle with them. Beauty-farm cooking requires "a touch of poetry" and spices and herbs can give that poetic touch.

The golden oils all bring their own subtle and agreeable flavors. Try them all, singly or mix two or three varieties and make your own blend.

Vegetable salt adds more flavor to cooking and is used on beauty-farms.

And for more flavor and savor, you will want several bottles of wine and cider vinegar to make your own special fragrant herb vinegars, as they do in France. Dr. Jarvis in his book, *Folk Medicine*, pointed out the many benefits of cider vinegar for your health. It is my desire to share with you the benefits of vinegars, as an inner and outer cosmetic.

YOUR REFRIGERATOR

You will always need a supply of lean milk and fresh sweet butter. If possible, use whipped butter; you will need less.

And now for your own cooking skills: You need to learn only how to short-cook your vegetables in a little liquid—three table-spoons—so that it is all gone when the vegetable is cooked. For more flavor you can also use a tablespoonful of vegetable or chicken broth. Your heavy cooking pot will conserve the flavor and mois-ture and prevent burning. Just before serving a fresh vegetable, you add a bit of vegetable salt and a bit of butter; whipped butter looks like hollandaise sauce, and you need very little. You have never tasted more delicious vegetables and, of course, when you sauté vegetables in golden oil as the Chinese do, you do not need any butter. I can tell a good cook by one sign: the height of the flame under her pot.

T.L.C.

Always remember, low temperatures give high quality in all cookery: boiling, sautéing, roasting; the simple exception is broil-ing. But the most important ingredient in beautyfarm cookery is: T.L.C.—Tender Loving Cooking! When the cook cares, the food remains tasty, full of beauty and health-giving goodness; it even looks good when it comes to the table and that is as it should be. Remember, we also eat with our eyes!

Good food is the everlasting pleasure that never fades. Enjoy your beautyfarm cooking and reap its benefits in health and good looks for you and your loved ones. They say that Frenchmen would rather marry a fine cook than a beautiful girl because the pleasures of good cooking go on long after other passions have diminished.

One more requisite will complete your private beautyfarm. On every beautyfarm there is one wise, inspired man or woman with a strong personality who gently, but firmly inspires the guests and the staff with the will to accomplish what they are there to do: to redesign bodies and spirits, both within and without. It used to be said of beautiful Ann Delafield, when she was directing the first Elizabeth Arden farm, that she handled the spoiled ladies with a silken glove and a steel hand. On your private beautyfarm that guiding, inspiring woman with the silken glove and the steel hand will have to be *you!*

BEAUTYFARMS UNLIMITED

You have learned how to turn your shining bathtub into a beauty spa. Now let me tell you how much more enjoyment you can have if you will take the next step in your beauty plan.

The more you become acquainted with the wonders of wise Mother Nature, the more you realize how generous she is with her earthly children. She gives her mightiest gifts: the sun, the soil, the air, the water, to produce the living foods that nourish us. We also know that we can derive great beauty-giving energy directly from the sun, by exposing ourselves intelligently to its healing and soothing rays, and from water in which we bathe and swim. And how comforting the earth itself can be!

You have surely discovered what a happy change it is to walk on soft, springy earth after hard, jolting pavements; to walk in the woods with soft moss underfoot, or just to lie on green grass and smell its fresh fragrance. These are some of nature's priceless gifts, and lucky are the people who still live among trees and grass in fresh air.

Millions of city dwellers, who live far from nature's beauties, look forward to their holidays when they can relax and recharge themselves in the quiet of fields and forests. The wholesome desire to get away from city tensions has given birth to the beautyfarm idea.

Thousands of people have discovered that they come back tired from their holiday; neither their bodies nor their minds have enjoyed a complete change. So many Americans spend their vacations traveling long distances, getting no closer to the countryside than seeing it through a car window, or perhaps from 30,000 feet above in a jet plane.

Only of late have we begun to appreciate the value of getting to the country, preferably to a farm, away from noise and irritations, to eat food that comes directly from the good earth to the dining table.

This can do wonders, especially for tense and harassed women. Elizabeth Arden was the first to see the possibilities of this idea when she turned her non-paying Maine farm into a beauty farm, inviting those who could afford it to come and relax for three or four weeks at a fabulous price. Now there are other beautyfarms and rest resorts springing up all over the world. But they are still only a drop in the bucket. There should be beautyfarms in every state.

The women have discovered the beautyfarms first, as they always do in matters pertaining to better looks and health. But the men will follow. I predict that one day soon we shall have VIP Hi-Vi farms for men. They cannot come too soon!

Perhaps next year I will be able to settle down in some spot where sun, soil, air and water are at their best; where modern farmers will supply us with home-grown produce: fresh milk, cheese, meat, grains, fruits and vegetables, all raised on healthy, rich soil, without harmful sprays and chemicals. I have offers to head beautyfarms everywhere: in California, Florida, Arizona and Nevada; also from England and France, in the fertile Dordognes district and from Germany, from one of the largest sanatoriums, specializing in nutrition.

As soon as I find an ideal place for a beautyfarm, I will invite you ladies who have followed me for so many years. Some of the women whom I would like to help are my friends, others are women who do not make enough of their beauty potential. Here are some of the ladies in my gallery of beautiful women.

GALLERY OF BEAUTIFUL WOMEN

Beautiful Princess Saroya, who since her divorce from the Shah of Persia has been frantically searching for inner happiness. I last saw her sitting in the bar of the Bayrischer-Hof Hotel in Munich, a bored look masking her natural beauty.

The Countess of Carnarvon, better known as Tillie Losch, the famous dancer, whose new career as a painter permits her to indulge sometimes unwisely in the too-rich food she learned to love in her native Vienna.

The Duchess of Windsor, an outstanding example of a woman of arresting individuality, whose intelligence, charm, chic and superb good taste have won the admiration of all who know her, and of millions who do not.

Queen Juliana of the Netherlands, who prior to her marriage to Prince Bernhardt delighted the world by transforming herself into a slim and chic princess, but today, unlike Queen Elizabeth of England, has forgotten that a queen should also be beautiful!

Ruth Dubonett, one of the twelve beauties invited by Lady Mendl to meet me in Paris in 1938, and who looked just as young and beautiful when I met her recently in New York. Ruth has become a food enthusiast and is busy from morning to night helping her friends on both sides of the Atlantic.

My dear friend, Dagmar Godowsky (about whom I could write a whole book!), whose bubbling wit and exuberant personality are only slightly dimmed by the pounds she has added since I first met her in the south of France thirty years ago.

Bea Lillie, the perennially young and slim English comedienne, who is proof that a clown can also be a lady. Just to see her walk into a room or onto a stage lifts my spirits.

Blanche Yurka, superb woman and actress, who admits to being over seventy, and whose interest in theatre, music and philosophy becomes more passionate with each passing year.

Ilka Chase, actress, authoress and lecturer whose crisp good looks, unerring chic and sparkling wit has kept her in the forefront of American women for more than twenty years. Ilka now writes a syndicated column, which is enjoyed from coast to coast.

Colette Lefort, career woman (she is the director of my Paris office), slim, chic and intelligent. After a busy day at her office, she returns to her apartment on the Quai de Passy and assumes the role of wife (she is married to Dr. Charles Cashin, a brilliant Paris surgeon) and hostess to their many friends in the worlds of art, medicine, literature and theatre.

Princess Grace of Monaco who should be the envy of every woman in the world. Beautiful, slender, soignée, elegant, she could not look more aristocratic had she remained just plain Grace Kelly. She lives in a castle, happily in love with her prince and their two beautiful children. May they live happily ever after!

Jessica Dragonette, beloved by millions as the "Princess of Song" during the golden years of radio; now happily married to Nicholas Meredith Turner. She has lost none of her good looks and her tiny figure is the envy of chic New Yorkers.

The Maharani of Jaipur who while sojourning in London proves that East and West *can* meet. She uses American lipstick and powder, but keeps the exotic touch of ancient Indian eye makeup, a pale gray powder which is applied around the edge of the eye. She has proved that Indian women *can* stay slender and lovely.

Hedda Hopper, who caused women to gasp when they saw how young and beautiful she looked in her recent television appearances.

Paulette Goddard, forever young and beautiful, full of the joy and excitement of living and always looking forward to tomorrow rather than backward at yesterday.

Anita Loos, a doll-like woman, who has not changed one iota in the many years I have known her. Her familiar boyish "hair-do" accents her big eyes and her "little girl" face, but under it is one of the cleverest and wittiest brains in the American theatre.

And last and best, I invite Ann Blodgett, schoolteacher, who has devoted thirty years of her life to teaching other people's children; Mary Mack, faithful secretary, who has for all these years put her boss before herself; Mrs. Jones, Mrs. Schmidt and Mrs. Stein, the wives of doctors, lawyers, merchants, scientists, mechanics and farmers; mothers of Johnny, Freddy and Susan who owe it to themselves and to their families to look younger and live longer, be happier and healthier and ever more beautiful!

A HAPPINESS ROOM

Orientals have such a room in their homes, and I should like to see one in every home of the Western world. This room would have a lock on the door so that you can shut out the world and be alone when you feel the need for solitude. The room should be cheerful with gentle colors, and the greens and yellows of growing things and sunshine, and it should have green growing plants (artificial plants are depressing, like artificial people) and if possible, a singing bird.

The Happiness Room should have music, a radio or better still, a hi-fi with a variety of records: lively ones, even rock and roll, to work off tension; some beautiful ones for quiet moments of happiness, and some Bach or Beethoven for reviving the spirit.

You will need a good chair, your thinking chair, and perhaps this should be a rocking chair to rock away tension while you catch up on your thinking. You will need a couch, firm and supporting, for refreshing moments of deep relaxation, and a small pillow for your head.

The floor should be inviting to stretch out on, too, with clean soft carpeting; as in a Japanese home, people should take off their shoes when they enter the Happiness Room. One or two exercise mats on the floor will invite you to do your stretching and firming exercises.

In your Happiness Room there should be all the devices that make exercise a pleasure and a reward: a great big mirror, your Beauty Slant board, dumbbells, a hanging bar to swing on and stretch and straighten your spine.

You can see that I think of this as the favorite room in your house. So many suburban homes have their rumpus or recreation or play room. Whatever purposes it may serve now, its value could be increased a hundred times if you used your imagination and redesigned it as a Happiness Room. Or you may have a porch, or an airy attic full of unused objects that would give more happiness to the Salvation Army than they now do to you. Get rid of them and give yourself real happiness instead by using the space creatively. Even if you have a small home with no extra room, or a city apartment, create a happiness corner, a place screened for privacy when you want it, where you can do the things you want to do, stretch, yawn, day-dream, laugh or cry, dance, sing, pray.

Your Happiness Room will become your tranquility retreat. And eventually, as you cultivate the spirit for which this room stands, you will carry your happiness room *within* you and retire to it wherever you may be, and whenever you feel the need for deep tranquility.

A BEAUTYFARM AFLOAT

And now there is a brand new beautyfarm idea, a floating beautyfarm. My Paris office informs me that a Greek ship has been offered to me, the same luxurious cruise ship on which Queen Frederika of Greece entertained her royal and distinguished friends and relatives.

The ship is to make a beauty cruise through the blue Mediterranean waters among the fabulous islands of Greece and westward, even to my beloved Sicily. The lucky ladies would sun, swim, eat the exotic fruits and beauty-full native foods of each land with picnics and banquets ashore. There would be sun, air, soil and sea water, all the gifts of bounteous nature. And the ancient beauties of those romantic islands: the temples and statues, the plane tree on the Isle of Cos where Hippocrates sat teaching medicine to his students 500 years before the Christian era; the waters where the thousand Greek ships sailed to recapture Helen of Troy. This would give me a chance to show you beautiful Taormina where I spend much of my time, the land of the Cyclops, the Pool of the Virgins, where only virgins traditionally could bathe, the Greek Theatre, 2,500 years old, and Mt. Aetna towering into the sky, looking down and giving strength and serenity to all.

All this, with constantly changing scenes and settings, and even constantly changing cuisine for the refreshment of body and spirit. It will be a dream of delight. And to make it come true there will be my capable staff under the direction of my friend, lovely

Colette Lefort, who has done so much to advance my work all over France and England.

A cruise on the floating beautyfarm will be no more expensive than the present beautyfarms in Florida, California or Arizona. It will be an experience that one carries in memory for life and an education in good and beauty-full living at its best. I hope you will begin now to save your money for your cruise on the world's first floating beautyfarm.

CHAPTER 24

Au Revoir

Once in my travels abroad I had the wonderful experience of meeting Dr. Carl Gustav Jung, the sage of Zurich. Recently, Dr. Jung celebrated his eighty-fifth birthday. He was still living fully in the beauty of the world around him, still "thinking along the lines of nature." Even at eighty-five he could say, "There are always things ahead, and . . . they are never quite the same. They are 'as good as new'—like human beings."

And here is further wisdom from this wise man. He said, "The more your actual life becomes routine and habit, the less it will be satisfactory. . . .

"New goals demand new eyes which see them and a new heart which desires them."

Now at the end of our little journey into the world of beauty that can be yours, I wish for you the new eyes to see yourself as you will be, and the new heart with which to bring your new beauty into being.

For you can have beauty if you have the wish for it, and the will to make your wish come true. Remember this: most of the things that make a woman beautiful cannot be bought. They come free.

You can buy a coiffure and wave and even hair color, but you cannot buy beautiful, shining, living hair, and without good hair, manufactured beauty aids can only make you look artificial. You can buy the most exquisite cosmetics but they will not give you the inner glow to wear them well. You can even buy a new figure, at a salon where you will be pommeled and exercised and taught to stand and walk beautifully. But you will not keep that beautiful figure and carriage unless you also cultivate them from within.

I have tried to show you in these pages not only that you can be beautiful but also *how* you can be beautiful. As Dr. Jung tells us in the wisdom of his years, think along the lines of nature.

Nature is benevolent and generous to those who trust her. Her gifts of sun, water, and beauty-giving foods are all free. Free, also, is the wonder of the body and the magic of its self-renewing cells. Never forget that if you do not like the self you see in your mirror today, you can create a new self for tomorrow.

BETTER THAN BEAUTY

I have talked about all the physical aspects of beauty, until now perhaps you say to yourself that Gayelord Hauser has been too long in Hollywood where all beauty has become standardized to an oval face, porcelain-capped teeth and sweeping eyelashes. But you would be wrong. External beauty is important. It is the card of introduction that opens doors to opportunity, even to friendship and love. But there are some things in our earthly lives that are better than physical perfection.

We all know some individuals among our friends who would never win any beauty contests, but who have an inner glow of warmth and tranquility that attracts people as sweet clover attracts bees. They are usually individuals who have lived eventful lives, and fortune has not always smiled on them, but they have not become cynical. They have made the best of their experiences, the bitter and the sweet. They possess understanding and compassion enough for all the world.

When such a person speaks, the face lights up with a radiance from within that beggars description. It is a radiance that surpasses physical good looks. But this inner quality is not inherited, and it cannot be bought. It is usually a quality that grows with loving and serving others, with giving and doing for others so that one forgets the self. Only selfishness and self-centeredness are really ugly. Remember the old saying, "Beauty is as beauty does." The beauty that comes from giving of oneself is the kind of beauty that remains, regardless of age.

Nothing can dim this beauty, for it depends on nothing material that can be lost, such as money and possessions. I think of Queen Nazli of Egypt, who once had fifteen castles, and who now lives simply and beautifully in Beverly Hills, enjoying her grandchildren growing up around her. Grandma Moses at the age of one hundred sits serenely painting the simple, beautiful world of her memories. I wish you could have seen her smile with wonder like a child when she said to the newspapermen, "They say I'm a millionaire!" It might be so or it might not, her smile said. Either way, it would make no difference. She would still love the world and paint it lovingly, as she has done during one of the most beautiful old ages the world has ever witnessed.

In my book, *Look Younger, Live Longer*, I spoke of some of these wonderful people who have been my friends and students, and who have made me very proud of them. Now in this book I want to make a cheerful report on two of them. Grandma Reynolds is still merry and brisk at ninety-seven; she appeared recently on television in Playhouse 90. Ann Astaire, mother of two world-famous children and still beautiful at eighty-one, recently crossed the ocean with me by jet plane in six hours. Nothing can daunt the eternal youth of these great ladies.

And no superficial good looks, not even youth, can compare with the beauty of such women. The values of the spirit transcend all externals.

Sunshine and shadow

Each day brings its joy and each day brings some sunshine which we could not appreciate, were it not for some shadows. Learn to accept the shadows with the sunshine. Worry is a profitless state of mind, and nothing is so damaging to your looks as the habit of worry. Let us never forget that the natural, wholesome tendency of the human mind is toward gladness and joy. All Nature is filled with gladness. Look around you, and listen: the birds sing, the leaves rustle, the trees sway, the smallest stream ripples and chuckles, and at night the stars shine steadily and faithfully. There is a constant inner hum which you can hear in your relaxed moments. Listen to it. It will help you to become quiet and to develop a sunny spirit and a joy in life. These are the essential qualities of heart and mind which are so necessary to inner beauty.

A person who lives only for financial security has missed the true purpose of living. Real security comes from an inner serenity, a feeling of fulfillment, which no stock market crash, nor even a threatening "A" bomb can take from us.

For this kind of security we need other, more important values than money—in particular, the value of service to others.

Never shall I forget the day I was privileged to spend with Albert Schweitzer. I sat entranced for hours while he played the organ in the little church at Gunsbach. We ate a simple delicious dinner and for those few hours we shared the serenity of his spirit. With me that day was Marian Preminger, who has done so much wonderful work since then for the Schweitzer Foundation.

In the presence of such people you have the feeling that this confused world is not lost, that all will be well again. Great people are simple people. With them one is relaxed, the spirit is calm and confident.

We can all cultivate this trust in life. Albert Schweitzer believes that every one of us, no matter what we do and who we are, can find full achievement to the very end of our lives. All that is required of us is that we do the best we can, take care of our health, live and eat simply, never stop working, and give the greatest part of our time to others.

"For remember," Albert Schweitzer tells us, "you don't live in a world all your own. *Your brothers are here, too.*"

Take heart from these wise men and women of our time. You can create beauty of body and mind from within, and you will create beauty for those around you, your man and your loved ones.

It is my great wish that through our meeting in these pages I have helped you to become the person you always wanted to be, a woman lovely, a woman beautiful, a woman ageless and serene.

238 East Sixty-Second Street
New York City, U.S.A.
Springtime, 1961

—◦◦⊰◘◦⊱◦◦—

Part Five

BEAUTYFARM

COOKERY

CHAPTER 25

Out of the Frying Pan

The Devil could not be everywhere so he invented the frying pan!

Not only I, but nutritionists all over the world agree that serving quantities of fried food dripping with saturated fats is the most devilish way to destroy health and good looks. Nothing, I believe, can do so much damage to skin, scalp and waistlines as gross, greasy fried food. So the first step in our Eat and Grow Beautiful plan is to throw away your frying pan or give it to your dearest enemy!

BEAUTYFARM COOKBOOK

My next book will be a complete beautyfarm cookbook with exciting recipes from all over the world. Testing and tasting these hundreds of recipes will take a long time. In the meantime, you can get your start in beautyfarm cookery with these recipes. Every recipe has to pass these tests:

1. It has to *taste* good because the more pleasure it gives, the more it satisfies and helps to curb overeating.

2. It has to *do* good, contributing to your health and good looks; no more empty foods.

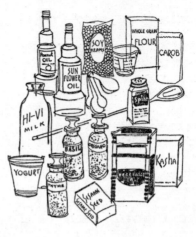

3. It has to *look* good, since we also "eat with our eyes" and beautifully prepared food nourishes the psyche.

NATURAL GOOD COOKS

If you are one of those fortunate Eves, a natural good cook, I congratulate you. You will have no difficulty in preparing beautiful and delicious foods in the modern *avant garde* manner. You need not give up any of your favorite recipes; you simply adapt them to meet these three beautyfarm tests: taste good, do good and look good. Also, remember that the Cosmetic Diet differs from ordinary diets in the following ways:

It is high in proteins.
It is high in vitamins.
It is high in minerals.
It is high in fatty acids.
It is high in fresh foods.
It is high in eye appeal.
It is low in carbohydrate (starches and sugars).
It is lowest in hard fat and grease.

Our first concern should be to muster up as many first class, or complete, proteins as possible. So let us begin with our fine meats and other good proteins.

HIGHEST QUALITY PROTEIN DISHES

Beef. North and South Americans prefer beef to any other kind of meat. I had not realized this until I saw cold statistics showing that 50 percent of all the meat eaten in the Americas is beef in the form of steaks, hamburger, roasts and stews. The next most popular meats (which I do not recommend in our beautyfarm cookery) are pork and pork products. And lamb, one of the meats I recommend highly, is one of the most neglected of all meats. Only 5 percent of Americans eat lamb regularly.

Unfortunately, beef is very high in fat and the prime and choicest steaks and roasts, which most of us prefer, contain approximately 30 percent of hard fat. The less expensive cuts of beef contain only about half as much fat and the same high-quality protein. You yourself—or your butcher—can cut off 40 or 50 percent of the trouble-making fat before cooking. Of all cooking methods, broiling reduces the fat content the most. For roasting, remove as much fat as possible and roast in a slow oven. If you make beef stew, prepare it the day before or in the afternoon and refrigerate it so all the undesirable fat comes to the top and solidifies; then remove it before reheating and serving. This may sound complicated, but it is not, and it can do a great deal to prevent middle age spread.

Veal. Veal makes many excellent dishes. It is probably the leanest of all meats, containing only about 10 percent of fat. The protein is every bit as good as that of beef. In addition veal is easier to digest, is cheaper than beef and can be prepared in a dozen different ways. Nothing can be better than a veal steak Paillard, a thin broiled veal steak prepared as the French women do it, or Vitello ala Salvia, as my cook makes it in Sicily. Very little beef is eaten in Southern Italy and I believe that is one of the reasons why they do not have many cholesterol problems. Broiled veal spiced with herbs makes a superb beautyfarm dish; I am most eager that you learn to eat more young, tender veal of all kinds. Also try stuffed veal breast and veal birds.

Pork. Pork contains as much as 60 percent of hard fat and has no place in healthful cookery nor on a beautyfarm. Smoked pork, lean ham and bacon are permissible, but always broil them until all fat is in the bottom of the pan. Never use any kind of pork fat in cooking, especially if you have trouble with your skin.

Lamb. Very young lamb contains only about 15 percent fat and makes many a delicious dish. Have your butcher cut off as much visible fat as possible and get rid of the rest of the fat by broiling the chops. Young tender lamb stew, cooked with a generous amount and variety of fresh spring vegetables can be a dish for the gods; prepare it the day before and place in the refrigerator; then, before reheating, the fat which has come to the top can easily be removed. Roast leg of spring lamb, a great favorite on beauty-farms, should be baked slowly. Experts have proved by repeated tests that slow baking best retains the goodness and tenderness of all roast meats. To make gravy, remove the fat easily by pouring it over three or four ice cubes in a sieve; most of the fat will cling to the cubes and can be discarded. Reheat the lean gravy and enjoy it to your heart's content.

Chicken. This popular meat is one of our festive and important foods, especially when prepared in the modern manner. Always remember that the younger the chicken, the less fat it contains. A spring broiler contains only about 10 percent of fat, but an old stewing hen can contain as much as 40 percent fat. This is hard fat, remember. Don't you dare serve your husband such an "early grave" stew without skimming off the fat. In preparing chicken, no lard or any solid fat should be used. Simply brush with one of the golden vegetable oils and broil, bake or roast. Do not use the chicken fat or any other meat drippings. Remember the woman who gave all her fat drippings to a neighbor she didn't like!

Turkey. This is another favorite and an excellent protein food. The fat content of turkey depends upon whether or not the turkey was fattened for the market, but most fowl contains only 10 or 15 percent of fat. If you are lucky enough to go hunting for wild fowl, I envy you. All wild game is richer in nutrients and has much more muscle than fat, a good example of the shining effect of exercise. If you enjoy wild duck, pheasant, quail or grouse, just be sure and remove the excess fat.

Fish. This beauty-full food has scored a "breakthrough," says the National Fishery Council, and they are right. For years we have been told to eat more fish for health, and at last Americans are following this good advice. To this I want to add: eat more fish for good looks. Fish contains about the same first class protein as meat, but fish has several other desirable qualities: It is richer in phosphorus and if it is from the ocean it contains an extra bonus of the beauty-giving mineral, iodine. Of late fish has gained another special merit: fish fats are proven to reduce cholesterol, and so the Fishery Council has coined another slogan: "Eat fish and live longer." On the average, fish is much leaner than other animal proteins. The fat content of beef is up to 40 percent and it is of the "unfriendly" variety, whereas the fat content of fish is only 15 percent, and of the "friendly" variety.

All seafood is of paramount importance in our Cosmetic Diet; here is a sample listing of first class proteins from the sea you can choose from. Try them all:

Flounder	Trout
Halibut	Tuna
Haddock	Clams
Red Snapper	Crabs
Salmon	Lobsters
Sardines	Oysters
Sole	Shrimp
Swordfish	

Fish lovers can have a different seafood every day of the week. Remember also, our great oceans are still relatively uncorrupted and free from sprays and additives. Do not make the mistake of using a quantity of grease in fish cookery. Brush fish with one of your golden oils to seal in all the goodness. If a butter sauce is desired, then make one with half butter and half oil and flavor it generously with chopped parsley. In Sicily, where they are great connoisseurs of all seafood, they cook it with olive oil and fresh lemon juice.

BROILED LOBSTER TAILS

If you use the quick-frozen African lobster tails, follow directions on the package. Usually one quick-frozen package makes two or more servings.

Oil broiler pan or grids with a bit of golden oil. Place lobster tails on broiler, flesh side up and season with a bit of vegetable salt. Broil in moderate oven (325-50° F) for about 8 minutes and baste twice during broiling period with a mixture of one tablespoon fresh lemon juice and one tablespoon of golden oil. If lobster tails are thick and larger than ordinary, broil for 10 minutes. Then turn lobster tails over, shell side up, and broil for two to three minutes more, basting once more with lemon and oil mixture. Remove from oven and turn lobster tails flesh side up and sprinkle each with a tablespoon of finely chopped watercress or dill. Serve at once.

Lobster tails can be served hot with a hot or cold hollandaise sauce or chill lobster tails and serve with cold hollandaise sauce.

CANTON GOLDEN SHRIMP SAUTÉ ON RICE

One pound quick-frozen deveined cooked shrimp. Follow directions on package for defrosting. Heat two or three tablespoons of golden oil in a saucepan or chafing dish and one teaspoon of sesame oil for flavor. Add two tablespoons of spring onion tops or chives. Sauté onion or chives about two minutes in hot oil; add shrimp. Stir enough to coat with oil and sprinkle lightly with vegetable salt. Sauté about six minutes or until all shrimp are a light golden brown and serve at once on brown rice.

If you use the deveined raw shrimp, increase cooking time to 8 or 10 minutes.

This makes 4 to 6 servings.

DELIGHTFUL LIVER DISHES

You can use calf liver or the less expensive beef or lamb liver for these simple, but good dishes. Select the freshest liver with dark red color.

Rinse, drain quickly and thoroughly, and remove outside skin and veins. To broil liver, which is the best cookery method, cut in slices about one-fourth to one-half inch thick. Place in oiled broiler pan, season lightly with vegetable salt and sprinkle about one tablespoon of golden oil over the liver. Broil under moderate heat about 5 minutes on each side. Season again lightly with vegetable salt and add finely chopped chives, or chopped capers and raw scallions.

LIVER AND ONIONS

You may want to serve liver in the traditional way, with either onions or apples added to the skillet. For these dishes cut the liver into thin, noodle-like strips; sauté lightly in about one and one-half tablespoons golden oil; stir lightly as it cooks, and sprinkle with vegetable salt.

In another pan sauté two medium-size onions, peeled and cut in rings, in one tablespoon golden oil, and season with a little white pepper. When the onions are golden and beginning to brown, serve them around the hot liver in a warm serving dish. Or stir the onions lightly through the cooked liver, and serve garnished with parsley and lemon sections.

LIVER AND APPLES

Cook liver, as described above for liver and onions. Core apples, do not pare, then slice them about one-half inch thick. Sauté apples in about one tablespoon golden oil about 5 minutes, or until almost tender. Season with a very little cinnamon and brown sugar, and vegetable salt. Turn slices, cook until lightly browned on other side. Apples should be tender, but not mushy. Serve the hot liver on a warmed platter surrounded by the apple slices. If there are good juices in the liver pan, stir a little yogurt into the pan, heat, and pour over the liver on the platter. One pound of liver makes four delightful servings.

FRESH CHICKEN LIVERS WITH MUSHROOMS

¾ lb. fresh chicken livers   3 tbsp. minced onion
¼ cup golden oil   ½ tsp. vegetable salt
  2 cups sliced mushrooms   ⅛ tsp. paprika

Wash, rinse, and cut the livers in pieces. Heat the oil in a heavy skillet and sauté the livers, mushrooms, and onion over low heat, stirring occasionally, for about 5 minutes. Add seasoning and serve on toast or boiled rice, or in the fold of an omelet.

No doubt you have your own favorite meat dishes. By all means enjoy them, but learn to cook them in the modern manner—lean,

lean! In place of the hard fats, learn to use the golden oils. Here are some beautyfarm favorites to start you on your way:

LAMB CHOPS GARNI

Golden oil	1 tsp. thyme, chopped
4 lamb chops	1 tsp. sweet basil, chopped
Vegetable salt	1 tsp. parsley, chopped

Brush lamb chops lightly with golden oil. Preheat the broiling oven about 5 minutes. Place chops on oiled broiling rack about two inches below the heat. Leave the broiler door open unless your range directions state otherwise.

Sear the chops on both sides under high heat. Then reduce the heat and continue cooking. Turn the chops occasionally.

For single chops about three-fourths inch thick, broil about 10 to 12 minutes. For double chops, of one to one-and-one-half inch thickness, broil 15 to 20 minutes.

When the chops are done, sprinkle a little vegetable salt on a hot serving platter, place the chops on the platter, add a dab or two of the herbs mixed with a few drops of golden oil. Serve at once. Makes four servings.

CHIPPED BEEF

This good beef is all protein, most of its fat having been removed before the meat was dried into the delicious flavorful morsel we serve too often as a richly creamed dish.

Instead of creaming this meat, here is a savory appetizer idea. Grind about one-half cup chipped beef, blend with about one-fourth cup lean cottage cheese, season with vegetable salt and add a few chopped capers. Moisten with yogurt to make a good spreading texture.

Spread the beef cheese mixture on half moons of pumpernickel or on sesame seed bread or crackers. Or spread on thin slices of whole wheat bread, cover with another slice of bread, and cut this sandwich in slender strips.

Use protein-rich chipped beef too, in an aspic of chicken or turkey; the red strips of dried beef alternating with the pale chicken and turkey slices add color and flavor.

BLANQUETTE DE VEAU

Veal stew at its best

2 lbs. breast or shoulder of veal
1 qt. water
1 tsp. vegetable salt
1 small carrot, sliced
1 onion, peeled and stuck with clove
Bundle of herbs (parsley, bay leaf, 1 small stalk of celery, sprig dried thyme) tied together

10 small onions, peeled
¼ lb. mushrooms, sliced
2½ tbsp. golden oil
Vegetable salt and grated nutmeg
2 fresh egg yolks
1 cup yogurt
1 tbsp. lemon juice
Chopped parsley

Cut veal into bite size pieces, cover with water in a deep stewing pot, add the salt. Bring to boil, then skim well. Add the carrot, onion and bundle of herbs, cover the pot and cook over low heat about 30 minutes. Add the small onions and continue cooking one-half hour longer, or until the meat is tender.

Sauté the mushrooms in the hot oil in another pan, about 5 minutes. Remove the cooked meat, carrot, and small onions to a warmed serving platter, cover, and place in a warm oven, leaving the oven door open.

Discard the bundle of herbs and the large onion used in the pot liquid; skim off all fat. Then add the mushrooms in the oil in which they were sautéed. There should be about three cups of pot liquid and mushrooms. Cook and stir 15 minutes, taste, correct seasoning, adding a little more vegetable salt if needed, and about one-fourth teaspoon of nutmeg. Beat egg yolks, mix with yogurt and lemon juice. Add a few spoonfuls of the hot pot liquid to the egg mixture, stir, then return all to the pot. Stir briskly all the time, cook just below boiling point. Do not boil.

Spoon the mushrooms over the top of the meat on the platter, pour the pot sauce over all. Add sprinkling of parsley. Makes six or more servings.

The sauce on this stew is not the classic thick creamed sauce made in French kitchens, because the French cooks use too much flour and cream. But this low-fat sauce is delicious, well-flavored and light.

VEAL SCALLOPINI

1 lb. veal round steak	1 clove garlic
2 tbsp. golden oil	1 tsp. lemon juice
1 tsp. vegetable salt	1 cup California sauterne

Cut veal into serving-size portions and dip in wholewheat flour. Heat oil with crushed garlic in heavy utensil. Sauté meat until it turns a golden brown. Remove garlic and add wine and lemon juice. Cover tightly and let simmer about 20 minutes or until meat is very tender. Remember, wine helps to tenderize and gives a delightful flavor; the alcohol evaporates.

CHICKEN AT ITS BEST

For this delicate, wonderfully flavored low-fat dish of chicken, select a bird not less than three and one-half pounds, or a capon of about five pounds. Have poultry dealer singe, clean and truss the bird.

Rub the bird inside and out with a little golden oil and lemon juice. Place the chicken breast side up in an uncovered roaster. Roast in a hot oven, 450° F. about 20 minutes, or until brown. Reduce the heat to moderately slow, 325° F. and roast, allowing 18 to 25 minutes per pound. For a plump chicken roast a little longer, to be sure it is well cooked through and not red around the bones.

While the chicken roasts, baste it at 15 minute intervals with the beautyfarm basting sauce. When the chicken is nearly done, turn it breast side down and let the underside brown evenly. To test a chicken for doneness insert a two-tined kitchen fork into the thickest part of the breast and the second joint. If the juices do not run red, the chicken is done.

Some prefer the moderate-temperature method of roasting. For this, heat the oven to 350° F. Roast the chicken at that temperature for 25 to 30 minutes per pound. A four-pound chicken requires 1 hour and 40 minutes to 2 hours.

For a good poultry stuffing, mix about three and one-half cups cooked brown or wild rice, and add four chopped cooked prunes, and one chopped whole orange, seeds removed. Stuff and bake as described, allowing a few minutes more per pound.

Or for the added pleasure of eating herbed roast chicken, add 1 teaspoon oregano and sweet basil to the stuffing. Or add these herbs to the hot oil and water with which you baste the chicken, or to the Beautyfarm Basting Sauce. A three and one-half pound chicken serves four or more.

VEGE-NUT STUFFING

2 cups shredded carrots
2 shredded apples
1 cup shredded celery
1 large onion, shredded
1 cup shredded summer squash
½ cup raisins, chopped fine

1 cup chopped walnuts
2 green peppers, chopped
Vegetable salt to taste
1 clove of garlic
2 eggs, well beaten

Combine all ingredients. This dressing is utterly delicious and was the pride of my cook, Anna Lee.

CELERY NUT LOAF

½ cup sliced celery
½ small onion
⅜ cup nutmeats
¾ cup tomato juice
½ tbsp. grated yellow cheese
1 tsp. vegetable salt

1 tbsp. vegetable oil
⅔ cup wholewheat bread
   crumbs or crumbled
   shredded wheat
   biscuit
2 fresh eggs, well beaten

Put the celery, onion, and nutmeats through the medium knife of a food grinder. Add all the ingredients except the eggs and mix well. Add the beaten eggs and mix in lightly. Pack into a loaf pan prepared with 2 teaspoons of vegetable oil and a thick layer of crumbs (2 or 3 tablespoons) evenly sprinkled on the bottom. Bake in a moderate oven (375° F.) about 35 minutes, until thick enough to be turned out. Remove from the oven and loosen the sides with a knife. Invert the pan over a platter and turn out the loaf. Garnish with wedges of ripe tomato and a generous sprinkling of chopped parsley. Preparation: 20-25 minutes.

BEAUTYFARM CURRY SAUCE

In India, curry powder is usually added to the stock in which the meat, chicken or vegetables have been cooked. No thickening is used. The amount of curry powder used depends on its strength and on your own taste. Some like it mild, some like it hot. However, most Americans prefer this curry sauce which is similar to a thin white sauce. (The original Indian version is recommended for reducers!)

1 tbsp. golden oil	2 fresh egg yolks
1 tbsp. fresh butter	½ pt. sweet cream
2 tsp. curry powder	½ tsp. vegetable salt
½ cup vegetable or chicken broth	

Melt the butter and oil, but do not brown, in heavy skillet. Blend in curry powder and stir until smooth. Add broth and simmer for three minutes. Beat egg yolks and mix them with the cream. Now reduce the heat (important) and pour egg and cream mixture into skillet. Do not let the sauce boil after eggs and cream have been added. This delicious basic sauce has been used successfully by thousands of my students. With it you can make a dozen different delicious curries and it takes only a few moments to prepare this Indian delight.

Lean Lamb Curry: Cook lamb in usual manner. Remove excess fat. When tender, pour curry sauce over lamb and let simmer for five minutes.

Seafood Curry: Put shrimp, crabmeat or lobster into the hot curry sauce before the egg and cream are added. When sea food is thoroughly heated, pour the egg yolk and cream mixture over and simmer for three minutes more.

Egg Curry: Cut six hard cooked eggs into quarters. Drop these carefully into the hot curry sauce. Heat thoroughly, sprinkle with paprika and serve very hot.

Avocado Curry: Peel two or three not over-ripe avocadoes. Cut into thick slices. Put into hot curry sauce for only a few minutes and serve at once.

All curries taste best when served over cooked, dry, flaky rice.

Beautyfarm basting sauces

You can prepare a delectable roast chicken, turkey, or duck without using any fat, even in the basting. Prepare the fowl, or separate pieces such as breast, halves, legs, for roasting. Roast as usual, but baste every twenty minutes of roasting time with the following sauce.

2 chicken or vegetable bouillon cubes	1 cup orange juice
	¼ cup lemon juice
1 cup boiling water	½ tsp. vegetable salt

Dissolve the bouillon cubes in the boiling water. Combine with the fruit juices. Add salt and mix well. Use for basting as described.

More Lean Basting Ideas: For a roast lamb, skim the fat from the roaster continually during the cooking period. Baste the roast frequently with a warm mixture of white wine, bouillon, and a few chopped fresh mint leaves.

Blend tomato or mixed vegetable espresso (see index) with bouillon. Add a crumbled bay leaf and a dash of dried rosemary. Heat slightly, and use to baste veal as it cooks. Wonderful flavor in the roast when you carve it onto warmed dinner plates.

Baste roasting chicken, turkey, and other fowl with a warm mixture of orange juice, lemon juice, bouillon, flavored lightly with oregano and a little dried rosemary. And, for superlative flavor in any roast, rub the meat thoroughly with vegetable salt before it goes into the oven. Basting washes some of the seasoning off, so add a light sprinkling of vegetable salt over the top of the roast after the last basting.

Eggs are a wonder food!

Eggs are a complete food, complete enough to make a beautiful chick! Eggs contain all the necessary amino acids and they are a treasure-house of vitamins and minerals, especially vitamins A, B-2 and iron. The raw egg yolk, beaten into orange juice, makes a splendid pep and beauty booster, but the white of raw eggs should not be used habitually. The raw egg white can cause all sorts of skin difficulties and allergies because the avidin in the white combines with the biotin, one of the B-vitamins, and so prevents it from getting into the blood stream. Biotin deficiencies can be responsible for many ugly skin conditions. Eggs are nutritionally at their best either hard-cooked or at least until the white is firm. Contrary to popular belief, hard-cooked eggs are not hard to digest. It is always wise to keep some hard boiled eggs in the refrigerator. Each one contains seven or eight grams of first class protein. Eggs also have tremendous satiety value, whether eaten with or between meals. They help to satisfy an overdemanding stomach. All healthy people should enjoy one or two eggs a day. They are high in cholesterol, but they are also high in lecithin and the B vitamins which help to keep cholesterol on the move. Unless your doctor has specifically forbidden you to eat eggs, I hope you will enjoy them daily. Eggs are also wonderful fortifiers of other foods. Try and obtain the freshest eggs possible. Beauty-farms can raise their own fertile eggs. These seem to have definite advantages over the mass-produced eggs from chickens which are never allowed on the ground.

EAT EGGS IN EVERY FORM

Soft boiled, hard boiled, poached, scrambled, even fried, but use the friendly golden oils, like sesame oil. This has a delightful flavor. Hard fried eggs in butter are definitely detrimental to good health and good looks. Raw egg yolks can be enjoyed in every form, especially mixed into fruit juices and broths.

MILK AND MILK PRODUCTS

Milk, like eggs, contains a first class tissue-building protein. It would be ideal if we could get fresh milk directly from the farmer, but only beauty farmers who have their own healthy certified herds are in this advantageous position. The fresh milk you buy in your market is also a first-class protein. Remember, one quart of milk contains about thirty-two grams of protein, therefore, any woman drinking a pint of milk gets sixteen grams of good protein, plus the necessary amount of calcium. Milk, when combined with other foods, makes them doubly valuable. In some parts of Italy they cook their spaghetti in milk to give it extra food value. Cooking cereals in milk at once makes them doubly a beauty-full food. Skim milk is preferable for all adults unless they are painfully thin. Half a cup of powdered skim milk contains around thirty grams of good protein, therefore, one of the most delightful and easy-to-fix beauty drinks is a half cup of powdered skim milk, stirred into a quart of fresh skim milk. Here you have at least fifty grams of fine protein. To vary this drink and for extra flavor, you can flavor it with a tablespoon of honey, molasses, licorice, carob powder, or if you are watching your waistline, add a bit of cinnamon or nutmeg.

LEAN COTTAGE CHEESE

The best cottage cheese today is made in America and in France, where the biggest dairies have learned to remove the cream from the milk and with special processes of fermentation use their millions of gallons of skim milk to make a delectable, creamy cheese, without the cream. Lean cottage cheese can be used in a hundred different ways. Its protein is a perfect protein, as good as that in filet mignon and much, much less expensive. Lean cottage cheese makes an ideal beautyfarm food; one half cup gives you twenty grams of complete protein; it also contains large amounts of lactic acid so valuable to the friendly bacteria in the digestive tract. In addition, cottage cheese contains some vitamin A, so important for smooth skin; vitamin B, the anti-dry skin vitamin, and a wealth of calcium and phosphorus, so important for good bones, teeth and proud posture. Most important, lean cottage cheese is probably the most versatile of all foods. It can take the place of meat, when meat is not available or too expensive, it can be used in place of butter as a spread, it marries well with any vegetable for salads unlimited. It mixes with all fruits and makes dozens of delightful desserts, it makes nourishing drinks, and salad dressings, and all can be enjoyed to your heart's content; there is no fat and no cholesterol.

In Germany, cottage cheese is called "*Lucullus Kaese*," named after Lucullus, the rich Roman, famous for his gourmet banquets. In Russia, where I saw more cottage cheese than any place, it is sold in the markets by the bucketful. It is called *"Tvoroge"* and devoured for breakfast, lunch, dinner and in-between. Then, of course, lean cottage cheese, whipped to a creamy consistency with another beauty-full food—yogurt—can take the place of sour cream in excellent desserts and nourishing between-meal drinks, especially when mixed in an electric liquidizer with fresh fruit such as berries or apricots.

MAKE YOUR OWN COTTAGE CHEESE

If you want to be sure that your cottage cheese is fresh, you can make your own. This is an inexpensive way to keep your protein intake high. Whenever you are tired of drinking milk, you can eat it in the form of delightful fresh cottage cheese.

Directions: Heat a quart of milk in a heavy utensil or double boiler. When warm, add one tablespoon of lemon juice. Stir and keep heat low. When milk curdles, remove from stove. Then pour entire quart into cheesecloth or muslin and drain. A bit of vegetable salt improves the flavor. If cottage cheese is too dry, mix it with yogurt.

Now that you have learned to make your own cottage cheese, there are endless ways to use it. No doubt you have your own recipes, but here are a few new ones:

Protein Salads Unlimited

Mix equal amounts of fresh cottage cheese with finely shredded carrots and top with yogurt dressing. Serve on crisp greens.

You can make dozens of complexion salads by mixing equal parts of cottage cheese with radishes, celery, green pepper, cucumber, onions, parsley. Try them all.

Hi-Vi Fruit Salads

Mix cottage cheese into gelatin salads and desserts. When meat portions are meager, serve cottage cheese as a side dish. As a change from plain cottage cheese, flavor it with herbs, seasonings or with a bit of Rocquefort cheese. You can mix cottage cheese with scrambled eggs or with chipped beef. These make a delightful breakfast dish:

COTTAGE CHEESE PANCAKES

3 fresh eggs	2 tbsp. golden oil
1 cup sieved cottage cheese	4 tbsp. sifted flour
Pinch vegetable salt	

Beat eggs light and frothy, then add cottage cheese and oil. Add flour to mixture and mix until smooth. Put heaping tablespoonful on hot oiled griddle. Bake both sides golden brown. Serve with honey or applesauce.

YOGURT

Yogurt is a type of cultured milk, like acidophilus milk with a virile strain of *bacillus bulgaricus*. The advantages of using yogurt in place of ordinary milk are many. The bacteria in buttermilk and ordinary sour milks cannot live at body temperature nor can they survive the hydrochloric acid of the stomach, hence they cannot live and multiply in the digestive tract.

One of the principle reasons for using real yogurt on beautyfarms is that its bacteria can live and multiply in the intestinal tract. Dr. Gustav Martin of the Warner Institute of Therapeutic Research proved that the bacteria in yogurt actually manufacture or synthesize vitamins of the B complex.

Yogurt has been popular for centuries, especially in Bulgaria. In France, yogurt is becoming increasingly popular. The French use it as a food, drink and dessert. Chambourcey, the leading dairy in Paris, now makes the best yogurt. It is made of lean milk so everybody can enjoy it. If you can buy ready-made yogurt in your city, by all means do so, but if you cannot, here is a million dollar beauty secret for making your own. Please remember that the ferment in yogurt makes milk easier to digest and by fortifying inexpensive skim milk with a cup of powdered skim milk, you have one of the finest protein-rich, easy-to-digest foods of the first order.

In just one quart of such fortified fat free yogurt, you have about sixty-five to seventy grams of first class, tissue-building protein.

How to Make Real Yogurt

The easiest way to make the above Hi-Vi yogurt is to heat one quart of fresh skim milk. Heat this mixture carefully until it is hot, but do not boil. This is important, boiling kills the *bacillus bulgaricus*. Into this hot, but *not* boiling milk, you stir one cup of powdered skim milk, plus three tablespoonsful of ready-made yogurt. Pour this mixture into a wide-mouthed thermos jar, cover and let it stand over night. It takes from four to six hours for yogurt to become solid. The next morning, remove top of thermos and place the yogurt in refrigerator.

A Yogurt Starter

If you are unable to buy ready-made yogurt in your city, write or go to your nearest health food store and purchase a bottle of real yogurt culture. With such culture you can make yogurt for a whole month. After your first initial batch, made with this culture, always save a half cup to make the next batch. If you make yogurt for a whole family, I suggest that you invest in a professional yogurt maker.

DELICIOUS HONEY YOGURT

Parisians and other real yogurt gourmets eat their yogurt "straight," but for variety's sake and to induce "milk haters" to enjoy yogurt, it can be made with many flavors: honey, molasses and any of your favorite fruit preserves. Flavored yogurts are already commercially available, but they are usually loaded with empty sugar. Once you have learned to make real yogurt, white and custardy, try making yogurt with different flavors.

Honey yogurt is made by stirring three tablespoonsful of honey into the milk before you heat it. The milk should be good and hot, but do not boil. If you have learned to make honey yogurt, experiment with other flavors, but always remember, the beauty value is in the protein-rich yogurt itself.

BLOODY MARY YOGURT!

For a delicious appetizer or between-meal lift, mix a half cup of yogurt with a half cup of thick tomato juice; season with a pinch of vegetable salt and a few drops of fresh lemon juice. (This is an excellent pick-up for the morning after and does much more good than a Bloody Mary.)

ORANGE YOGURT

Place a tablespoon of fresh frozen orange juice concentrate on top of a glass of thick chilled yogurt. Serve in crystal goblets.

You can make dozens of different desserts by adding any of your favorite fruit concentrates to chilled yogurt.

RASPBERRY YOGURT

Fill dessert glasses with thick chilled yogurt and top with a tablespoon of fresh, canned or frozen raspberries.

Take your choice of any and all fresh or frozen fruits. They "marry" very well with fresh yogurt and make beautyfarm desserts unlimited.

ELEGANT YOGURT PIE

A Polish count brought this nutritious recipe to America. Yogurt pie is one of the favorite desserts in Hollywood. I ate it for the first time at a glamorous party given by Cobina Wright, Hollywood's beloved First Lady. This is a rich dessert and should be reserved for special events.

Fill a lean eight-inch crisp pastry shell with the following:

1 cup thick yogurt	½ tsp. vanilla
½ lb. fresh, mild cream cheese	Dash salt
1 tbsp. honey	

Whip the filling nice and smooth; pour into pastry shell and place in refrigerator until served.

A Hundred Ways To Use Yogurt Cream Cheese

As a spread on bread. Remember it is protein, not fat and you can use it generously. It is even good with your breakfast toast; pears and peaches stuffed with this delightful cheese make nutritious and delicious desserts. You can also make a variety of delightful protein-rich salad dressings and, of course, this lean yogurt cheese makes the most delicious cheesecake you ever ate.

I dedicate this million-dollar beauty recipe to beautyfarms every-

where. In my beautyfarm cookbook there will be many exciting recipes from all over the world. Perhaps some of my new readers will send me some of their new and unusual recipes.

Make Your Own Cream Cheese

If you like cream cheese and your waistline cannot afford it, here is a million-dollar tip: simply dump a cup of your yogurt into a piece of muslin or fine cheesecloth and hang it above your sink to drain overnight. The very next morning you have a white ball of the tenderest, creamiest cream cheese you ever ate; protein-rich, calcium and vitamin B-rich, but no fat! To give this beauty treat more flavor and savour, season the cupful of yogurt with a pinch of vegetable salt and the smallest pinch of brown sugar.

THE SOYA BEAN, A POTENT
VEGETABLE PROTEIN

Soya beans are the cheapest source of protein of high quality. They can be served in many different ways: cooked, baked, toasted, sprouted, as milk, in soups and many other ways. Unfortunately, Americans in the past failed to adopt this Oriental "meat," perhaps because they used to be difficult to prepare, but now there is a new easy-to-cook soya bean grown right in the United States. This new soya bean, served occasionally, will be a welcome change for many. If you are too busy to cook soya beans, I recommend the canned ones. They are a fine and inexpensive protein. Try them baked.

BAKED SOYBEANS

1 cup dried large soybeans	1 onion, thinly sliced
Hot vegetable broth	1¼ tsp. vegetable salt
4 tbsp. golden oil	¼ lemon cut in thin slices
2 tbsp. unsulphured molasses	Juice of ¼ lemon

Wash the soybeans and put them in a kettle in which you can boil them next day. Pour 3 cups of water over them and soak overnight. Bring to a boil in the same water and cook slowly, adding hot vegetable broth as needed to keep the beans covered. Simmer for 3 to 4 hours, until the beans are a light tan. Transfer to a covered baking dish and add the oil and molasses. Bake in moderate oven (325° F) for 1-2 hours, depending on the age and quality of the beans, until they are brown and well done. Stir occasionally during the baking and keep the beans in liquid until the last half-hour. At that time add the onion, salt, and the lemon juice and slices. Return to the oven until the top is brown. Serve in the baking dish and garnish with chopped parsley or onion tops. 4 servings.

You can save yourself the above work by buying canned soya beans. They are delicious and nutritious. Into a utensil containing two one-pound cans of baked soyabeans, mix the following:

¼ cup unsulphured molasses	1 tomato sliced
1 tbsp. prepared mustard	1 onion sliced on top
1 tbsp. vinegar	

Makes 6 delicious servings.

Soybean Flour

This is one of the most nutritious foods of all. One tablespoon of soya flour has approximately the same food value as an egg. Soybean flour should be added to muffins, biscuits, waffles and breads. Using soya products for breakfast makes it easy to get sufficient proteins into this most important meal.

How to grow bean sprouts

Among the finest vegetables used by Orientals are the potent little bean sprouts. They furnish not only protein but rich amounts of vitamin C. They are so easy to grow:

Cover the bottom of a four-cornered Pyrex dish with one layer of soy or mung beans. Cover with lukewarm water and soak overnight. In the morning, pour off excess water from the corner of the dish. Cover glass dish with another one of the same size and place in a corner for even temperature. Add fresh water twice daily. Rinse and pour off all excess. Tender sprouts will appear the second day

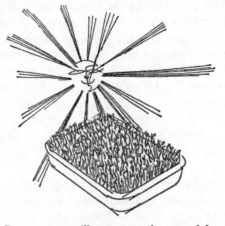

Bean sprouts will appear on the second day

and they are usually ready to eat on the fourth day. The hulls of the beans will rise to the top or sink to the bottom and are easily removed. These bean sprouts are another natural, rich source of vitamin C and you derive the most benefit when sprouts are eaten raw and mixed into salads or sandwiches. They are also excellent sprinkled over cooked vegetables and, of course, are wonderful when mixed into chop suey. Bean sprouts are a "wonder food." After you have learned to sprout soy beans, you should also try wheat, lentil, alfalfa and other edible seeds. In an emergency sprouts could become real life savers! Mung and soy beans are for sale at your diet and health food shop.

BEAUTYFARM VEGETABLE COOKERY

Short-cooking is the beautyfarm way. The quicker vegetables are cooked, the less is the loss of beauty-giving vitamins B, C and P. These vitamins, like salt, dissolve in water so we use very little or no water, and never is any of the vegetable cooking water poured off because with it the beauty-giving vitamins go down the sink.

There are two ways of short-cooking. I have taught the first method for several years: you simply cut up or shred the vegetables into thin slices with a vegetable shredder. Such shredded vegetables are cooked in a very few minutes' time. Put cut up shredded vegetables into a heavy cooking utensil, and to prevent any possibility of burning, put two or three tablespoons of liquid into the cooking utensil. When liquid steams you add your cut up vegetables and cover tightly. Cook the vegetables until tender, but not mushy, and all you add is a pinch of vegetable salt and, if your waistline permits, a small amount of butter—whipped butter goes further, it looks and tastes delightful and is easier on the waistline. Cooking the vegetables in two or three tablespoonfuls of fat-free vegetable or chicken broth enhances the flavor.

Chinese Cookery

Palm Springs, California, is the home of several exclusive beautyfarms and health spas. It is also famous for its very fine restaurant, the *Beachcomber*. In this restaurant vegetable cookery has become a fine art. While watching the Filipino chef, I wished that all beautyfarm cooks might see how simply and how deliciously fresh vegetables can be turned into flavorsome dishes. The fresh vegetables come directly from the Imperial Valley. They are scrubbed painstakingly and cut into bite-size pieces. (This is the second method of short-cooking.) This chef uses golden sesame oil. It is mild and does not overshadow the fresh taste of the vegetable itself. The golden sesame oil is heated in a heavy steel cooking utensil and when it is very hot, but not smoking, the cut-up tender vegetables are sautéed for just a few minutes in this good oil. All the goodness is sealed in and nothing is poured off. I suggest that beautyfarms everywhere adopt this simple way of sautéeing fresh vegetables in golden oils. With such sautéed vegetables, there is no need for extra butter. All you need do is add your favorite herbs, a bit of vegetable salt or, if you prefer, you can spike the vegetables with a bit of soya sauce.

BEANS, CARROTS, TURNIPS

All root vegetables can be short-cooked in minutes in this easy manner: Select the youngest and tenderest vegetables available. Wash and scrub, then shred on medium-size shredder. In a small heavy utensil prepare two or three tablespoonfuls of vegetable water or chicken broth. When this steams, put in your shredded vegetables. Cover tightly for five minutes. Shake occasionally to

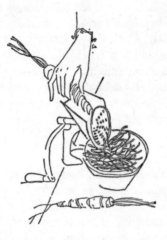

prevent sticking. As soon as shreds are tender, add vegetable salt to taste, a bit of whipped butter or a tablespoon of golden oil.

P.S.: If you shred your vegetables, even cauliflower and broccoli can be cooked in a matter of moments.

BEAN SPROUTS SAUTÉ

1 lb. fresh bean sprouts	1 tbsp. soy sauce
2 tbsp. golden oil	¼ tsp. vegetable salt

Put two tablespoons peanut or sesame oil in heavy cooking utensil. When very hot, add bean sprouts, stir and mix in soy sauce and salt. Then cover utensil tightly, reduce the heat and cook four minutes more. Bean sprouts taste best when served very hot.

BRAISED ENDIVES

6 Belgian endives	Juice 1 lemon
¼ cup golden oil	3 tbsp. finely minced watercress
½ tsp. vegetable salt	

Rinse the endives in cold water. Cut off any damaged outer leaves. Slice off root end and tips of top end.

Heat oil in shallow heavy utensil. Add endives, sprinkle with vegetable salt and lemon juice. Cover the utensil, lower the heat to the minimum for cookery and cook 5 minutes. Increase the heat and cook 15 to 20 minutes, depending on the thickness of the endives. Shake the casserole from time to time. Add a very little hot water or bouillon if needed.

Serve hot as a vegetable, or serve cold Vinaigrette as a salad. Makes 6 servings.

CHINESE SNOW PEAS

1 lb. Chinese snow-pea pods	1 tsp. vegetable salt
3 tbsp. sesame oil	½ cup chicken broth

Only Chinese grocers, or gourmet food shops specializing in this delicacy, can supply you with the most tender and young pea pods which go by the fairy-tale name of snow peas.

To prepare them, wash the pods, clean them like string beans by pulling off any strings and breaking off any obvious tips. Heat the oil and seasoning in heavy utensil. Stir the pods in, add the chicken broth, cover and cook 2 minutes. Then stir, and cook 2 minutes more. Add more chicken broth if needed.

Usually 4 to 6 minutes' cooking is as much as the Chinese cook allows for this tender vegetable. The peas should still be a bit "chewy," as are all Chinese vegetables. Serve them hot with rice and chicken, or any meat. Makes four servings.

SUMMER SOUP FROM PERSIA

In Iran, Lebanon, Turkey, and all over the Near Eastern world, there are wonderfully cooling and delicious soups made with cold yogurt and chopped iced vegetables.

These soups are served as the main dish of luncheon, with sesame seed bread, and afterwards a small cup of hot coffee or a tall cool fruit drink.

One of the most flavorful and delectable of these cold yogurt soups is this one:

1 cup chopped peeled onion	Vegetable salt
½ cup diced unpared cucumber	Freshly ground pepper
½ cup chopped water cress	Garnish
2 cups very cold yogurt	

Combine the vegetables and chill them until very cold. Then mix them with the cold yogurt. Pour into chilled soup bowls, adding one or two ice cubes to each bowl. Add a dash of pepper. And for garnish, place a slice of one of the bright red miniature "marble" tomatoes on each serving, or a spoonful of diced lemon peel, or of diced stuffed olives. Makes two to four servings.

Some Lebanese hosts simply serve to each guest a bowl of yogurt and a platter of iced, chopped vegetables. Everyone chooses the vegetables he likes best, spoons them into his yogurt, stirs and enjoys the dish for its cooling and its fine flavor. Try this on your overweight friends.

COOLING APPLE SOUP FROM STOCKHOLM

For luncheon on a hot day or supper on a warm night the Scandinavian fruit soups are becoming popular. You may prefer to add a small amount of gelatin to the fruit mixture instead of the traditional potato flour or cornstarch used by Swedish cooks. If gelatin is added, use 2 teaspoons unflavored gelatin to one quart soup. Soften the gelatin in one-fourth cup cold water, then stir it into the hot soup after removing the soup from the heat. Stir gelatin in well to dissolve evenly. Let the soup cool, then chill as usual. It should be stirred well before serving to break up any suggestion of jelly.

Here is the traditional recipe for Swedish Apple Soup:

3 cups diced pared apples	⅛ tsp. vegetable salt
1 qt. water	1 tbsp. potato flour, cornstarch
¼ cup honey	or preferably gelatin
2 inch stick cinnamon	¼ cup cold water
Grated peel 1 lemon	¼ cup white wine or sherry

Combine the fruit, water, honey, cinnamon, and lemon peel and salt in an enamelware saucepan. Cook gently until the fruit is soft. Let cool a little and pass through a fine sieve. Reheat. Mix the potato flour or cornstarch with the cold water, stirring smoothly. When the soup is boiling, stir the cornstarch in slowly. Stir and cook 10 minutes. Add wine or sherry and mix. Remove from heat. Let cool, then chill thoroughly.

Serve in cold glass bowls, the soup garnished with a spoonful of grated raw apple and a mint leaf. Makes four servings.

CHERRY SOUP FROM COPENHAGEN

This clear, refreshing ruby soup is a feast for the eyes as well as the palate. It is made from great black or deep-red ox-heart cherries. Prepare it well ahead of the luncheon or supper at which you want to serve it, and let it chill thoroughly.

2 lbs. ripe ox-heart cherries	2 cups Burgundy, claret or a rosé wine
2 cups water	
2 inch stick cinnamon	1 tbsp. Cognac, or cherry brandy
2 cloves	
¼ tsp. vegetable salt	2 tbsp. honey, more if desired

Pit the cherries into an enamelware kettle. Add water, cinnamon, cloves and salt. Cook slowly until the cherries are soft. Rub them through a sieve. Add the wine, brandy, and honey to taste. Reheat slowly, but do not boil. When steaming hot, remove from the heat. Let cool, then chill thoroughly.

Serve in chilled glass bowls, each set deeply in a larger bowl of cracked ice. Makes six or more servings.

In place of the whipped cream which the hardy Danes serve on this soup, you may like to stir a tablespoon of snowy cold yogurt through each bowl, or swirl a little yogurt on top of each serving.

PORTUGUESE GASPACHO

I first became acquainted with this unusual cold soup when I visited Portugal, but I have since learned that it is also popular in Spain, Mexico and South America. It is an ideal dish for hot weather. There are dozens of variations of the basic recipe. You can add garlic, parsley, chives or fresh herbs such as basil or tarragon when available, and experiment with small amounts of paprika and a dash of cayenne. A cup of stock can be substituted for tomato juice:

4 good sized ripe tomatoes peeled and chopped
1 large unpeeled cucumber, diced
1 onion minced
1 green pepper without seeds finely minced
1 cup tomato juice
½ cup French dressing (⅓ cider vinegar, ⅔ olive oil, vegetable salt).

Mix all ingredients in a bowl and put in the refrigerator to cool. Serve in soup dishes over a cube of ice.

TOMATO MADRILÈNE

To make a flavorful, delicious Madrilène, you must first prepare a simple tomato bouillon by combining equal amounts of fresh or canned tomato juice, and fat-free chicken stock or bouillon from cubes. Season this mixture with lemon juice (about one tablespoon), vegetable salt and a pinch of brown sugar.

For each four cups of this juice-and-bouillon mixture add one-half teaspoon basil, one tablespoon chopped peeled onion, two cloves, one-half teaspoon celery seeds.

Heat gently in a stainless steel kettle. Simmer, do not boil. When thoroughly hot remove from the heat, let cool, then strain. Serve as a simple soup, reheated and garnished with chopped parsley or a paper-thin slice of lemon.

Or use it in this delightful Madrilène recipe:

2 tbsp. unflavored gelatin	¼ cup chopped, cooked shrimp,
½ cup water	chicken or mixed raw vege-
4 cups tomato bouillon	tables if desired
Thin slices lemon, or	Vegetable salt, to taste

Soften the gelatin in the water. Heat about one cup of the bouillon and stir the softened gelatin in until dissolved. Then combine this with the remaining three cups of bouillon. Taste, and season with your favorite herbs. Stir well. Chill.

When the gelatin is firm, break it up lightly with a fork into good-sized chunks. Serve heaped in very cold bouillon cups with a thin slice of lemon in the bottom of each cup, or a spoonful of chopped cooked shrimp or chicken. Or add a spoonful of mixed finely chopped raw green pepper, chives, and cucumber. Makes four servings.

VEGETABLE ESPRESSOS ARE POTENT BEAUTIFIERS

For quick pick up, for more verve and radiant good looks there is nothing more refreshing than a tall, cool glass of vegetable espresso.

Everybody knows that the potent cafe espresso came from Italy. It is the concentrated fragrance of coffee steamed into a small cup. Cafe espresso has become an after dinner favorite all over the world. Only a few people know that vegetable espresso originally came from Czechoslovakia where they first called it vegetable juice because that is what it was, until a brilliant inventor perfected a vegetable espresso machine which not only extracts the watery essence but also breaks up the vitamin-laden inner cell structure of all vegetables and turns them into vegetable juice that is rich and fullbodied. The result is no more flat-tasting watery juices. *Instead we can now make vegetable espresso unlimited!*

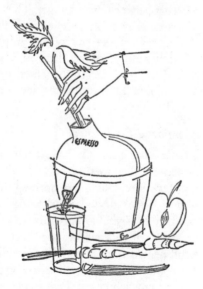

It has been a long slow progress since I had Harold, the butler on the Elizabeth Arden Beauty Farm, extract the juice of celery, carrots and apples with a little handpress I brought from Germany. In those days it was a real labor of love to make fresh juices; most of the liquid leaked down to the kitchen floor, and in the cumbersome process and exposure to air the juices lost their appetizing color. Today, anyone in a matter of moments can make appetizing, vitamin- and mineral-rich vegetable espresso.

I learned about the potency of fresh vegetable extracts as long ago as the early twenties, in the sanatorium in Carlsbad, where the head nurse, Sister Karoline, prepared what she called "*Pflanzen-blut*," which means the blood of the plant. All the patients in this sanatorium were given three glasses of these fresh "live" vegetable extracts.

These concentrated extracts from the freshest and crispest vegetables obtainable (on beautyfarms they can grow their own) are nature's most potent beautifyers, a rich source of vitamins, minerals, and enzymes and—what is so very important—vegetable espressos taste delicious. Beautyfarms here and abroad were first to make use of these fresh cocktails; they serve them between meals, since the natural sugar content helps to raise the blood sugar level and prevents between-meal hunger. They are also served as a first course because they make excellent appetizers and help to prevent overeating toward the end of the meal. In England, France, Germany, Italy and, of course, here in our own country, thousands of my students have greatly benefited from these fresh vegetable espressos and now I ask you to include them in your *Eat and Grow Beautiful Program*.

Doctors Now Recommend Fresh Juices

For years vegetable juice cocktails have been treated as stepchildren, perhaps because they used to be so hard to make. Some bars served tired, watery juice, which had nothing in common with the sparkling fresh espressos of today. Nowadays many doctors strongly recommend fresh vegetable juices to patients who dislike eating vegetables or to patients whose poor teeth prevent them from getting the full benefit from uncooked vegetables. Some doctors recommend a combination of fresh carrot extractive, mixed with milk, for those patients who cannot eat roughage.

Dr. Garnett Cheney of the Department of Medicine at Stanford University in California caused great excitement when he announced that with plain, fresh cabbage juice, he cured ulcers in a few weeks time! His cure was based on giving his patients a quart of fresh cabbage juice or 75 percent cabbage juice and 25 percent celery juice. This was the first time that freshly made vegetable juice, or the "blood of the plant," as Sister Karoline called it, was recognized in medical circles.

Here we are mainly concerned in the beauty-giving qualities of the fresh extractives. If you have a health problem and are interested in the many health-giving and curative properties of fresh vegetable juice extractives, I suggest you read the book, *Vegetable Juices for Health,* by Dr. H. E. Kirschner, a practicing physician who has had years of experience in every phase of nutrition. In this book Dr. Kirschner gives many remarkable case reports of what fresh vegetable juices can accomplish.

How To Make Fresh Vegetable Espresso

Wash all vegetables carefully. Do not soak any vegetables in water for any length of time, as this will leach out vitamins B and C which dissolve in water as salt does, but wash them under running cold water. Do not peel carrots and other root vegetables. Instead, scrub them with a stiff brush and cut them in pieces to fit into your vegetable juicer.

If you are buying a new vegetable juicer, buy the most modern one you can find, one that does not vibrate and get out of balance and one that gives you vegetable *espresso*, not just the watery liquid. A good efficient juicer is a good investment for the entire family. There are several on the market since I introduced the drinking of vegetable juices; some are made for bars and some for home use. The one I take with me all over the world weighs only about six pounds. It is easy to operate because it has only three parts. Also, and this is important, if you buy a new device, the juice must not be watery and it must not touch tin, lead or aluminum; the juice must flow into a bowl of stainless steel which cannot possibly affect the color, taste or chemistry of the juices.

When you have scrubbed your vegetables sparkling clean, put them into the juicer and drink your first glass right from the spout. If you make extra juice, be sure to put it at once on ice and cover tightly to stop enzyme action or the juice will loose its appetizing color. Never expose fresh vegetable extractives to the air a moment longer than you have to. Work fast! DRINK THEM FRESH AS THEY COME FROM THE ESPRESSOR AND, FOR MAXIMUM BENEFIT, DRINK TWO CUPS EACH DAY AND SIP THROUGH A STRAW.

Removing Poisonous Sprays

Some vegetable sprays are poisonous to people who lack the normal digestive acid. For these people, and for everyone in

Mexico and the Orient, it is wise to wash all vegetables in the following solution: Buy from your druggist, one ounce of chemically pure hydrochloric acid and pour it into three quarts of water. This makes a one percent solution and is entirely harmless. Put this solution in a porcelain or glass vessel. It can be used for a week or more. Simply place the vegetables in the solution for five minutes; then remove and rinse with ordinary water. Your health food stores also have a ready-made solution to make vegetables scrupulously clean.

GOLDEN CARROT ESPRESSO

This is the great favorite with everybody. The dark California carrots are best. Drink this to your heart's content. Remember, a cup of carrot espresso is rich in vitamin A, B, C, and B-2, plus a good combination of the minerals calcium, iron and even iodine. Carrot espresso helps complexions to glow, helps the eyes, soothes the "inner man" with its vegetable mucilage. But more than anything else, it tastes so good, straight or mixed with practically all other juices.

FRESH CARROT CAPUCINO

Half a cup of carrot espresso with half a cup of milk makes one of the finest "builder-uppers," rich in vitamins and double rich in calcium. It makes an ideal between-meal drink and is a favorite on beautyfarms. Waistline watchers should use skim milk.

CELERY ESPRESSO

This is a favorite in England. It is a natural digestive and one of the best appetizers. By all means use the dark-green outside stalks. They contain more beautifying chlorophyll. Do not use many of the dark-green leaves; they make the juice too bitter, and they may have been sprayed heavily. Mixing a few drops of lemon or grapefruit juice adds to the flavor and prevents the juice from turning dark. Celery espresso contains vitamins A, B, C, and some E, also the minerals sodium, potassium, and chlorine. This makes it an ideal cocktail for reducers. Celery juice can be mixed with many other juices; try celery and carrot espresso, half and half. This is the combination I served at the famous press party at Maxim's in Paris.

Fresh apple espresso

Nothing tastes better than a fresh apple espresso. Cut up juicy ripe apples, peeling and all, into slices to fit your juicing machine. This espresso cannot be compared with ordinary watery apple juice or cider. It is the whole apple, peeling, seeds and all, in easy, digestible liquid form. It contains the whole aroma and goodness of the apple, including beauty-giving vitamins A and B, plus fair amounts of vitamin C. The minerals include good amounts of sodium. Drink this liquid apple for its sheer deliciousness. Apple growers should get together and install juicing machines in every drugstore and sell apple espressos as the citrus growers have done with oranges. There will never be any surplus apples once Americans have tasted apple espresso. Here is a slogan for the apple growers: "Drink an apple a day, keep troubles away."

My favorite cocktail

Put equal amounts of golden carrots, dark green spinach and rosy apples into your juicer. The result is an unusually delicious cocktail. Serve it chilled as a first course or between-meal drink.

Fresh cabbage espresso

Cut tender young cabbage in slices to fit your juicer. This makes a sweet-tasting light green juice. Add a few dark green stalks of celery to improve the flavor and give more character.

Plain cabbage juice, besides vitamins A, B, and C, contains the new Vitamin "U" factor, as Dr. Cheney calls the healing factor in cabbage juice. If you tire of cabbage juice you can always flavor it with an extra carrot or an apple. Cabbage juice discolors quickly. To prevent this, add some grapefruit juice before storing it in the refrigerator.

Fresh watercress

This dark-green liquid, like spinach and parsley juice, is better mixed than alone. Use both leaves and stems. Watercress juice contains practically all vitamins and minerals, including iodine, and thus a small amount fortifies other juices. Straight watercress juice, because of its sulphur content, can become an irritant and should therefore always be mixed with other juices. Try pineapple and watercress, half and half.

FRESH TOMATO ESPRESSO

Like fresh liquid apple, fresh tomato espresso tastes unbelievably delicious. Put unpeeled ripe tomatoes into the juicer, and you will see for yourself that fresh tomato espresso bears no resemblance to ordinary watery canned tomato juice. You will be delighted with the flavor, the color, but above all, the valuable contents of this fresh juice. There is plenty of vitamins A and C, some vitamin B. Spiced with a bit of lemon and a dash of vegetable salt, it makes one of the most delicious appetizers. Tomato espresso can take the place of citrus fruits in countries where these are unavailable or too expensive. Tomato espresso makes delicious beautyfarm sauces and soups.

FRESH PINEAPPLE ESPRESSO

Remove the tough outside fibers from a ripe pineapple, and cut in slices to fit your electric juicer. The resulting foamy drink is fit for a duchess. Pineapple juice contains an excellent digestive called bromelin and is therefore most helpful before or after a meal of heavy foods. Fresh pineapple juice also contains the vitamins A, B, C, and some B-2, plus nine necessary minerals including iodine. At your next dinner party, serve chilled fresh pineapple juice flavored with a bit of watercress juice or fresh mint. This is the combination the Duchess of Windsor liked when I served it to her in Paris. I dedicate this appetizer to Her Highness.

FRESH GRAPE ESPRESSO

All fresh grapes contain the important vitamins A, B and C plus large amounts of minerals. The large amount of inert sugar makes grapes an ideal food for elimination and reducing diets. Thousands of tired and overweight people take the "grape cure" in Meran,

Italy, and other resorts. There you eat grapes to your heart's content, but the peeling and seeds are not used. You can take your own "grape cure" right at home by drinking all you want of fresh grape espresso while grapes are in season. Be sure to wash grapes carefully to remove all sprays.

BEAUTYFARM ESPRESSO

Peel tender young rhubarb, wash fresh ripe strawberries, and put them through the vegetable juicer. Two-thirds rhubarb and one-third strawberries make a good combination. Sweeten this beautiful rose-colored extract with two teaspoons of honey. I served this combination on the beautyfarm in Maine and it became very popular. This combination is mildly laxative and not more than one glassful a day should be taken.

FRESH RHUBARB AND MOLASSES

Mix one tablespoon of unsulphured molasses into a glass of fresh rhubarb juice and drink before or with breakfast. One glassful a day for two weeks makes an excellent "spring tonic" for those with "liverish" complexions.

FRESH CUCUMBER ESPRESSO

Cut tender unpeeled cucumbers into strips and put through vegetable juice extractor. The juice alone is flat-tasting and must be mixed with apple juice, pineapple juice, or carrots and celery. Cucumbers are believed to have a flushing action upon the kidneys, and the juice is recommended in reducing and cleansing diets. Cucumbers also contain vitamin A, B, and C, plus chlorophyll and many minerals. Whenever making fresh cucumber espresso, make enough extra to use externally on the face. It is a mild bleach for freckles and makes the skin velvety soft.

Liquid Salad For Adam

Liquid salads are an important part of the diet therapy used at the famous diet sanatoriums in Switzerland. Old and young are given two glasses of vegetable juices a day. I recommend this "liquid salad" idea, especially if your husband will not eat whole salads. Put any combination of vegetables into your juicer, dressing and all. Delicious combinations are celery, carrots, and tomatoes, or watercress, celery and tomatoes. A great favorite is a mixture of celery, apples and a bit of parsley, You can make a "liquid salad bowl" by putting head lettuce, a bit of cabbage, celery, a small cucumber, tomatoes, and half a green pepper through the extractor, and spice it with a bit of vegetable salt. Such a liquid salad taken before a meal is a wonderful way of breaking an addiction to over-rich desserts.

Eat, Drink and Be Beautiful!

Distinguished hostesses all over the world now serve at least one cocktail without alcohol for guests who do not wish martinis and for those who watch their waistlines. One of the most elegant parties I ever attended was at the French Embassy in Constantinople on the Bosporus. Madame de Saint Hardouin, the Ambassadress, served cool carrot and celery espresso and chilled peach and mint cocktails in high-stemmed champagne glasses, side by side with the other cocktails. A king and his queen, many princesses and diplomats from many lands enjoyed these refreshing drinks and asked for seconds. It is no wonder that Madame de Saint Hardouin is one of the most beautiful women of our time. Her blond hair and skin have long been the envy of every diplomat's wife. Ily de Saint Hardouin, I am happy to say, is a longtime friend and student and because of her, the entire French Embassy had the benefit of beauty-full eating.

APPETIZERS OR SALADS

The Ever-New Green Salad

Salads are so familiar and essential in our meals today that almost every woman has become a salad inventor. Here are some ways to glamorize salads as they do on some of the elegant beauty-farms.

Use any crisp good leafy green, and add a pungent herb to the salad bowl. Cut the herb fine with scissors, or rub it between your fingers. Chervil and thyme are favorites in America.

When the good summer sun has made your garden mint patch

fragrant and leafy, cut some of the leaves with the kitchen scissors into a half cup of finely cut chives, parsley and onion tops. Toss all into a big bowl of lettuce or romaine. Use your favorite golden oil dressing and toss with spoon and fork until the whole bowlful shines like green gold.

For another luncheon, instead of the loud-mouthed garlic bud or crouton dipped into garlic oil, add a tablespoon of minced fresh basil and watercress to a tossed salad. Dress all salads with your favorite golden oil dressing and season with vegetable salt. Serve at once, while the herbs are still speaking to you.

Luncheon Salads

You can make these luncheon salads a complete meal. Make a bed of your favorite salad vegetables; break them into bits or if chewing is a problem, chop the vegetables. To these greens you can add any of your favorite proteins, depending upon your taste and pocketbook: Half a cup or more of cottage cheese, salmon, tongue, lean ham, chicken, tuna fish, hard boiled eggs, leftover meat, all make splendid salad combinations. Blend them with a tablespoon of your favorite salad dressing. With such a salad bowl, all you need is one slice of good bread. Any one of these salads is fit for a beauty queen.

LEAN COTTAGE CHEESE SALAD

½ cup lean cottage cheese
½ cup sliced small radishes
½ cup diced celery

2 tbsp. chopped green pepper
Pinch vegetable salt

Mix the vegetables and chill. Add the cottage cheese to any desired salad dressing and fold this into the mixed vegetables.

COMPLEXION SALAD

1 cup finely chopped carrots
1 cup finely chopped celery
1 cup finely chopped cabbage

¾ cup diced apple
8 tbsp. pineapple juice

Mix and saturate ingredients with pineapple juice. When thoroughly chilled and crisp, serve on lettuce or escarolle with sprigs of watercress. Top with your favorite dressing.

BRIGHT EYE SALAD

Break up a bunch of fresh watercress, dark green lettuce leaves, half a cup chopped carrots and half a cup of unpeeled cucumber. Marinate the whole with French dressing.

SALADE APHRODITE

Equal amounts of: Apples, finely chopped
Celery, finely chopped
½ cup yogurt
Vegetable salt

The beauty of this salad depends entirely on how quickly the apples and celery are stirred *into* the bowl of yogurt. This prevents their becoming brown. To be served on the crispest lettuce leaves.

RAISIN CARROTTE

Soak half cup seeded raisins in one-fourth cup lemon juice. When raisins are plump, combine with 1½ cup shredded carrots. Moisten mixture with beautyfarm mayonnaise and serve on bed of crisp lettuce.

Refreshing Fruit Salads

You can make delicious mixed raw salads with fresh ripe fruits by giving attention to freshness, texture, taste, and arrangement of the fruits. The choice of fruits which blend well is a matter of individual taste, limited only by what the market and your pocket-book afford. The best fruits are always those which are in season, preferably ripened in the sun. A combination of no more than four, one of which should be of the citrus group, makes a more palatable mixture than a hodge-podge of many fruits.

Here are some favorite beautyfarm combinations:

Apple and mint	Persimmon and orange
Avocado and citrus	Pear and cream cheese
Banana and raisins or dates	Pineapple and cream cheese
Orange and ripe banana	Pineapple and date
Orange and black mission figs	Pineapple and mint
Orange and onion	Pineapple and strawberry

Among fruits, orange and apple are basic ingredients. They supply sweet juiciness, crisp substance, and color. Orange has the added advantage of lending itself to preparation in various shapes: slices, whole or cubed, skinned sections, or small wedges cut across the sections from the core out.

The fruit should be prepared in large, neat slices, cubes, wedges, or balls—and with only the sharpest of tools—to avoid crushing or tearing. Include at least one fruit which will give a touch of harmonizing color, or use as a garnish a few cherries, grapes or berries. Always chill cut fruit and do not mix until just before serving time.

GREEN-GOLD DRESSING

Use the French dressing recipe and spice it with two tablespoons of mixed, finely minced fresh herbs and greens: chives, parsley, thyme, scallion tops, green pepper; beat all into the French dressing. Serve on hearts of lettuce, or a slice of Chinese cabbage, or on a bowl of mixed greens; on thin, thin, thin slices of unpared cucumber and grated carrot on a base of Chinese cabbage; on whole ripe tomatoes, scooped out and half-filled with diced raw cauliflower, turnip and avocado.

Serve this green dressing with broiled fish fillets and lean steaks. Serve a chilled bowl of this dressing with sliced cold turkey, chicken and veal for Sunday night buffets.

BREAD AND OTHER HIGH ENERGY FOODS

"HIS Bread" is what Sicilians call bread made from the wholewheat flour with all its goodness as it comes from the field. Here is such a bread in its modern version, as you can make it in your own modern kitchen. One loaf of such bread is all you need for a week; it is so nourishing and satisfying you will only want to eat one slice at a time.

Directions: Into a large bowl put 2½ cups of wholewheat flour, preferably stone ground; 3 tablespoons of fresh wheat germ; 3 tablespoons soya flour; 4 tablespoons powdered skim milk; 2 teaspoons brown sugar and 1 teaspoon vegetable salt. Dissolve ½ cake of yeast (½ oz.) in a cup of lukewarm water and add this to your dry ingredients; also add 1 tablespoon of golden oil. Mix thoroughly until you have a smooth dough, put it in an oiled bowl and cover. Let rise in warm place one and one-half hours; punch down and let rise 20 minutes more. Finally knead into compact loaf and put into a large bread pan, cover, and let stand in a warm place. When dough has again risen to top of bread pan, bake for about 40 minutes at 400° F.

Sensational EL MOLINO Bread

There is no longer any excuse for not baking your own bread once a week when it can be done as quickly and neatly as with the El Molino ready bread mix. This is a delightful mixture containing stone-ground wholewheat flour, unbleached flour, sesame flour, honey, skim milk, natural sugar, plus a fast-acting yeast and even a bright and shining bread pan. All you do is add water.

In this combination of ground fresh sesame seed with whole, high-protein wheat, an entirely new experience in bread-eating awaits you. For real honest-to-goodness bread, I invite you to bake your own with the El Molino ready bread mix.

Most health food stores and special diet shops carry this exciting new bread mix. If yours does not, drop a card to the El Molino Mills, Alhambra, California.

BEAUTYFARM SOYA MUFFINS

Take 1½ cups soya flour, 2 teaspoons baking powder, 1½ teaspoons vegetable salt, 2 fresh eggs, 3 tablespoons brown sugar, 1 tablespoon grated orange rind, 1 cup milk, 1 tablespoon golden oil, ¼ cup floured raisins, and ¼ cup floured walnut meats. Sift together the flour, baking powder, and salt. Separate the eggs and beat the yolks until very light and frothy. Beat the sugar into the egg yolks, add the orange rind, milk and oil and mix well. Pour the egg mixture into the dry ingredients and mix. Add the raisins and nut meats and mix thoroughly. Fold in the egg whites beaten stiff. Pour into small muffin tins and bake in slow oven, 300° F, for about 35 minutes. The glamorous Mrs. Eric Remarque (Paulette Goddard) calls these "the most."

CORN BREAD CARROTTE

1 cup yellow corn meal	1 tsp. vegetable salt
1 cup grated golden carrots	2 tbsp. golden oil
1 tbsp. brown crystal sugar	2 fresh eggs

Combine in mixing bowl: corn meal, carrots, golden oil, brown crystal sugar and vegetable salt. Mix well, then stir ¾ cup boiling hot water into the mixture. Add 2 tablespoons cold water to 2 egg yolks. Beat until thick and add to the mixture. Finally fold in stiffly beaten egg whites. Pour into a warmed oiled pan and bake at 400° F for about 25 minutes.

FRESH WHEAT GERM MUFFINS

1½ cups milk	1½ cups wholewheat flour
½ cup golden oil	1 cup fresh wheat germ
1 tsp. vegetable salt	2 fresh eggs
1 tsp. brown crystal sugar	

Separate eggs. Beat yolks, add vegetable salt, brown sugar and golden oil. Stir in the milk and add flour plus fresh wheat germ. Last, fold in stiffly beaten whites of eggs. Bake in hot, oiled muffin pan at 350° F for about 35 minutes.

LIGHT-HEARTED BAKED POTATOES

Fragrant, delicate potatoes baked by this recipe need not add ounces to anyone's weight. Select medium sized baking potatoes. Scrub them thoroughly and remove any blemishes. Wipe them dry, then rub the skin with a little golden oil.

Bake the potatoes on a rack in a moderately hot oven, 425° F for 40 to 60 minutes, or until the potatoes feel soft when pressed with your towel-protected fingers.

Remove the potatoes from the oven and break open the skin immediately to let the steam escape.

Blend, for each potato, one tablespoon yogurt, one-fourth teaspoon vegetable salt, one teaspoon finely cut chives.

Scoop the hot potato out into a bowl, blend quickly with the yogurt mixture. Return to the potato shells. Serve at once, or reheat for a few minutes in a slow oven.

BEAUTYFARM POTATO CHIPS

You can eat these with a clear conscience. Simply scrub potatoes until they shine. Do not peel, but slice very thin. Spread out thinly on a cooky sheet and sprinkle lightly with a bit of vegetable salt. Place in moderate oven for about 40 minutes or until potatoes turn into brown chips. Then turn off heat, but leave in for 15 minutes longer to make them extra crisp.

WHOLEWHEAT PILAF

¼ cup golden oil
2 shallots or small onions, peeled and minced
3 cups cracked wholewheat
6 cups fat-free chicken broth, or bouillon from cubes
1½ teaspoons vegetable salt

1½ teaspoons dried sweet basil, thyme, or crumbled sage
½ cup chopped sunflower seeds
½ cup small white soaked raisins

Use three-quart flameproof casserole or saucepan. Heat the oil, and sauté the shallots or onions about 3 minutes. Add the wheat, stir and cook until hot and golden. Stir in the broth, add vegetable salt and herbs, seeds and raisins.

Cover the casserole, cook slowly 20 minutes; the wheat should absorb the bouillon.

Serve this dish with meat or chicken. Makes three to six servings.

KASHA, A HI-VI GRAIN

Kasha or buckwheat groats are an almost forgotten grain in America. In Russia it is one of the most important staple foods. It is high in energy and fairly high in protein, but most of all it is delicious and makes a welcome change from rice and potatoes.

Kasha is easy to cook. The whole kernel takes only about twenty minutes; the cracked ones take only five minutes. The Russian method is the simplest and leanest:

1 cup whole buckwheat groats
2 cups water (if used for breakfast, otherwise chicken or beef broth).

Use heavy cooking utensil, stir the cup of unwashed buckwheat groats into the boiling liquid. Add salt, let boil for one or two minutes; then cover the utensil; turn heat to low and let simmer for fifteen minutes or until all liquid is absorbed. Every grain should be separate. Kasha must never be mushy!

Beautyfarm Method: Put two tablespoons of golden salad oil into heavy skillet. When oil is very hot, stir in one cup of buckwheat groats which has been mixed previously with a raw beaten egg. Add a teaspoon of vegetable salt. Finally add two cups of fat-free chicken broth or vegetable water. Bring to a boil, then reduce heat, cover tightly and let cook until all liquid is absorbed.

STUFFED GRAPE LEAVES À LA GREQUE

This is a delightful combination of the flavorsome leaf of the grape vine and nutritious brown rice. It is new to most Americans, but actually it is a very old and respected dish among the Greeks and Armenians. Stuffed grape leaves are an ideal beautyfarm dish, tasty, nutritious and very appealing to the eye. Stuffed grape leaves make a nutritious first course or as an accompanyment to meat. If you can't get fresh grape leaves you can always buy them canned in Greek and Armenian communities. Here is my recipe:

18 grape leaves
1 cup raw brown rice
2 tbsp. finely chopped parsley
1 medium-size onion, peeled and grated

2 tbsp. golden oil
1 tsp. vegetable salt
Juice ½ lemon
Yogurt

Wash grape leaves. Boil in very little water until soft. Cook brown rice as directed on package. Combine parsley and onion and sauté five minutes in olive oil. Mix the cooked rice, parsley and onion and vegetable salt. Add the lemon juice and mix well. Place about one to two tablespoons of the rice mixture on a grape leaf, fold the bottom of the leaf up over the rice, then fold the top of the leaf down, then fold over each end, making a neat, tight roll.

Place leaf rolls in rows close together in a wide, shallow baking dish. Cover with chicken or vegetable broth. Cover the dish and cook in a moderate oven, 325° F for 30 minutes. Or cook them on top of the stove, over a low heat, about the same length of time. It is important that the tightly wrapped leaf rolls be placed snugly together, so that each helps the other to hold its shape.

When the rolls are done, lift them carefully to a warmed serving dish. Mix a little yogurt with the liquid in the baking dish, stir, heat two minutes, and pour over the rolls. Serve hot. Makes six or more servings.

Natural Brown Rice

White rice, with much of its flavor and food value polished away, has no place in beautyfarm cookery. We use the natural brown rice, which consists of the whole kernel with only the outer husk removed. Brown rice is a high energy food which should replace the foodless white rice in every modern kitchen.

QUICK WILD RICE

½ cup wild rice
½ cup boiling water

½ tsp. vegetable salt
1 tsp. butter

Add the rice to the boiling, salted water. Cover and cook over a slow fire without stirring, if possible, for 15 minutes. Take off the cover, dot the butter over the top, and let stand a few minutes on a warm grid to dry out the steam. Serve with fowl or chops.

BEAUTYFARM DESSERTS

Fresh, ripe fruits are Nature's choicest *sun*-cooked desserts. The Chinese ate fresh peaches a thousand years before the Christian Era, and Homer sang of pears in the days of Helen.

In those days fruit was a rarity; today it is a necessity. Fruits make the best and most delicious desserts after meals. Serve big bowls full whenever possible and occasionally make fresh fruits into lightly honeyed compotes. Your favorite fresh fruits can also be sliced into delicate, thin pie shells; since these are made with the golden oils we can eat them with good conscience.

Sparkling Fruit Gelatin

Gelatin desserts, when prepared correctly, are naturals for beautyfarms. Let us remember that the sweet, colored gelatins are not to be used in beautyfarm cookery. We use only the pure white gelatin which you can buy by the pound, and for color and flavor we add pure, unsweetened fruit and vegetable juices. Follow the simple directions on the gelatin package.

Unsweetened grape juice makes a delightful and decorative gelatin dessert. When it is partially set, remove it from the refrigerator and beat it until it is light and foamy. Then pour into a mold which has been rinsed in cold water. Chill. Serve with double-strength lean milk or a spoonful of Honey Custard.

Orange juice flavored with a little sherry makes a golden jelly. For variety's sake, try this orange sherry gelatin. Whip it as described above; pour it into a mold and chill. Serve this garnished with thin sections of fresh orange. Sprinkle with a bit of coconut. Pour it into a square pan and chill. When firm, cut in small cubes. Pile the sparkling golden squares into dessert glasses and garnish with a few cherries.

Very important: To make gelatin dishes into first-class, tissue-building protein, whenever possible combine or serve with milk, cheese, or meat.

WINE JELLY DELIGHT

There is an elegant aura about wine jelly. The color captures the sparkle of dinner table candles, the flavor reminds one of summer and the vineyards of France. Incidentally it is a nutritious and easy-to-make beautyfarm dessert and a favorite of weight watchers.

4 tbsp. unflavored gelatin
1 cups cold water
3 cups boiling water
2 tbsp. honey
Juice 1 orange

Grated peel and juice 1 lemon
2½ cups sherry, Madeira or port wine

Soften the gelatin in the cold water about 5 minutes. Then add the boiling water and honey and stir until gelatin dissolves. Stir in fruit juices and peel, and let cool. (Some cooks strain out the peel after a few minutes.)

When the gelatin mixture has cooled, add the wine. Pour into a two-quart mold which has been rinsed with cold water. Chill until firm.

Unmold onto a chilled serving dish. Garnish it with grape leaves and small clusters of grapes. Makes eight to twelve servings.

FRUIT COMPOTE À LA LADY MENDL

Make a moderately sweet syrup of about one cup of honey to one cup of water. While it is cooking, pick over your favorite fresh fruit: berries, cherries, halved apricots, pears, etc. Pour the hot, hot syrup over the fruit. Cover immediately to prevent the delicate aroma from escaping, and when cool, put covered fruit in refrigerator until served.

I have seen princes and statesmen devour this delicious compote. I dedicate this recipe to Lady Mendl's chef, Monsieur Fraise, who first served it to me.

HONEY CUSTARD

4 egg yolks	4 egg whites
¾ cup honey	⅛ tsp. salt
3 cups milk	

Beat the egg yolks until lemon colored, adding honey gradually as you beat. Then add the milk gradually, beating the mixture smooth. Whip egg whites with the salt until they are stiff and stand in peaks when the beater is withdrawn. Fold the yolk mixture into the whites.

Pour into six or eight individual custard cups. Place the cups in a shallow pan, and add about one inch hot water to the pan around the cups.

Bake in a moderate oven, 325° F until the custard is firm. This should be about one hour. To test, insert a silver knife blade and if the custard does not adhere to the blade, it is ready to be removed from the oven. Let the cups cool a little, then chill in refrigerator.

Serve the custard in these cups. Or turn each out into an individual dessert dish. You can feed the eye and the palate when you garnish this high protein custard with thinly sliced strawberries, or a few fresh blueberries, or small mandarin orange or tangerine sections. To the top add a little oasis of grated pistachio nuts. Makes six to eight servings.

HONEY RASPBERRY SHERBET

To serve this fragrant frozen dessert, heap it in large wine glasses instead of the usual dessert dishes. Place a geranium or grape leaf under these stem glasses on their dessert plates.

2 tsp. unflavored gelatin	¾ cup honey
¼ cup cold water	2 egg whites
1 qt. fresh or quick-frozen red raspberries	⅛ tsp. salt
	Few additional whole berries
¼ cup lemon juice	and fresh mint leaves
1¾ cups water	

Soften the gelatin in the one-fourth cup cold water. Press the berries through a sieve or ricer, or use a blender. Add lemon juice to the berries and mix.

Combine the one and three-fourths cups water and the honey in a saucepan and boil 10 minutes. Remove from the heat and stir the soaked gelatin into this hot syrup to dissolve. Let the syrup cool. Add the sieved berries and mix to combine smoothly. Pour into refrigerator tray. Chill about one-half hour.

Whip egg whites with the salt until stiff and they stand in peaks when the beater is withdrawn. Fold whites into the chilled berry mixture. Pour back into the refrigerator tray. Freeze for one-half hour, then beat well. Freeze three hours or more, beating the sherbet at half-hour intervals. Beat again before serving. Makes five or more servings. Garnish the sherbet with a few whole berries and a mint leaf.

PASADENA APRICOT WHIP

Wash dried apricots. Soak overnight in orange juice until apricots are large and plump. Sweeten to taste with orange blossom honey. Fold soaked apricots into one cup of lean whipped cream. This is also delicious when frozen.

P.S.: You can make this same delightful dessert with large prunes soaked overnight.

FIVE MINUTE APPLESAUCE

Select juicy apples. Do not peel, but shred on medium shredder. Put one tablespoon sesame oil in heavy skillet. When oil is very hot, place shredded apples in oil and stir for one minute. Then turn heat very low and leave to steam for three more minutes. Sprinkle top of applesauce with honey and toasted sesame seeds. This makes an elegant and quick dessert.

APPLE SNOW

Cut up five large unpeeled juicy apples and make apple sauce. Sweeten with a bit of honey. When apples are soft, strain through sieve. Then mix thoroughly with one or two whites of eggs beaten very stiff. Serve in high-stemmed dessert glasses.

BEAUTYFARM PIE CRUST

Delightful and flaky crusts can be made with the light golden oils, and fresh fruits of all kinds can be piled high into these tender pie shells. Individual small pie shells also make a welcome and elegant dessert, especially when filled with fresh ripe fruits or honeyed fruits and sprinkled with toasted sesame seeds.

½ cup sesame oil	2 cups wholewheat or
⅓ cup cold water	unbleached flour
	1 tsp. vegetable salt

Mix the sesame oil with the water, quickly add the flour and the salt. Mix ingredients quickly as possible with a fork. Shape into a ball and place mixture between two large sheets of wax paper and roll thin. Bake shells to a golden brown.

This pie mixture can be kept in the refrigerator and every time you serve beautyfarm pie you can add new delightful touches to the crust. Before baking pie crust, sprinkle a tablespoon of sesame seeds, poppy seeds or chopped sunflower seeds over the pie shell and press into buttom of crust. Such small tender pie shells are unbelievably delicious.

WHEAT GERM PIE CRUST

1 cup sifted wholewheat flour	¼ cup golden oil
⅛ tsp. grated nutmeg	2 tbsp. milk or water
¾ tsp. vegetable salt	¼ cup wheat germ

Sift the flour, nutmeg and vegetable salt together into a mixing bowl. Pour over all at once, without combining, the oil and milk or water. Stir all ingredients lightly together. Add wheat germ, and continue stirring until blended. Form mixture into a ball. Place the dough on a large sheet of waxed paper, flatten slightly, cover with another sheet of waxed paper, and roll until the dough is nice and thin. Remove the top paper. Invert the rolled dough and its bottom paper into a pie pan. Remove the paper. Shape the dough into the pan as usual, trim the edge, and make a decorative rim with thumb and forefinger or by pressing with a fork. Prick the bottom of the crust well with a fork. Bake in a hot oven, 475° F about 10 minutes, or until golden and crisp looking.

Let crust cool. Pile high with sliced ruby-red strawberries or pour Honey Custard in to half-fill the crust. Chill. Then fill with fresh fruit slices or red raspberries or blueberries. This is also wonderful with fresh plums prepared this way: Cut them in halves, do not peel. Remove stones. Simmer halves in a mixture of equal parts water and honey, to cover, about 7 minutes. Let cool in honey mixture. Then spoon the fruit carefully in rows around the custard filling in the baked pie crust. One pie makes five or six servings.

Special Recipes for Special People

A basic diet, such as the Cosmetic Diet, is of primary importance in our *Eat and Grow Beautiful* program. However, within the last twenty years we have discovered that there are certain foods and food combinations which can give extra vitality and which have proven extremely valuable in overcoming certain beauty defects.

Here are some of the newer combinations which thousands of my students have found helpful.

HI-VI LEAN MILK

Here is more kitchen magic. Put one cup of dry skim milk into a quart of fresh milk (skim milk if you are watching your weight). This tastes like real milk or cream and not like the watery blue skim milk which no one enjoys. Here, within one quart of milk, you have the nourishment of two quarts—70 grams of good protein, rich in calcium and the beautifying B vitamins. The only nutrient missing is the vitamin A of cream, and this you supply in your vitamin concentrate. Drink this basic lean Hi-Vi milk. Use it in your coffee, over your cereals, make cream gravies with it, have a bottle of it in your refrigerator at all times and before retiring at night, check up on your protein intake (not less than 70 grams). You can always make up any deficiency with this Hi-Vi milk.

A TOAST TO YOUR CROWNING GLORY

1 cup Hi-Vi lean milk	1 tsp. honey, molasses or fruit
1 tbsp. pure gelatin	flavor
1 tsp. sesame oil	

Adding milk to gelatin doubles its potency. This single cup provides about 15 grams of first class protein, vitamin B and calcium, plus the anti-dry-hair fatty acids of sesame oil. This potent combination will also be kind to troublesome fingernails.

SCHOOL GIRL COMPLEXION

1 cup yogurt	1 tsp. food yeast
2 tsp. honey or molasses	1 tsp. wheat germ flour

Mix in one cup and eat with spoon or put in liquidizer and make a frothy drink. Also be sure to drink two glasses of carrot espresso every day.

TOOTH OR CONSEQUENCES

Here is a high protein, high calcium and high vitamin C drink.

1 cup orange juice

2 tbsp. cottage cheese (heaping)

1 tsp. very fine bone flour or 2 calcium tablets

Liquidize all three into a smooth drink and drink daily; also make sure that your daily vitamin concentrate contains vitamin D. For exercising the teeth, enjoy a daily handful of sunflower seeds, and of course check with your dentist.

COOKED CEREALS IN THE MODERN MANNER

On cold days cooked whole grains give added nourishment. Only the whole grains are worthwhile cooking, especially: wholewheat, brown rice, buckwheat (kasha), oats, barley and soya bean grits. All these are nutritious and contain their normal amount of beautifying vitamins and minerals, but you can triple their food value by adding half a cup of wheat germ to the cooking cereal just before removing from the heat. Eating cooked cereals with half a cup of hot Hi-Vi lean milk makes them higher in protein and more appetizing.

PEP BREAKFAST IN A CUP

When pressed for time, beat one or two fresh egg yolks (not the whites), one or two teaspoons of fresh wheat germ and one teaspoon of food yeast into a glass of fresh or frozen orange juice.

APPLE BREAKFAST

Put one cup of creamy white yogurt into a breakfast bowl. Add two teaspoons of fresh wheat germ, one teaspoon of honey and into it shred one juicy apple and mix. You can have a different yogurt breakfast every day of the week by adding any one of your favorite fruits to the yogurt with the wheat germ and honey.

COLD CEREALS À LA MODE

You can fortify any one of your favorite cereals by covering them with a tablespoon of fresh wheat germ, half a cup of fortified Hi-Vi lean milk and a lacing of honey.

SWISS COFFEE

One cup of this delicious beverage can add eight grams of protein to your breakfast. It has the aroma of coffee, plus the nutrition of good protein and minerals of milk.

Fill the largest cup with one-half freshly made hot coffee and the other half with hot lean milk. In Switzerland they pour hot coffee and hot milk simultaneously in twin streams into their large coffee cups and watch it foam. Unfortunately, rich Swiss milk is only for the skinnies. In its place we use fortified lean milk which tastes like cream, but contains only the protein sans fat—half hot coffee, half hot milk is ideal!

LEAN MILK SHAKE

Whip 2 tablespoons of instant skim milk crystals and 1 teaspoon of food yeast into a glass of fresh or frozen orange juice. If you like extra sweetening, add 1 teaspoon of orange blossom honey.

You can make dozens of different and delightful lean milk shakes by using all the different fresh, frozen and canned fruit juices.

MILK SHAKE FOR SKINNIES

1 cup vitamin D milk	1 tbsp. peanut oil
½ cup unsweetened pineapple juice	1 tbsp. food yeast
	1 tbsp. honey
1 tsp. wheat germ	1 very ripe banana

Put the ingredients into liquidizer and whip until smooth. Very ripe bananas are rich in digestive enzymes and are a wonderful food for underweighters.

REDUCERS' DELIGHT

Mix one pint thick California tomato juice, one pint sauerkraut juice and four tablespoons food yeast in a quart mason jar, and keep in refrigerator. Excellent lean, before or between meal drink.

"E" BOMB FOR ENERGY

1 cup Hi-Vi lean milk
1 tsp. golden honey
1 tsp. carob powder

1 tsp. mild-tasting food yeast
1 tsp. dark molasses

Here is a most potent combination of inexpensive Hi-Vi foods. This can be mixed quickly in one glass. Many are amazed at the quick burst of energy derived from this potent combination. One of my students was so delighted with the results of this combination he called it his "E Bomb."

INSTANT SWISS BROTH

1 tbsp. skim milk powder
    (heaping)
1 tsp. food yeast

½ tsp. mixed dried herbs
Vegetable salt to taste

Stir above mixture into a cup of hot skim milk. This Hi-Vi drink is delicious as a hot broth, a between-meal refresher or as a relaxing good nightcap.

TRANQUILLO

1 cup tomato juice
1 tbsp. food yeast

Pinch salt

Beat food yeast and salt into a cup of very hot tomato juice and sip slowly. When upset or on edge, wait, do not eat a big meal, have a Tranquillo!

INSTANT PICK-UP

Put two tablespoons of powdered skim milk crystals, two teaspoons of unsulphured molasses and one teaspoon of food yeast into a cup of Hi-Vi lean milk. Mix or beat until frothy.

HOT MILK LASSIE

Whip one teaspoon of clover honey and one teaspoon unsulphured molasses into a cup of fortified hot milk. Delightful night-

18 CARAT GOLDEN DRINK

Mix one pint of golden carrot espresso with a pint of golden orange juice. Serve in chilled glasses with a sprig of fresh mint.

ALONE AT LAST!

Here is a strong "sleeping potion" that many of my students swear puts them to sleep. Put ¼ teaspoon of pure garlic powder and a pinch of salt into a cup of hot milk or take three fresh, cut-up cloves of garlic and place in cold milk and let come just to a boil (do not boil). Strain and sip slowly. This draught is best taken when alone!

SMORGASBORD FROM THE SEA

Take 10 quarts of fresh ocean water and boil down into one quart. The concentrated salt water tastes quite salty, but only a teaspoon needs to be taken every day. It can be mixed into soup, cereals, tomato juice or any other food. If you live far away from the ocean, your best source for getting some of the benefits from the deep sea is to use fresh or dried sea plants or tangy sea greens in tablet form. These too are saturated with the ocean's many minerals.

If you smoke too much: You know you should not. Dermatologists say nicotine is bad for the skin, so cut down and in the meantime, double up on your vitamin C supply. According to Dr. W. J. McCormick of Canada, cigarettes use up the vitamin C in the body.

If you drink too much, in spite of good intentions, at least double up on your vitamins, especially the B complex. According to Dr. Roger J. Williams of the University of Texas, the craving for alcohol requires far greater quantities of vitamins than normal diets supply.

Golden Oils Galore

How lucky we are to be able to choose among so many varieties of golden vegetable oils! These are our beauty-full, friendly fats which metabolize so much more easily than the hard facts. These oils are also a weapon against excessive cholesterol.

Sunflower oil, soya bean oil, safflower oil, sesame oil, wheat germ oil, peanut oil, corn oil, olive oil: these are the great favorites. Use any one of them. Still better, combine two or three in your salad dressings. Sesame oil has the mildest flavor and sunflower oil is a close second. These two oils are also used as the favorite fats in beautyfarm cookery. Try to get these oils very fresh and cold pressed. They are worth looking for and your local health food store has a supply of all of them. Make your dressings fresh and keep them refrigerated. Rancid oils are deadly to good looks as well as taste.

FAVORITE GOLDEN OIL SALAD DRESSING

½ cup sunflower oil
½ cup peanut oil
½ cup olive oil
½ cup herbal vinegar

2 tsp. honey
2 tsp. vegetable salt
1 clove garlic

Directions: Place all ingredients into covered jar and shake vigorously whenever you use this basic and delicious golden oil dressing. Give it a different flavor every time you make it. Here are some choices: add 2 tablespoons of chopped fresh parsley, fresh chives, fresh mint, mild onion or dried herbs; half a teaspoon oregano or curry powder; 1 teaspoon dried mustard; 2 tablespoons of Roquefort cheese; 2 tablespoons chopped ripe olives. Use your imagination; there is absolutely no limit to the number of delightful salad dressing combinations, especially if you learn to use some of the pungent herbal vinegars.

HONEY-MINT VINEGAR

1 cup golden honey
3 cups chopped-up fresh mint

1 quart cider vinegar

Let vinegar come to a boil, then slowly add honey and mint. Let simmer on low flame for 7 minutes. Strain and pour into clean bottles. This can be used at once.

GOLDEN FRUIT SALAD DRESSING

Juice of two oranges, juice of two lemons, two tablespoons cider vinegar, one teaspoon honey, one teaspoon vegetable salt, one pint peanut oil.

Directions: Put all ingredients in air-tight jar and shake before using.

LEAN, NO-OIL DRESSING FOR OVERWEIGHTS

½ cup finely chopped vegetables
1 cup liquid from canned okra
Juice, 1 lemon

1 cup thick tomato juice
½ tbsp. honey
¼ tsp. vegetable salt
Dash of garlic

Use celery, parsley, onion, and green pepper for the chopped vegetables, or any other vegetables in season. Add the okra liquid and thin with lemon juice and tomato juice. Season with honey and vegetable salt and add a dash of garlic, or onion if you prefer, unless onions are among your chopped vegetables.

YOGURT SALAD DRESSING

Combine one-half teaspoon cider vinegar, one-fourth teaspoon honey, a pinch of vegetable salt and one-half teaspoon grated lemon rind. Mix this into one-half cup of thick yogurt. This delightful salad dressing can also be varied with chives, watercress or parsley.

GOLDEN YOGURT MAYONNAISE

Combine four tablespoonsful of beautyfarm mayonnaise with four tablespoons of thick yogurt. Whip into consistency of cream and add a tablespoon of finely chopped golden carrot.

HOMEMADE FRENCH MUSTARD

Pound in a mortar:

1 tbsp. dried parsley
1 tbsp. chopped tarragon

1 tsp. chopped chervil
½ cup mustard seeds

When reduced to a powder, strain through a fine sieve and slowly add:

1 tbsp. golden oil   1 tbsp. herb vinegar

Mix thoroughly and keep refrigerated.

OLD FASHIONED DILL PICKLES

Scrub 200 very fresh, medium sized cucumbers. Soak them overnight in cold water. Next day prepare mason jars. Place a small handful of fresh dill on bottom of each jar, next a layer of cucumbers. Alternate these layers of dill and cucumber until each jar is filled. Top with dill, a clove of garlic, and three thick slices of fresh horseradish. Then fill up the jars with following brine.

Directions for Brine: Mix 2 quarts cider vinegar, 4 quarts water, 1 pound plain salt, 1 pound brown sugar in large kettle. Bring to boil and let boil for three minutes; pour this hot mixture into jars. Be sure that all pickles are covered. Seal tightly. Let stand for ten days and then enjoy. (Note: The fresh horseradish keeps the pickles firm.)

MEXICAN GUACAMOLE

Mash a peeled ripe avocado with fork and stir in two tablespoons of lemon juice. Add a teaspoon of minced onion and a mashed clove of garlic, ½ teaspoon vegetable salt and if you want to be real Mexicano, a dash of cayenne. Diced fresh tomato and crumbled crisp bacon can also be added. Serve guacamole immediately to prevent discoloration. It is used as a salad, a sandwich spread or as a dip for finger salads.

BEAUTYFARM PEANUT BUTTER

¼ cup peanut oil   Pinch of salt
2 cups shelled peanuts

Place oil in liquidizer. Turn on high speed and add peanuts gradually. Blend until smooth. If chunks are wanted, turn blender off as soon as butter thickens. Just a pinch of vegetable salt brings up the flavor.

GOLDEN GRAIN MAGIC

Here is an old-new cooking magic for all grains. Simply stir half a cup of your favorite wholewheat cereal (try cracked wheat) into two cups of boiling water. Let simmer for two minutes, then add a pinch of salt and pour the boiling mixture into a wide-mouthed (pre-heated) thermos bottle. Close tightly and lay thermos on the side. Next morning you wake up to a fragrant hot cereal, cooked by a genie while you slept peacefully. All you add is half a cup of Hi-Vi lean milk and a bit of honey.

LEAN WHIPPED CREAM

With plain ordinary skim milk you can make a delectable and protein-rich whipped cream to be used over your favorite desserts. Try it on berries, apricots or over fruit pies:

1 cup skim milk	½ tsp. vanilla
2 tbsp. pure gelatin	Pinch salt
1 tbsp. honey	

Warm milk to dissolve gelatin. Add honey, vanilla and salt. Whip to consistency of whipped cream.

KUMISS FROM THE ORIENT

1 quart lean milk	¼ yeast cake
2 tbsp. brown sugar	2 tbsp. warm water

Place yeast in warm water, heat the milk until warm, not boiling; add sugar and yeast. Put in air-tight bottles or cork very tightly. Let stand overnight in pantry. Serve chilled the following day.

IF YOU DON'T LIKE MILK

In case of allergies or where there is a definite dislike for milk, I suggest that you use Dr. Irvine McGuarrie's formula. Dr.

McGuarrie, who is head of the Department of Pediatrics at the University of Minnesota, created this formula for babies after weaning, but this combination makes a potent beautyfarm dish:

½ cup stewing beef	2 tbsp. honey
½ tsp. veal bone ash (very fine bone flour)	1 tbsp. rice (heaping)
1 tbsp. soya oil	Enough water to make one pint

Put ingredients in liquidizer until very fine. According to Dr. McGuarrie this formula is nutritionally equal to a pint of fresh milk.

BEAUTYFARM LAXATIVE

Here is another old-new recipe. Grind up three cups of laxative dried fruits: one cup black figs, one cup stoned prunes and one cup seedless raisins. To prevent sticking, pour boiling water through grinder, then put fruits through grinder once, sprinkle three teaspoons of Swiss Kriss, the laxative herbs, over the fruit. Mix well and put through grinder for the second time. Then form fruit mixture into balls the size of a small walnut. Roll in brown sugar crystals and keep in refrigerator. This is the most delicious-tasting and effective laxative.

BEAUTYFARM BROTH

This old potassium broth formula has given pleasure and comfort to thousands. It is a part of my Seven Day Elimination Diet which has become to popular here and abroad. It is a one-week "housecleaning" spring diet and is especially pleasant and very successful when taken in the spring when all nature turns green and glad and vegetables are at their best. This diet is given in detail in my book, *Be Happier, Be Healthier*. Here is the recipe for my mineral-rich, lean, beautyfarm broth:

1 cup finely shredded celery, leaves and all	1 tsp. vegetable salt
1 cup finely shredded carrots	1 qt. water
½ cup shredded spinach	1 cup tomato juice
1 tbsp. shredded parsley	1 tsp. brown sugar or honey

Put all shredded vegetables into a quart of water, cover and cook slowly for about 30 minutes, then add tomato juice, a teaspoon vegetable salt, and a pinch of brown sugar or honey. Let cook for a few more minutes. Strain and serve. This lean, hot broth can be drunk all day long. If served for dinner, stir in a fresh egg yolk.

POTAGE HIPPOCRATES

Here is the original vegetable broth recipe around which I built my famous Beautyfarm Broth. The Greek physician Hippocrates, who lived five hundred years before Christ, recognized the health and beauty-giving value of clear vegetable broth. He recommended a broth made with carrots, celery root, parsley and especially leek.

1 cup chopped carrots	1 cup chopped leek
1 cup chopped celery root	½ cup chopped parsley

Into 1½ quarts water put carrots, celery root, leek and parsley and cook for 30 minutes. This makes a rich combination of the beauty-giving, water-soluble vitamins. The finer the vegetables are cut, the more flavor there will be in the broth. Whenever you make "the soup of Hippocrates," add some other flavorsome vegetables like onions or tomatoes and a bit of vegetable salt.

Double Your Protein in waffles, pancakes, muffins, biscuits and bread without changing your favorite recipe. Simply add 2 tablespoons of low-fat soya flour to each cup of flour and double-sift. This will double the protein value and give added richness, much as milk and eggs do. Baked goods with added soya flour keep fresh longer because soya flour holds moisture and adds an appetizing golden brown to all baked things.

CRISP WHEAT GERM STICKS

2 cups wholewheat flour	2 cups fresh wheat germ
1¼ cups fresh milk	1 tbsp. honey
½ cup golden oil	1 tsp. vegetable salt

Mix and knead all ingredients, then cut dough and roll in the form of sticks ¼ inch thick and five inches long. Put on oiled cooky sheet; sprinkle with sesame seeds and bake about 40 minutes or until a golden brown at 350° F.

POPPED WILD RICE

Put one teaspoon of golden oil into electric popper. On top of it sprinkle one tablespoonful of wild rice. After it pops, season with vegetable salt and serve as a festive appetizer or between-meal snack.

HONEY ICE CREAM

3 fresh eggs	3 cups fresh cream
¾ cup unheated honey	1 tsp. real vanilla

Separate eggs. Beat yolks creamy thick, then slowly add honey, cream and vanilla. Put in freezer until solid, then return to mixing bowl and add stiffly beaten egg whites. Stir this mixture until smooth. Return mixture into freezing trays until firm.

Beauty Holiday

A famous English writer, returning from his American lecture tour, was asked by the press to give his impressions of the United States, and his answer was: "In America you are wined, dined and harassed to death." It was not in very good taste for a guest to make such an ill-natured report. Surely there are many wonderful things to be said for our hospitable country. But the British author was right about our being overindulgent with food and drink.

Drinking, like eating, becomes harmful only when done to excess. No serious scientist will criticize you if a cocktail relaxes you or if you enjoy a glass of wine with your dinner. Millions of Europeans have enjoyed these simple pleasures for hundreds of years without ill effects. Our main problem, however, is that we are "dripping in fat," as Carl Sandburg expressed it. One purpose of this book is to encourage you wives to cook leaner. In my chapter on reducing I present the shortest shortcut for permanently reducing excess weight, but it is so much wiser and easier to *prevent* overweight, with all its hazards. Here are some suggestions for busy, harassed, over-wined and over-dined people to protect themselves from this greatest of beauty enemies.

Once a week, stop and declare a beauty holiday. If you are a career woman this can be Saturday or Sunday. If you are married you can give yourself and your husband a health holiday and both of you will benefit tremendously. If you are a lady of leisure you can choose any day of the week, perhaps Monday. Whatever day you choose, make it *your* day, once every week.

In Germany nowadays thousands keep what they call their *Gesundheits Tag*, their Health Day. On that day they live chiefly on *Rohkost*—fresh fruits and vegetables and some milk product. The whole day is devoted to relaxing and re-charging the body, and it ends with a long walk and an early bedtime. The newly industrialized Russians are now facing a tremendous obesity problem since their physical labor has decreased and their rations have increased. Soviet doctors recommend what they call "unloading days." In order to get rid of excess weight accumulated during the week, one unloading day a week is recommended, on a simple diet. They have a choice of five different "menus": an Apple Day, on which one can eat three pounds of apples; a Vegetable and Apple Day, combining green vegetables and apples; a Rice Day with Fruit, two pounds of fruit and one dish of boiled rice; a Milk Day, which is very popular, allowing 1½ quarts of skim milk plain or in the form of yogurt; and a Fruit and Meat Day of two pounds of fresh fruit, usually apples or plums, and a helping of lean meat.

HOLIDAY FOR BEAUTY

We lucky people of the Free World can make our "unloading days" much more pleasant and derive the same benefits. All we need to do is eat lean foods and as many fresh ones as possible, to give the digestive tract a rest. While resting the inner man, we can also relax, sleep more, take leisurely baths and walk in good fresh air. Here is one such Holiday For Beauty:

Sleep a little longer; take it easy all day

BREAKFAST: Sliced orange, ½ grapefruit or half a melon

Black coffee, if you insist, but a fragrant herb tea is preferable

Do your seven-minute stretches

Take a long, relaxing bath

MIDMORNING: Your choice of any fresh fruit (except bananas)

LUNCHEON: Clear vegetable broth

Chopped carrot and cottage cheese salad, sprinkled with a very little golden oil dressing

Tea or coffee

MIDAFTERNOON: Your choice of any fresh fruit (except bananas)

A long walk in the fresh air

DINNER: Glass of vegetable espresso

One or two short-cooked vegetables

Yogurt with fruit

Hot beverage

BEFORE RETIRING: If hungry, eat some fruit or drink a glass of Hi-Vi lean milk.

Take a fragrant rose geranium oil bath

HOLLYWOOD LIQUID DIET

Making Sunday a "Juice Day," is a habit for many of the film stars. After a strenuous week at the studio, they devote the week-end to relaxing and dieting. They prefer the liquid day because it is easy to follow and there is very little cooking to do. Here is a simple all-liquid day:

Stay in bed as long as you like

BREAKFAST: Large glass of orange or grapefruit juice

Coffee or mint tea with honey

Do your seven-minute stretches

MIDMORNING: Your choice of a large glass of vegetable espresso: carrot, celery, apple—singly or mix all three. Drink through a straw. Or drink large glass of tomato juice fortified with a tablespoon of food yeast and a teaspoon of lemon juice

LUNCH: 2 cups of hot Beautyfarm Broth
1 large glass yogurt or buttermilk
English tea, mint tea or coffee

MIDAFTERNOON: Take leisurely walk
Your choice of large glass vegetable espresso: carrot, celery, apple—singly or mix all three. Drink through a straw

DINNER: Beautyfarm Broth with egg yolk beaten in it
1 large glass yogurt straight or with a teaspoon honey
Your choice: coffee, papaya or mint tea

BEFORE RETIRING: Check on your elimination
Take luxurious hot milk bath
If hungry, have a cup of hot or cold milk before retiring

IF YOU LIKE GRAPES

Thousands of European women habitually take a day or two of their famous "grape cure," originated in Merano, Italy. Women in the northern part of Italy are convinced that this traditional natural regime, followed at intervals, is responsible for their fair skins. Here is how you can take the one day "grape cure."

BREAKFAST: 1 large glass of freshly made grape juice
1 slice of Zwieback
Hot mint tea with honey

MIDMORNING: 1 pound fresh grapes, eat everything but the seeds

LUNCHEON: Baked potato
                       Large helping green salad
                       ½ pound bunch of grapes
                       Herb tea with honey

MIDAFTERNOON: Large glass fresh grape juice; drink
                       through a straw

DINNER: Hot vegetable broth
                       ½ cup cottage cheese
                       Large bunch of grapes
                       Hot mint tea with honey

BEFORE RETIRING: If hungry, more grapes can be eaten. To
                       get the benefits of this century-old
                       grape cure, you are asked to eat at least
                       two pounds of grapes a day
                       Melons, berries, cherries, apricots or
                       peaches, in fact, *any* fresh ripe fruit can
                       be used for a day of beauty. Follow the
                       above meal plan and have at least two
                       pounds of the fresh fruit or its juices.
                       One day of your favorite fruit is a re-
                       freshing change and an excellent pre-
                       ventive for expanding waistlines

ONE DAY WONDER DIET

If you like milk shakes or eggnogs, you will like this protein-
rich one day diet. You can prepare the entire menu in fifteen
minutes and keep it in the refrigerator to be enjoyed throughout
the day. Be sure to measure the ingredients correctly.

4½ cups lean milk   3 tbsp. golden oil
   3 fresh eggs   ½ cup orange juice

Pour all ingredients in liquidizer and mix well. Keep cold and
always shake before drinking. Take a glassful whenever hungry.
Or divide into six or seven portions, and take the first glass for
breakfast, another at midmorning, a third for lunch; space three
more glasses throughout the afternoon, and save the last one for

a nightcap. There is a load of concentrated protein in each glass which prevents hunger. Many women prefer this concentrated easy liquid day because there is nothing to cook and it is so easy to follow. You can include some celery, carrots, green peppers or an apple in the diet if you feel the need for bulk.

SENSATIONAL CARUBA DIET

The caruba tree played already an important part in Bible times. The fruit of the caruba tree, the caruba bean, also called honey locust or St. John's Bread, is still a new food to most people, but in the countries along the Mediterranean the honey locust bean to this day is the favorite sweet and is eaten in place of candy.

The dried fruit of the caruba tree is now ground into a very fine flour. It is alkaline, high in beauty-giving calcium and natural sugars, low in starch, very low in fat—only 2 percent as compared with 52 percent fat in chocolate. What makes the caruba bean sensational is the fact that it looks and tastes like chocolate and is rich in pectin. It seems to fill the stomach without overloading it and gives a sense of contentment. Here let me introduce you to a foamy, delightful, chocolate-tasting drink which you can make in a jiffy.

5 cups skim milk	1 tbsp. gelatin
3 tbsp. carob powder	1 tbsp. sesame oil
1 fresh egg	1 tbsp. honey

Mix all ingredients in large bowl. Whip with rotary beater until foamy or place contents in liquidizer; fill only half way because carob powder and gelatin puff up and make the mixture light and foamy.

If you like chocolate milk shakes, the caruba mixture will appeal to you. Keep it in the refrigerator and always stir or shake before using. Drink a small glass whenever you are hungry or you can divide it into six or seven glasses, as in the Wonder Diet.

You Can Drink One Meal A Day

This is not a whole day of liquids. This is my new idea of making *one* meal a nutritious liquid meal, which has become tremendously popular. The difficulty with most formulas is that after a few days, they become boring; the pleasure of novelty is gone. On beauty-farms this is avoided by creating a new and different liquid meal every day of the week. The single liquid meal is a wonderful device when you are pressed for time or whenever the contours need whittling down. The recipe is simple: put all the nutrients in a liquidizer and beat them together until the mixture is smooth and foamy. But do not gulp it down, just because it is smooth and liquid; drink your liquid meal slowly through a straw and you will derive twice as much pleasure and benefit. Your liquid meal can be cold or hot and it can take the place of breakfast, lunch or dinner.

Liquid Meals à la Carte: Unlimited Choice

GOLDEN EGGNOG

½ cup Hi-Vi lean milk   2 drops vanilla
 1 fresh egg   ½ tsp. honey
½ cup orange juice

LIVER AND—

 1 cup hot boullion   1 tsp. parsley
 2 tbsp. sautéed liver
 1 tsp. onion

Serve this tangy drink hot.

HI-VI BOOST

 1 cup Hi-Vi milk   2 slices pineapple
 2 tbsp. cottage cheese

CHICKEN AVOCADO

 1 cup lean chicken broth   1 tsp. parsley
 1 heaping tbsp. avocado

CREAM OF MUSHROOM   (Serve hot)

 1 cup Hi-Vi lean milk   Pinch vegetable salt
½ cup small white mushrooms
 1 tsp. onion

CHICKEN DINNER (Serve hot)

1 cup chicken broth
3 tbsp. boned chicken

1 tsp. chives or parsley

EYE BRIGHT

½ cup orange juice
½ cup carrot espresso

1 fresh egg yolk
1 tsp. food yeast

GREEN-GOLD

1 fresh egg yolk
½ cup parsley

Whip ingredients into cup of
hot chicken broth

CLEAR COMPLEXION

½ cup sauerkraut
1 cup yogurt

1 dill pickle

BEAUTYFARM SPECIAL

1 cup Hi-Vi lean milk
1 fresh egg yolk

4 ripe apricots

BOUILLABAISSE

1 cup hot clam juice
2 tbsp. boned fish

1 tbsp. shrimp
Pinch garlic powder

CARUBA DELIGHT

1 cup Hi-Vi lean milk
1 tbsp. carob powder

1 tsp. brown sugar

With any of the above liquid meals, you may eat some fresh celery, carrot sticks, slices of sweet green pepper, radishes or an apple.

CHAPTER 26

Cosmetics from Your Kitchen Shelf

You know that oils, lotions and perfumes have been used by women since the beginning of history. What you may not know is that there are some excellent cosmetics right on your kitchen shelf. Many of these are good as food as well as cosmetics. The many kinds of golden oils, milk baths, honey masks, herbal concoctions have always been popular. In the 15th Century Caterina Di Sforza, a great Italian beauty, wrote her *Ricettario di Bellezza*, "Recipe for Beauty." It was the beauty bible for lovely ladies of that time. In it she gave 543 of her beauty secrets for hands and face. They are amusing, but if you try them it is at your own risk. I print them only to show you that this beauty mistress of 500 years ago knew that many of the simplest foods were also good for external beauty. To make men swoon over a fair *signorina* complexion, Caterina recommends this concoction:

Thirty egg whites, mixed with equal amounts of cold pressed olive oil, three cups of wine vinegar and enough cottage cheese to make a thick paste. Fair ladies were advised to apply this mask one hour before the grand ball.

351

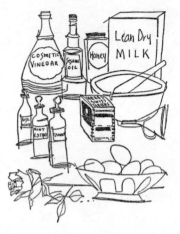

For a hand lotion Caterina gave this formula: Take the soft inside part of a fresh loaf of bread and knead it with 2 egg whites, then soak in vinegar overnight. Make into emulsion and apply to rough red hands to make them smooth and lily-white.

Today we rightly laugh at such complicated *ricettarios*, but women of the past did know about the beauty effect of olive oil, egg white, cottage cheese and, of course, vinegar.

In all the old herbals and recipe books, no matter whether Greek, Roman or German, I have found hundreds of cosmetic recipes using herbal steams, oils, milk, cottage cheese, honey and always vinegar.

Within the last few years the Vermont doctor, D. C. Jarvis, has sung the praises of two old fashioned foods, honey and vinegar. His formula is extremely simple: two teaspoons of vinegar and two teaspoons of honey in a glass of water once or twice a day is what Dr. Jarvis prescribed to his many patients for years.

Whether or not vinegar does contain all the health-giving properties that are claimed for it, only biochemists of the future will be able to prove. Here I am interested in the beauty-giving properties of all vinegars.

Vinegar is familiar as a mild antiseptic; physicians to this day recommend dilute vinegar solutions for female hygiene. But vinegar also contains other beauty-giving and protecting ingredients which we have completely forgotten. Caterina Di Sforza knew it from experience, Dr. Culpepper knew it from his medical practice, your grandmother surmised it, and today we know scientifically that the mild acidity of vinegar solutions helps to protect the acid mantle of scalp and skin. This is why the old alchemists concocted vinegar formulas, and the famous beauties of all ages had their chemists compound vinegar rinses, vinegar douches and vinegar baths; and in England to this day I have found cosmetic vinegar on the shelves of apothecaries, and herb shops and in Germany you can buy *Gesichts-essig*—face vinegar—in many *Drogerien* or drug stores. Even in barber shops after you have been shaved, the barber pats your face with *cosmetic vinegar*.

What can cosmetic vinegar do: We know that the scalp and skin normally exude a mild acid that protects them against infection. Every time you shampoo your hair you remove that protection; every time you wash and soap your face you wash off that acid veil and every time you take a bath with soap and hard water you destroy nature's safeguard. I believe innumerable scalp and skin troubles, including the two arch-enemies of beauty, dry scaly scalp and dry scaly skin, can be helped by protecting the natural acid mantle of scalp and skin. To restore it, after shampooing, washing, bathing and shaving you need only use a bit of cosmetic vinegar. You don't have to be afraid that you will smell like a salad. The herbs transform vinegar into delightful tonics. I suggest that each beautyfarm make its own specific herbalized cosmetic vinegars; all the ingredients can be grown right on the farm. You can make your own, from your pantry shelf, by this formula:

COSMETIC VINEGAR

Put two heaping tablespoonfuls of dried peppermint leaves into a pint of water. Let come to a boil and simmer for two minutes, then strain and mix hot infusion with a pint of cider vinegar. Let stand for 48 hours before using. One-half cup in ½ a tub of water makes a delightful refreshing bath, especially recommended for those with dry itching skin.

P.S.: If the above is too much trouble, then mix a pint of hot water with a pint of vinegar. Let cool off then add one teaspoon of rose geranium oil and keep in tightly corked bottle. Never use straight vinegar for cosmetic purposes. It is much too strong and irritating to the skin.

MAYONNAISE FOR THE FACE

Several years ago it suddenly occurred to me that ordinary mayonnaise, consisting of golden vegetable oil, fresh egg yolks and a little vinegar should make a perfect cosmetic. Several of my friends tried it and came back with enthusiastic reports. About that time I was interviewed by Arlene Dahl, one of Hollywood's true beauties, who also writes a syndicated beauty column. Arlene was very enthusiastic about my facial mayonnaise and devoted one of her columns to this new idea. Since then I have received hundreds of letters from women all over the country telling me of the wonderful results they have obtained by using this simple cosmetic. One lady wrote: "It did my face so much good I decided to use it on my body. Now my skin is soft all over and for the first time in my life I was able to acquire an even golden tan without drying up like a baked potato. My husband says I smell like a salad but I don't care and neither does he. He likes salad!"

A few months ago, while doing research for this book, I learned that my idea of using mayonnaise as a cosmetic was not an original one after all. Dr. Leo Kumer, the famous dermatologist of Vienna, Austria, mentions it in a book which was first published in 1952.

I have worked out the following recipe which utilizes oils which are smooth in texture and rich in unsaturated fatty acids (which are called vitamin F in Europe). The egg yolks supply vitamin A, plus valuable lecithin, and the herb vinegar is mildly acid and antiseptic. The addition of a few drops of perfume will prevent you from smelling like a salad!

FACIAL MAYONNAISE (OR FACIALAISE)

2 fresh egg yolks	1 tbsp. herb vinegar
½ cup sunflower oil	2 drops of rose geranium oil or
½ cup sesame oil	your favorite perfume
1 tbsp. wheat germ oil	

Mix three oils in a measuring cup. Place fresh egg yolks in cold bowl and beat slowly. At first add oil very slowly and beat with rotary beater. Gradually add more oil. As mixture thickens, add vinegar and perfume. Beat until thick and golden. There is no better cosmetic for dry skin, for cleansing and removing makeup. Use it generously all over the body before bathing. It is also ideal for sunbathing.

BEAUTYFARM COSMETIC OILS

Here is a combination of the finest and richest fatty acid oils. No combination of oils can do more to keep the face softer and smoother. You will be amazed how a dry skin will gratefully drink in the combination of these purest and wax-free golden oils. Mix in a measuring cup the following seven oils:

3 tbsp. safflower oil	1 tbsp. olive oil
3 tbsp. sesame oil	1 tbsp. wheat germ oil
2 tbsp. sunflower oil	5 drops oil of rose geranium or
2 tbsp. avocado oil	your favorite perfume
2 tbsp. peanut oil	

In one bottle of this seven oil blend, you have one of the finest 100 percent natural cosmetics to be found anywhere. In connection with this seven oil formula, many of my students use a daily face bath with mild yogurt soap and lots of cold water.

EFFECTIVE ASTRINGENT FACE LOTION

¾ cup rose water	Pinch alum powder
¼ cup witch hazel	¼ tsp. glycerine
1 tsp. honey	½ tsp. spirit of camphor
½ tsp. white vinegar	½ tsp. extract of mint

Mix all in one bottle and shake. Apply this effective astringent all over face before applying makeup. Use cotton pads. To reduce under eye tiredness, soak cotton pads with astringent lotion and apply under eyes. Rest for five minutes.

FOR LARGE PORES AND OILY SKIN

⅓ cup powdered castile soap	⅓ cup almond meal
⅓ cup corn meal, white	

Mix dry in bowl and keep in jar. Fill palm of hand with mixture and make a paste with a bit of water, then with fingertips scrub area around nose and other oily and blackhead spots. Rinse off with warm water and follow with very cold water to close pores.

MILD SKIN BLEACH

Mix in one cup:

1 tbsp. lemon juice   1 tsp. glycerine
1 tbsp. regular peroxide

Massage gently into darkened skin areas, especially the neck. This helps to lighten old summer tan. Apply several times over dark brown spots.

SPOT LOTION

Purchase a small bottle of calamine lotion and ask your druggist to add one percent of phenol. A famous French beauty has given me this simple formula which has been a blessing to thousands of my students. Apply it to any trouble spot with clean fingers several times during the day. To discourage an oncoming pimple, soak a piece of cotton in Spot Lotion and apply over pimple. This lotion has amazing drying up qualities.

HONEY EGG MASK FOR DRY SKIN

1 fresh egg yolk   1 tbsp. fresh milk
1 tbsp. dry skim milk   ½ tsp. honey

Mix all four ingredients in cup. Beat into consistency of mayonnaise. Apply thickly over face and throat. Leave on for fifteen minutes, then wash off with warm water and finish with cold water.

YOGURT-MINT MASK

To wake up and freshen up the face, try this excellent easy-to-make combination.

Take one tablespoon of thick yogurt and one tablespoon of Fuller's Earth and stir into this one teaspoon of extract of mint from your kitchen shelf. Apply this creamy cool mixture all over the face, not too close to the eyes. Let dry and relax for fifteen minutes. Wash off with mild yogurt soap and rinse with cool water.

Fabulous face tightener

1 fresh egg white	½ tsp. honey
1 tbsp. dry skim milk	

Mix all three ingredients in cup. Whip with fork until smooth. Apply over face and throat as thick as possible. Lie quiet for fifteen minutes, preferably with head lower than feet (Beauty Slant). Wash off with warm water, then cold water and apply face lotion. Watch fine lines and droopiness disappear.

Neck tight

Here is a marvelously effective neck tightener. The whole idea is to bring the beautystream to the loose neck tissues.

Mix in a cup, two tablespoons dry skim milk, one egg white, one teaspoon of camphor, and one teaspoon of mint extract. Whip smooth with fork. Apply thickly all over neck (not face). Lie down and relax for 15 minutes. When dry, wash off with mild soap and rinse with cold water.

Lily-white hand lotion

¾ cup rose water	¼ tsp. white vinegar
¼ cup glycerine	¼ tsp. honey

The oldest, and still the best, hand protector. Keep bottle handy and rub a few drops into hands every time after you wash them. The results are surprising, but remember that both glycerine and honey are the oldest moisturizers known. This lotion is not sticky. Use it generously. If you are too lazy to make the entire lotion, let your corner drugstore mix the rose water and glycerine and you add the vinegar and honey.

A *Queen's Secret*. In the beautiful city of Budapest, before it was over-run by the Communists, the art and science of bathing for health and beauty equaled that of the ancient Greeks and Romans. No other place has so many different kinds of springs and soothing waters as Budapest. It is even said that Hungarian women have such beautiful complexions because of the fine, magnetic waters springing from the earth, and their many varieties of beauty baths. Hungarians will also tell you that their own Queen Elizabeth of Hungary, a famous beauty, was so attractive even at the age of seventy that she inspired a young man of 26 with "a burning passion." She ascribed her extraordinary beauty to her secret beauty bath, and only after her death was her recipe discovered. It is called "Budapest Water," a luxurious toilet water which you can prepare in your own kitchen. Here is all you need to make this fabulous cologne:

BUDAPEST WATER

2 oz. dried rosemary leaves	1 oz. dried lemon balm
1 oz. fresh lemon peel	1 pt. strong rose water
1 oz. fresh orange peel	1 pt. spirit of wine (alcohol)
1 oz. dried mint leaves	

Put ingredients into a large jar. Let the mixture stand for three weeks and then filter. This Budapest Water has one of the most delightful fresh odors you have ever experienced. It can be used as a cologne or added to the bath water. You can obtain the dried herbs in any gourmet shop and the rose water and spirit of wine, an alcohol available at your drugstore. Be sure and ask for the non-smelling alcohol. Do not use Iso-propynol.

THE LUXURIOUS OIL BATH

Golden oils in your food and golden oils for your bath. Here is a million dollar beauty trick which I pass on to every lady who loves luxury, but whose purse does not permit it.

You can make a wonderfully soothing bath oil that will make you feel like an heiress, but costs only pennies.

Pour one pint of peanut or corn oil into a bowl. Add two tablespoons of your liquid shampoo (detergent type) and whip with egg beater (if made for beautyfarm, use liquidizer). Right in front of your eyes you will see the detergent break the large golden oil globules into millions of finely divided oil atoms which will cling and cling to the skin and make it velvety soft. To make this bath unguent more luxurious, add a few drops of your expensive perfume to the mixture or add half a teaspoon of oil of rose geranium. Keep in bottle. Add 2 tablespoons to a warm bath and imagine you are on a luxurious beautyfarm. To combine the luxury of this oil bath with a thorough cleansing bath, all you need is a bar of rich yogurt soap.

To highlite your hair

Simply add one tablespoon of cosmetic vinegar to a quart of warm water and rinse thoroughly. Leave on scalp and hair for three minutes, then rub dry with warm coarse towel. For dark hair use dark vinegar; for blonde or gray hair white vinegar is more desirable.

For stubborn dandruff

Mix two tablespoons of cosmetic vinegar with one tablespoon of warm water. Dip cotton pads into solution and rub over entire scalp. Do not rinse. Two or three of these vinegar and water scalp rubs have given excellent results. Always use vinegar rinse after shampooing.

Swiss herb rinse

When hair is hard to manage and dull looking, make this simple herb hair rinse. Place three teaspoons of Swiss Kriss herbs into a pint of water. Let come to boil and simmer for five minutes. Strain and apply the herb lotion all over scalp and hair. Do not rinse.

Eyebright lotion

A combination of three old fashioned dried herbs makes one of the best and simplest lotions for the eyes. Simply put one heaping teaspoonful each dry herb, eyebright, camomile and fennel, into a pint of boiling water. Let simmer for only three minutes and turn off the heat. When cool, strain and filter and put in sterilized bottles. Use solution in clean eye cup as refreshing eye wash. For relaxing tired eyes, cover them with cotton pads soaked in the herbal solution.

Eliminating ugly liver spots

Adelle Davis, the popular California nutritionist, offers a very simple inside remedy to help get rid of these ugly blemishes. She says that for years she has watched for liver spots on all persons who come to her for dietary advice. She recommends that 100 units of vitamin E be taken after each meal and, she adds, that months or years later many of these people return with the ugly spots gone. If you are worried and have a few of these disfiguring liver spots on your face and hands, it is certainly a simple procedure to take the vitamin E capsules internally, and you might even get speedier results by rubbing a few drops of castor oil into the brown spots every day. According to Dr. Jarvis, with this simple Vermont formula the brown spots disappear gradually. Should you be so unfortunate as to have many deep-seated brownish, almost black spots all over your face and hands, I suggest that you investigate the simple and very effective peeling of the face or hands given by doctors, especially in Hollywood. Another successful method for removing brown spots, scars or freckles is to plane the skin away with a drill that looks very much like a dentist's drill. This process is used especially by New York physicians and can be done in one sitting.

Cosmetic patch test

If you suspect any of your 57 varieties of cosmetics of irritating your scalp, face, eyes, lips or hands you can make a simple patch test. Apply the suspected preparation to a piece of gauze and tape it to the inside of your upper arm where the skin is white and sensitive. Leave the patch on for 48 hours, then remove it. If there is no irritation or red spot the cosmetic is safe, but if there is a red spot and irritation (under the *patch*—not under the tape). then that particular cosmetic is not for you, no matter how touted it may be. If you seem to be sensitive to many cosmetics, you better stick to the simplest lotions or creams or, better still, use a combination of pure vegetable oils inside and outside.

Beautyfarm Listings

Here I present my first international list of beautyfarms, spas and health resorts. For more information, write directly to the addresses given below. For best accommodations, make reservations well in advance.

The Golden Door, Escondido, California. Luxurious and most glamorous of all beautyfarms. Accent on beauty, reducing and relaxation. Ladies only. Expensive. Address: The Golden Door, Highway 395, Escondido, California.

Rancho la Puerta, Tecate, Mexico, near San Diego, California. Modest ranch style accommodations. Serious, somewhat cultish regime, with accent on physical and mental fitness. Caters to both men and women. The Rancho produces its own organically grown grapes and features a grape cure. Inexpensive. Address: Rancho La Puerta, Tecate, near San Diego, California.

Springboard Farms, La Quinta, California (near Palm Springs). Delightful luxurious establishment surrounded by spacious gardens in picturesque grove of palm trees. Under personal direction of Dr. Charles Benson and his attractive wife, who supervise everything themselves. A paradise of a place to relax, reduce and recharge. Large swimming pool, soft lawns, exquisite beautyfarm cuisine by expert chef. Caters to both men and women. Most reasonably priced of all de luxe beautyfarms. Address: Springboard Farms, La Quinta, California.

Mainchance, Mount Vernon, Maine (near Augusta) and Mainchance West, Phoenix, Arizona. De luxe establishments with accent on beauty and glamor. Luxurious accommodations. Ladies only. Very expensive! Address: Elizabeth Arden, 691 Fifth Avenue, New York City, attention of Mrs. Versteeg.

HIDDEN VALLEY HEALTH RANCH, Escondido, California. Under the direction of Dr. Bernard Jensen. Beautifully situated. Comfortable ranch-type accommodations. Emphasis is on physical fitness and natural living. Both men and women accepted. Moderate prices. Address: Dr. Bernard Jensen, Route 4, Box 184, Escondido, Calif.

COMANCIAS GUEST RANCH, Thousand Oaks, California. Located in a secluded wooded cove near Los Angeles. Was originally a multi-millionaire's luxurious hide-a-way. Beautiful natural surroundings. An ideal place to escape from tensions. Features diet, massage, exercise, sports and relaxation. Both men and women accepted. Fair prices for excellent accommodations. Address: Comancias Guest Ranch, Box 457, Thousand Oaks, California.

LYTTON-BERNARD HEALTH CENTER, Guadalajara, Mexico. Specializing in the "Papaya Diet." Many other exotic tropical fruits are served. Ideal year round climate. Both men and women accepted. Inexpensive. Address: Dr. Lytton-Bernard, P.O. Box 1187, Guadalajara, Mexico.

ANN ROBINSON'S SUNSHINE TERRACE, Croton-on-Hudson, New York (near New York City). Private home atmosphere in a beautiful garden overlooking the Hudson River. Accent on diet for reducing, rest and relaxation. Ladies only. Moderate prices. Address: Ann Robinson, Croton-on-Hudson, New York.

CLINIQUE DIETETIQUE, Champigny, France. A country house near Paris converted into a well-equipped establishment. Accent on diet, exercise and physiotherapy. Ladies only. Not expensive by American standards. Address: Clinique Dietetique de Champigny, Champigny, France.

BEAUTY FARM, Knebworth, Hertfordshire, England. About 25 miles north of London. Efficient establishment. All comforts, but not as luxurious as American beautyfarms. Moderate prices. Accent on diet, rest and relaxation. Caters to both men and women. Address: The Secretary, Beauty Farm, Knebworth, Hertfordshire, England.

BIRCHER-BENNER SANATORIUM, Zurich, Switzerland. Pioneer diet establishment. Home of "Bircher Muesle." Serious, somewhat spartan regime. Beautiful hillside location overlooking the city. Not expensive for Americans. Address: Bircher-Benner Sanatorium, Zurich, Switzerland.

DR. BUCHINGER'S SANATORIUM, Uberlingen, Germany (on Lake Constance). Ultra modern, semi-luxurious establishment specializing in fasts. Beautiful situation. Excellent staff of doctors, nurses and therapists. Both men and women accepted. Inexpensive according to American standards. Address: Dr. Buchinger's Sanatorium, Uberlingen-am-Bodensee, Germany.

I hope that with the publication of this book many more new beautyfarms and spas will spring up everywhere. After investigating, there will be new listings from time to time which I will gladly send to new readers via my Newsletter.

WHERE TO BUY YOUR BEAUTY-FULL FOODS

If you wish to have a beautyfarm in your own home you must make certain that everything which comes into your kitchen is as fresh and vital as possible: fresh young vegetables grown in good soil, juicy tree-ripened fruits, fresh milk, eggs, cheese, butter, fish, meat and poultry and freshly-ground whole grain cereals.

Many cities now have "Farmers" markets, where the growers bring their fresh produce each morning. The most famous of these is the Farmers Market in Hollywood. If your community has such a market, by all means seek it out. If not, then shop around and find a grocer who prides himself on having the freshest, youngest and choicest produce available. Some of the large new supermarkets do an amazingly good job and can supply you with most of your daily needs, including some of the special foods such as brown rice, buckwheat groats (kasha), soybeans, herbal seasonings and vinegars.

I hope you will also find in your community or city a special diet shop, formerly known as Health Food Shops of which there are now about one thousand spread across the country. These diet shops or dietary food shops specialize in natural, unprocessed foods; whole grain products, unsulphured dried fruits, vegetable oils and a dozen varieties of unheated honeys with their natural flower flavors. They also carry a variety of seasonings, including my favorite one which is a combination of twenty-seven spices and herbs with which you can spike your salads, soups and sauces with one shake. Other staple items include a vegetable salt which contains seventeen different California vegetables, plus that necessary bit of iodine, in combination with earth and sea salt. Another product which should be in every beauty pantry is brewer's or food yeast, which can be used to fortify so many foods. My favorite one is celery flavored and is especially good when stirred into tomato juice. You will also find vitamin and mineral tablets, including one rich in calcium (very fine bone flour) and vitamin D; a special iodine-rich one, made from sea greens; and many varieties of herb teas, including strawberry leaves, peppermint, and rose hips, which is our richest source of vitamin C.

These special diet shops will supply you with many of the newer beauty-full foods which you will not find elsewhere, such as sunflower and pumpkin seeds, sesame seeds and chocolate-like carob flour, made from St. John's bread, which is excellent for reducers when combined with lean milk. The new is El Molino whole-wheat ready bread mix which will make it possible for you to bake beauty-full bread in your own kitchen.

When Dr. Norman Joliffe addressed the Dietary Food Association, he said: "Modern diet therapy demands that someone, some place in your community, establish a dependable diet food center to supply the requirements of the doctor and patients."

If you have never been to a special diet shop you have a pleasant surprise awaiting you. I hope there is one in your neighborhood.

You will have to rely on the corner drugstore to supply you with some of the ingredients for your beautyfarm cosmetics, such as rose water, witch hazel, glycerine, almond meal and oil of rose germanium. Swiss Kriss, the laxative herbal mixture which you will also use for your facial sauna bath, is available at most drug stores and at all special diet shops.

Most special diet shops also sell durable cooking utensils, shredders, liquidizers and juice extractors.

Index

A Guide to Recipes appears on page 368

Abrahamson, E. M., 36
Adrian, 172
Ageless Youth, 221
alcoholic beverages, 343
Alexander, Franz, 22
amino acids, 14, 16, 32, 36
Anatomy of Dessert, The, 78
Ann Robinson's Sunshine Terrace, 362
Arden, Elizabeth, 30, 271, 362
arteriosclerosis, 248–249
Askander, Alfred, 193–194
Aspasia, Princess of Greece, 119
Astaire, Adele, 118, 119, 120, 151
Astaire, Ann, 151, 166, 279
Astaire, Fred, 151
astringent face lotions, 355–356, 357
Atkinson, Donald T., 177
aura, 170
avocados, 79–80

baldness, 253–255
Baruch, Bernard, 95, 241
Baruch, Simon, 95, 241
Bates, William H., 179, 181
bathing, 235 ff.
bath oil, 358–359
Bean, William Bennett, 202
beauty bar, 50
Beauty Farm, 362
beautyfarm afloat, 275–276
beautyfarm back yard, 265–266
beautyfarm kitchen, 267–270
beautyfarms, 262
    list of, 361–363
Beauty Slant, 105, 135, 161, 263–264, 266
beds, 213–215
Belasco, David, 49, 167
Benson, Charles, 361
Benson, Ezra Taft, 109
Bergman, Ingrid, 136
Bernhardt, Prince of the Netherlands, 272
biotin, 70
Bircher-Benner, Dr., 45
Bircher-Benner Sanatorium, 87, 363
blood, 13–14
blood sugar, 40–42, 121
Body, Mind and Sugar, 36
body structure, 101
bones, 107–110
bosom, 133–135
Brady, William, 91–92
bread, 64–65, 80–81, 321–322
breakfast, 39–43, 259
Budapest Water, 358
Bunnell, Sterling, 15
Bunyard, Charles, 87
bustline, 133–135

butter, 38, 269
buttocks, 116–117, 135

calcium, 13–14, 72, 108–109, 177–178
calcium pantothenate, 70
Calver, George W., 249
Cannon, Walter B., 21
carbohydrates, 34–37
Carnarvon, Countess of, 119, 272
carob, 81
Carol, Martine, 136
caruba, 348
Cavendish, Lady, 119
cells of body, 9, 10, 14–17
Chase, Ilka, 272
Cheney, Garnett, 312
Chesterton, G. K., 23
Chevalier, Maurice, 136
chewing, 11, 123, 124, 125, 126, 196
Chittenden, R. H., 88–89
choline, 69–70
Churchill, Winston, 213
cleanliness, 221–224

Clinique Dietetique, 362
cocktails, 51
Comancias Guest Ranch, 362
complexion, 154–157
    See also skin
contact lenses, 181–182
Conway, Herbert, 162
cooking pots, 267, 269
Cooper, Lady Diana Duff, 119
Corbett, Margaret D., 181
Cosmetic Diet, 29 ff., 53 ff., 107, 187
cosmetic oils, 355
cosmetic vinegar, 353–354
cosmetics
    astringents, 355–356, 357
    Budapest Water, 358
    hand lotion, 357–358
    honey egg mask, 356
    mayonnaise, 354–355
    neck tightener, 357
    oils, 355
    skin bleach, 356
    spot lotion, 356
    vinegar, 353–354
    yogurt-mint mask, 356–357
    See also makeup
Crane, George W., 92–93
cress, 81–82

Dahl, Arlene, 354
dandruff remover, 359
Davis, Adelle, 360
Deane, Martha, 124
Delafield, Ann, 30, 105, 161, 263, 270

365

dentistry, 196–197
derrière, 116–117, 135
De Wolfe, Elsie, *see* Mendl, Lady
dieting, 118 ff., 343 ff.
Dietrich, Marlene, 136
diets
   caruba, 348
   grape cure, 346–347
   holiday for beauty, 344–345
   Hollywood liquid, 345–346
   liquid meals, 348–350
   one day wonder, 347–348
digestive system, 11–14
dinner, 50–53, 260–261
Di Sforza, Caterina, 351–352, 353
Douglass, Mrs. Kingman, 118
Dragonette, Jessica, 199, 273

Drobil, Rudolf, 161
dry skin, 143–146
Dubonett, Ruth, 272
dumbbells, 266

electrolysis, 165
Elizabeth, Queen of Hungary, 239, 358
Elizabeth II of England, 24, 272
Ellene, Madame, 154
El Molino bread, 322, 364
energy, 34–37
exercise, 112–117, 120, 127 ff.
eyeglasses, 180–182
eye opener, 54
eye operation, 163–164
eyes, 173 ff.
eye wash, 360

face, 149 ff.
face lift, 162–163
facial hair, 164–165
facial masks, 356–357
family life, 227 ff.
farmers markets, 363
fats, 14, 37–38
feet, 205 ff.
fingernails, 201–203
flaxseed, 94
fluorine, 74
Foldes, Eugene, 254
Fontanne, Lynn, 136, 151
Frederika, Queen of Greece, 275
Freud, Sigmund, 23, 119
Fromm, Erich, 6

Gabor, Eva, 172
Gabor, Zsa Zsa, 172
Garbo, Greta, 105, 135, 166–167, 169, 172
garlic, 82–83
Goddard, Paulette, 273
Godowsky, Dagmar, 272
Gofman, John W., 249
Golden Door, 361
golden oils, 37–38, 45, 46–47, 268, 336–337
Goldzieher, M. A., 157
Grace, Princess of Monaco, 273
grape cure, 346–347
Green, Harold, 192
Gumpert, Martin A., 108

hair, 185 ff.
hair brightener, 359
hair coloring, 191, 192
hair rinse, 359
Halla, Franz, 254
hand lotion, 357–358
hands, 200 ff.
happiness, 18–20
Happiness Room, 274–275
Health Day, 344
health food shops, 363–364
heart disease, 245, 248–249, 252–253
herb rinse, 359
Hidden Valley Health Ranch, 362
holiday for beauty, 344–345
Hollywood liquid, 345–346
honey, 35–36, 83–85
honey egg mask, 356
Hopper, Hedda, 166, 273
hormone creams, 157
Hunt, Terry, 133–134
Hunter, Ann, 170
husbands, 243 ff.
Hutschnecker, Arnold A., 23
Huxley, Aldous, 237
Hydro Face Molder, 158
hygiene, 221–224
Hyman, Harold Thomas, 143, 248–249

inositol, 69
iodine, 9–10, 72–73, 91–92, 189, 287, 364
Irene, 172
iron, 73

Jacobson, E., 218
Jaipur, Maharani of, 273
Jarvis, D. C., 352, 360
Jensen, Bernard, 362
Johnson, Lady Bird, 250
Johnson, Lyndon B., 249–250
Jolliffe, Norman, 75, 364
Jordan, Sara, 20–21
Juliana, Queen of the Netherlands, 272
Jung, Carl Gustav, 218, 277

Karputhala, Princess of India, 94, 119
kasha, 85
Kaufman, William, 232–233
Kellogg, John Harvey, 89
Kelly, Grace, 273
Kirschner, H. E., 313
Kleitman, Nathaniel L., 210
Kollath, Werner, 45
Korb, Donald R., 182
Kumer, Leo, 354

Lane, Lydia, 134–135
Langford, Frances, 49
Laszlo, Erno, 142, 154
laxative foods, 223–224, 341
lecithin, 85–86, 252–253
Lee, Anna, 165–166
Lefort, Colette, 273, 275–276
licorice, 86
Lillie, Bea, 272
liquidizer-blender, 267

liquid meals, 348–350
liver spots, 360
Loos, Anita, 273
Losch, Tilly, 119, 272
love, 6, 24–26, 243
Lubowe, Irwin I., 187, 254
lunch, 46–49, 260
lysine, 33, 34
Lytton-Bernard Health Center, 362

McCarrison, Robert, 30
McCollum, E. V., 64–65
McCormick, W. J., 336
McGuarrie, Irvine, 340–341
Mack, Mary, 273–274
Mack, Pauline Berry, 230
Mackenzie, Gertrude, 167
Mainchance, 361–362
makeup, 165–170
  See also cosmetics
Marañon, Gregorio, 255
margarine, 38
Markova, Alicia, 83
Marusia, 172
Mayer, Jean, 127
mayonnaise facial, 354–355
Mead, Margaret, 53, 231
Mechnikov, Ilya, 96
melon seeds, 93
Mendl, Lady, 49–50, 119, 165–167,
  171, 272
Menshikov, Dr., 222
metabolism, 9, 20
milk bath, 240
Miller, Fred D., 195
moles, 165
Morehouse, Laurence E., 250
Morrison, Lester M., 86, 252
Moses, Grandma, 279
mouth, 169–170, 193 ff.
Mueller, Erich A., 116
Murray, Alan E., 207
muscles, 101–102, 106–107, 110,
  115–117
muscle tensing, 116–117
My Love Affair with the State of
  Maine, 167

nagging, 246–247
Nazli, Queen of Egypt, 279
neck tightener, 357
nervous system, 15
niacin, 69
nose operation, 163
Nutrition and Physical Degeneration,
  108
nuts, 87–88

oil bath, 358–359
oils, golden, 37–38, 45, 46–47, 268,
  336–337
one day wonder diet, 347–348
On My Own, 83
Open Door to Health, 195

papaya, 88–89
para amino benzoic acid, 69
parsley, 89–90
patch test, 360–361

peanut flour, 88
peanuts, 88
perfume, 170
Philip, Prince of England, 24
phosphorus, 73
Pickford, Mary, 166
pillows, 215–216
plastic surgery, 153–154, 161–164
poisonous sprays, 313–314
posture, 99 ff.
Preminger, Marian, 280
Price, Weston A., 31, 108
proteins, 14, 32–34, 36, 259
pumpkin seeds, 93

Rainer, Jerome, 256
Rainer, Julia, 256
Rancho la Puerta, 361
reducing, 118 ff., 153–154, 343 ff.
Roosevelt, Eleanor, 83
rose hips, 90, 110
Rubin, William, 75

Saint Hardouin, Mme de, 119
St. John's Bread, 81
Sandburg, Carl, 124, 343
Saroya, Princess of Persia, 271–272
sauna face bath, 154–157
Schweitzer, Albert, 183, 280
sea greens, 91–92
sea water, 92–93
seeds, 93–95
selfishness, 6, 25
Senz, Eddie, 166
sesame seeds, 94–95
Sexual Pleasure in Marriage, 256
sexual powers, 255–258
shampoo, 188–189
Shapley, Harlow, 16
Shaw, George Bernard, 34
Shaw, Morton, 182
Sherman, Henry C., 66, 109
shredder, 267
Shriber, Donald, 232
sitz bath, 242
skin, 66, 67–68, 138 ff.
skin bleach, 356
Slaughter, Frank G., 138
sleep, 210 ff.
sleepwear, 216
Space shoes, 207–208
Spain, David M., 245
sports, 128–129
spot lotion, 356
sprays, poisonous, 313–314
Springboard Farms, 361
Stare, Frederick, 74
Steinhaus, Arthur H., 116
sulphur, 74
sunbathing, 146–147, 266
sunflower seeds, 93
Swanson, Gloria, 171
swimming pool, 266
Swing-Sway-Slump, 112–115, 212–
  213
Swiss coffee, 42, 43

teen-agers, 233–234
teeth, 193–198

tension
    and beauty, 18–19, 110–111
    and emotions, 22
    and exercise, 112–115, 212–213
    and eyes, 173–174, 179
    and hair, 189–190
    and laughing, 18, 20–21
    and nerves, 67
    and posture, 106–107
    and sexual fulfillment, 25
    and sleep, 210–211, 212–213
thyroxin, 9
Toklas, Alice, 38
Toumanoff, Princess Marusia, 172
tupelo honey, 84
Turner, Nicholas Meredith, 273

Uris, Dorothy, 198

vegetable salt, 364
vinegar, 47–48, 269, 352–354
Virchow, Rudolf, 45
vitamin A, 66, 175–176, 195
vitamin B-1, 64, 67
vitamin B-2, 64, 67–68
vitamin B-6, 68
vitamin B-12, 68
vitamin B complex, 66–67, 143, 176, 217
vitamin C, 70, 110, 176–177, 195, 364
vitamin D, 71, 109–110, 146, 177–178, 195, 217, 364

vitamin E, 71, 252, 360
vitamin F, 47, 71–72
vitamin K, 72
vitamins, 16, 63 ff.
voice, 198–199

walking, 135–137, 263, 264
Warner, Ann, 166
watercress, 81–82
weight table, 126
West, Charlotte, 221
Weyhbrecht, Hans, 159
wheat germ, 252
White, Paul Dudley, 5–6
white blood corpuscles, 45
Williams, Mrs. Harrison, 119
Williams, Roger J., 244, 336
Will to Live, The, 23
Windsor, Duchess of, 119, 171, 272
Wolf, Richard E., 229
Wolff, Charlotte, 200

yeast, 143
yogurt, 12–13, 95–96, 268
yogurt-mint mask, 356–357
You Are Younger Than You Think, 108
Young, M. Wharton, 254
Yurka, Blanche, 272

Zukor, Carl, 105

Guide to Recipes

almond milk, 87–88
Alone At Last, 336
Aphrodite salad, 320
apple
    breakfast, 333
    espresso, 315
    soup, 308
applesauce, 330
apricot whip, 329
avocado
    chicken, 349
    curried, 294
    guacamole, 339

basting sauces, 295
beans
    cooking of, 305–306
    soya, 302–303
    sprouts, 303–304, 306
beautyfarm special, 350

beef
    chipped, 290
    liver, 288, 289
    protein in, 285
Bloody Mary yogurt, 300
bouillabaisse liquid meal, 350
bread
    El Molino, 322
    Sicilian, 321–322
    wholewheat, 321, 322
bright eye salad, 320
broccoli, cooking of, 306
broth
    beautyfarm, 341–342
    Swiss, 355
brown rice, 326
buckwheat, 324–325

cabbage espresso, 315
carrots
    capucino, 314
    cooking of, 305–306

in cornmeal muffins, 323
espresso, 314, 336, 350
and raisins, 320
caruba delight liquid meal, 350
cauliflower, cooking of, 306
celery espresso, 314–315
cereal, 333
cherry soup, 309
chicken
  avocado, 349
  basted, 295
  liquid meal, 349, 350
  liver, 289–290
  protein in, 286
  roast, 292–293, 295
  stuffing for, 293
Chinese cooking, 305
chipped beef, 290
chop suey, 304
clear complexion liquid meal, 350
coffee, Swiss, 334
complexion
  drink for, 332
  liquid meal, 350
  salad, 319
corn bread carrotte, 323
cornmeal muffins, 323
cottage cheese
  making of, 298
  pancakes, 299
  and salads, 298, 319
  value of, 297–298
cream cheese yogurt, 301–302
cream of mushroom liquid meal, 349
cucumber espresso, 317
curry, 293–294
custard, honey, 328–329

desserts
  applesauce, 330
  apricot whip, 329
  fruit compote, 328
  gelatin, 327
  honey custard, 328–329
  honey raspberry sherbet, 329
  pie crust, 330–331
  prune whip, 329–330
  snow apple, 330
  wine jelly, 327–328
  See also yogurt
dill pickles, 339
dressing, salad, see salad dressing
duck, 295

"E" bomb, 335
eggs
  curried, 294
  value of, 295–296
18 carat golden drink, 336
El Molino bread, 322
endive, braised, 306–307
espresso
  apple, 315
  beautyfarm, 317
  cabbage, 315
  carrot, 314, 336
  celery, 314–315
  cucumber, 317

grape, 316–317
  pineapple, 316
  rhubarb, 317
  tomato, 316
  vegetable, 310 ff.
  watercress, 315–316
eye bright liquid meal, 350

fish, 286–287
flour, soybean, 303
fruit
  compote, 328
  salad dressing, 338
  salads, 320–321

golden eggnog liquid meal, 349
golden fruit salad dressing, 338
golden grain magic, 340
golden oils, 336–337
golden oil salad dressing, 337
grape espresso, 316–317
grape leaves, stuffed, 325–326
green-gold dressing, 321
green-gold liquid meal, 350
green salad, 318–320
groats, 324–325
guacamole, 339

Hi-Vi boost liquid meal, 349
Hi-Vi lean milk, 332
honey
  custard, 328–329
  ice cream, 343
  mint vinegar dressing, 337
  raspberry sherbet, 329
  yogurt, 300
hot milk Lassie, 335

ice cream, honey, 343
instant pick-up, 335
instant Swiss broth, 335

kasha, 324–325
kumiss, 340

lamb
  basted, 295
  chops, 290
  curried, 294
  protein in, 285, 286
  liquid meals, 349–350
  liquid salad, 317–318
  liver
    beef, 288, 289
    chicken, 289–290
    lamb, 288, 289
liver and—liquid meal, 349
lobster tails, 287–288

Madrilène, tomato, 310
mayonnaise, yogurt, 338
milk
  Hi-Vi, 332
  hot, 335, 336
  kumiss, 340
  powdered, 297
  sesame, 95
  substitute for, 340–341

milk (cont.)
    value of, 296–297
    as whipped cream, 340
milk shake, 334
muffins
    cornmeal, 323
    soya, 322–323
    wheat germ, 323
mushroom, cream of, 349
mustard, 338–339

orange yogurt, 301

pancakes, cottage cheese, 299
peanut butter, 339–340
pep breakfast, 333
pickles, dill, 339
pie, yogurt, 301
pie crust, 330–331
pilaf, wholewheat, 324
pineapple espresso, 316
popped wild rice, 343
pork, 285–286
Portuguese gaspacho, 309–310
potage Hippocrates, 342
potato chips, 324
potatoes, baked, 323–324
prune whip, 329–330

raisin carrotte, 320
raspberry
    honey sherbet, 329
    yogurt, 301
reducer's delight, 334
rhubarb juice, 317
rice
    brown, 326
    in grape leaves, 325–326
    popped, 343
    wild, 326, 343

salad
    Aphrodite, 320
    bright eye, 320
    complexion, 319
    cottage cheese, 319
    fruit, 320–321
    green, 318–319
    liquid, 317–318
    luncheon, 319–321
salad dressing
    golden fruit, 338
    golden oil, 337
    green-gold, 321
    honey-mint vinegar, 337
    no-oil, 338
    yogurt, 338
school girl complexion, 332
seafood
    curried, 294
    lobster tails, 287–288
    protein in, 287
    shrimp sauté, 288
sesame milk, 95
shrimp sauté, 288
Smorgasbord from the sea, 336
snow apple, 330
snow peas, 307

soup
    apple, 308
    beautyfarm broth, 341–342
    cherry, 309
    Madrilène, 310
    potage Hippocrates, 342
    summer, 307–308
    tomato Madrilène, 310
soybeans
    baked, 302–303
    flour, 303
    muffins, 322–323
    sautéed, 306
    value of, 302
sprouts, soybean, 303–304
stew, veal, 291
stuffing, 293
summer soup, 307–308
Swiss broth, 335
Swiss coffee, 334

Toast to Crowning Glory, 332
tomato espresso, 316
tomato Madrilène, 310
Tooth or Consequences, 332–333
Tranquillo, 335
turkey, 295
turnips, cooking of, 305–306

veal
    protein in, 285
    scallopini, 292
    stew, 291
vegetables
    cooking of, 304–305
    espresso, 310 ff.
    juices of, 310 ff.

watercress espresso, 315–316
wheat germ
    muffins, 323
    pie crust, 331
    sticks, 342–343
whipped cream, 340
wholewheat
    bread, 321–322
    cereal, 340
    pilaf, 324
wild rice
    boiled, 326
    popped, 343
wine jelly delight, 327–328

yogurt
    in baked potatoes, 323–324
    Bloody Mary, 300
    in cherry soup, 309
    cream cheese, 301–302
    honey, 300
    making of, 299–300
    mayonnaise, 338
    orange, 301
    pie, 301
    raspberry, 301
    in salad, 320
    salad dressing, 338
    starter for, 300
    in summer soup, 307–308
    value of, 299

Beauty

Appetizers Cool and Crisp

VEGETABLE ESPRESSO—CARROT, CELERY, TOMATO
FRUIT ESPRESSO—APPLE, PINEAPPLE, GRAPE; also CARROT STICKS
CAULIFLOWER KNOBS, CELERY HEARTS, GREEN-RIPE OLIVES
HOME-MADE DILL PICKLES

Soups and Broths from Many Nations

HOT—CHICKEN BROTH WITH KASHA, POTAGE HIPPOCRATES
BEAUTYFARM BROTH
COLD—YOGURT AND VEGETABLES PERSIAN STYLE
SWEDISH APPLE, DANISH CHERRY, PORTUGUESE GASPACHO

Salads of the Four Seasons

KENTUCKY LIMESTONE, ESCAROLLE, DANDELION, RAW SPINACH
ONION TOPS, COTTAGE CHEESE AND FRUIT, GELATIN AND FRUIT
GUACAMOLE MEXICAINE, RED CABBAGE AND RED APPLE
AVOCADO AND GRAPEFRUIT
DRESSINGS—GOLDEN OIL, GOLDEN FRUIT, GREEN GOLD YOGURT

Golden Grain High Energy Breads

EL MOLINO, WHOLEWHEAT ROLLS, SESAME STICKS
SOYBEAN or WHEAT GERM MUFFINS, CORNBREAD CARROTTE
RYE BREAD

Beverages Old and New

SWISS COFFEE ESPRESSO, CHINESE TEA, MINT TEA, PAPAYA TEA
LEAN MILK, CARUBA MILK, KUMISS, LIQUID APPLE

Delightful Desserts

FRESH FRUITS, FRUIT COMPOTE LADY MENDL, APPLE SNOW
HONEY CUSTARD, GRAPEFRUIT CARIBBEAN, HONEY ICE CREAM
RASPBERRY SHERBERT